Seminars in Child and Adolescent Psychiatry

College Seminars Series

Series Editors

Professor Hugh Freeman, Editor, *British Journal of Psychiatry*

Dr Ian Pullen, Consultant Psychiatrist, Royal Edinburgh Hospital

Dr George Stein, Consultant Psychiatrist, Farnborough Hospital, and King's College Hospital

Professor Greg Wilkinson, Professor of Psychiatry, The London Hospital Medical College

Other books in the series

Seminars in Psychology and Social Sciences. Edited by Digby Tantam & Max Birchwood

Seminars in Mental Handicap. Edited by Oliver Russell

Seminars in Basic Neurosciences. Edited by Gethin Morgan & Stuart Butler

Seminars in Adult Psychiatry. Edited by George Stein & Greg Wilkinson

Seminars in Forensic Psychiatry. Edited by Derek Chiswick & Rosemarie Cope

Seminars in Drug and Alcohol Abuse. Edited by Jonathan Chick & Roch Cantwell

Seminars in Psychiatry for the Elderly. Edited by Brice Pitt & Mohsen Naguib

Seminars in Psychopharmacology. Edited by David King

These titles are all currently in press. Another five titles are in preparation.

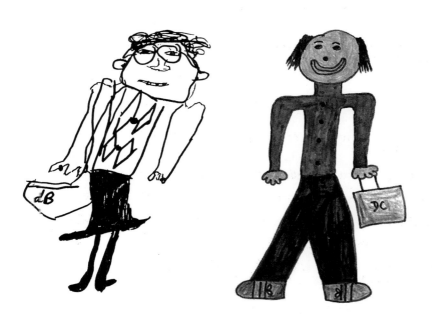

The editors

Seminars in Child and Adolescent Psychiatry

Edited by

Dora Black & David Cottrell

GASKELL

British Library Cataloguing-in-Publication Data

Seminars in Child and Adolescent
Psychiatry.—(College Seminars Series)
  I. Black, Dora II. Cottrell, David
  III. Series
  155

ISBN 0-902241-55-9

Distributed in North America
by American Psychiatric Press, Inc.
ISBN 0-88048-620-1

Gaskell is an imprint of the Royal College of Psychiatrists, 17 Belgrave Square, London SW1X 8PG

The views presented in this book do not necessarily reflect those of the Royal College of Psychiatrists, and the publishers are not responsible for any error of omission or fact. College Seminars are produced by the Publications Department of the College; they should in no way be construed as providing a syllabus or other material for any College examination.

Phototypeset by Dobbie Typesetting Limited, Tavistock, Devon
Printed in Great Britain by Bell and Bain Ltd., Glasgow

Contents

Plates

Contributors

Dr Mark Berelowitz, Consultant Child Psychiatrist, Maudsley Hospital, and Camberwell Child Guidance Clinic, London

Dr Dora Black, Consultant Child and Adolescent Psychiatrist, Royal Free Hospital, Honorary Senior Lecturer in Child and Adolescent Psychiatry, Royal Free Hospital Medical School, London

Dr David Cottrell, Senior Lecturer in Child and Adolescent Psychiatry, London Hospital Medical College, London

Dr Mary Eminson, Lecturer in Child and Adolescent Psychiatry, University Department of Child and Adolescent Psychiatry, Royal Manchester Children's Hospital, Manchester

Professor Ian Goodyer, Professor of Child and Adolescent Psychiatry, University of Cambridge, Cambridge

Dr Latha Hackett, Senior Registrar in Child and Adolescent Psychiatry, Royal Manchester Children's Hospital, Manchester

Dr Jean Harris Hendriks, Consultant Child and Adolescent Psychiatrist, South Bedfordshire Community Health Care Trust, and Honorary Consultant Child and Adolescent Psychiatrist and Senior Lecturer, Royal Free Hospital, London

Dr Brian Jacobs, Consultant Child and Adolescent Psychiatrist, The Maudsley Hospital, London

Dr Robert Jezzard, Consultant Child and Adolescent Psychiatrist, Guy's and Lewisham NHS Trust, London

Dr Tony Kaplan, Consultant Child and Adolescent Psychiatrist, Enfield Child Guidance Service and Chase Farm Hospital, Honorary Senior Lecturer in Child and Adolescent Psychiatry, Royal Free Hospital Medical School, London

Dr Ann Le Couteur, Consultant Child and Adolescent Psychiatrist, Enfield Child Guidance Service and Chase Farm Hospital, Honorary Senior Lecturer in Child and Adolescent Psychiatry, Institute of Psychiatry and Royal Free Hospital Medical School, London

Dr Julia Nelki, Consultant Child and Adolescent Psychiatrist, Royal Liverpool Children's NHS Trust (Myrtle Street), Liverpool

Dr Christopher Phillips, Consultant Child and Adolescent Psychiatrist, St Albans Child and Family Clinic, and Visiting Teacher, Tavistock Clinic, London

Dr Les Scarth, Consultant Child Psychiatrist, Royal Hospital for Sick Children, Edinburgh, and Honorary Senior Lecturer in Child Life and Health, University of Edinburgh

Dr Michael Wieselberg, Consultant Child and Adolescent Psychiatrist, University College and Middlesex Hospitals, and Honorary Senior Clinical Lecturer in Child and Adolescent Psychiatry, University College and Middlesex School of Medicine, London

Foreword
Series Editors

The publication of *College Seminars*, a series of textbooks covering the breadth of psychiatry, represents a new venture for the Royal College of Psychiatrists. At the same time, it is very much in line with the College's established role in education and in setting professional standards.

College Seminars are intended to help junior doctors during their training years. We hope that trainees will find these books useful, on the ward as well as in preparation for the MRCPsych examination. Separate volumes will cover clinical psychiatry, each of its subspecialties, and also the relevant non-clinical academic disciplines of psychology and sociology.

College Seminars will also make a contribution to the continuing medical education of established clinicians.

Psychiatry is concerned primarily with people, and to a lesser extent with disease processes and pathology. The core of the subject is rich in ideas and schools of thought, and no single approach or solution can embrace the variety of problems a psychiatrist meets. For this reason, we have endeavoured to adopt an eclectic approach to practical management throughout the series.

The College can draw on the collective wisdom of many individuals in clinical and academic psychiatry. More than a hundred people have contributed to this series; this reflects how diverse and complex psychiatry has become.

Frequent new editions of books appearing in the series are envisaged, which should allow *College Seminars* to be responsive to readers' suggestions and needs.

Hugh Freeman
Ian Pullen
George Stein
Greg Wilkinson

Acknowledgements

The picture of Dr Dora Black in the Frontispiece was by Leanne Butler, aged seven. Dr David Jones kindly provided Plate VII.

Introduction

The opportunity to work in a child and adolescent psychiatric team is an exciting but sometimes rather alarming prospect for the psychiatric or paediatric junior doctor, or for that matter trainees in any of the professions which make up the multidisciplinary team usually found in such placements. All the carefully acquired skills and knowledge of the trainee concerning adult function and dysfunction and all the skills in physical examination can seem redundant in the face of new techniques of assessment, new diagnoses and new treatment methods. There is a whole host of new professionals to liaise with – child psychotherapists, health visitors, teachers, educational psychologists and social workers, community paediatricians and many more.

This book aims to help the trainee new to the field chart a safe course through these sometimes confusing waters. Far from being redundant, a basic grounding in general medicine and adult psychiatry is an essential precursor to child psychiatric training. However, there is much that is new to be learnt.

Child and adolescent psychiatrists have a different concept of disorder from many adult psychiatrists. The most commonly accepted definition of childhood psychiatric disorder (see Chapter 5) describes behaviour which is developmentally inappropriate and which causes the child to suffer or the child's development to be impaired. Although some children do exhibit symptoms which are qualitatively different from the norm (e.g. children with infantile autism or with early-onset adult-type psychoses such as schizophrenia or bipolar affective disorder) the majority of disorders seen consist of behaviour, thoughts or feelings which are quantitatively different from the norm. Thus, most children with psychiatric disorder behave the same as all other children – but to a greater or lesser degree. They have more temper tantrums or go to school less, or have more fears and anxieties.

Children develop rapidly, so new skills can be acquired between one out-patient appointment and the next. When considering whether a child's behaviour is abnormal it is therefore essential to have a clear knowledge of normal child development. Behaviour which is quite appropriate at one age may be highly unusual at another. This can apply to both child and parental behaviour. Thus bedwetting and constant parental vigilance are both quite normal in a two-year-old and her parents but abnormal in a teenager and her parents.

A further complication for the newcomer is that when it comes to the 'presenting complaint', while the child may have the disorder, it is usually somebody else who is doing the complaining. Parents may want the psychiatrist to 'fix' their child without having to become involved themselves in treatment. A crucial skill which all newcomers have to master is the ability to engage parents and other relatives in assessment and treatment, and to be able to encourage parents, if necessary, to behave differently towards their children without making those parents feel blamed.

While parents may be the most concerned adults in many referrals, it is often the case that referrals are made by other adults who come into contact with the child and that parents may be unaware of or unwilling to acknowledge any problems. More than most medical subspecialties, child and adolescent psychiatrists have to work in close contact with other disciplines. The local social services have a statutory obligation to safeguard the welfare of children, the local education department to educate them. Many referrals will come from these sources as well as from general practitioners and other hospital consultants such as paediatricians.

We hope that this book will make clear the role of the child and adolescent psychiatrist in relation to all these other disciplines and organisations. Furthermore, we hope it will provide enough knowledge in areas such as child development, epidemiology, assessment, the disorders themselves, treatment and prognosis to enable the trainee to feel confident in his or her ability to begin seeing child and adolescent patients and their families.

Dr Dora Black
Dr David Cottrell
February 1993

1 A brief history of child and adolescent psychiatry
Dora Black

Training for child psychiatry • Organisation of services

Child psychiatry, as a specialty, separated from general psychiatry about 50 years ago although before that many general psychiatrists had treated children and adolescents, and some paediatricians had taken an interest in the whole child, considering the mind as well as the body as legitimate subjects of study. The history of the treatment of children's deviant behaviour goes back to ancient times (Wardle, 1991*a*) but the founding of the first child guidance clinic in Boston in the early 1920s for delinquent children marked the beginning of the application of 'scientific' methods to the study and treatment of deviant children.

The first child guidance clinic in the UK, and indeed in Europe, was founded in the East End of London by the Jewish Health Organisation in 1927 and a psychiatrist, Emanuel Miller, was appointed as honorary director together with a psychiatric social worker who had trained in Boston and a psychologist (Renton, 1978). This was followed closely by the London Child Guidance Centre (later called the Child Guidance Training Centre) in 1928 under the direction of Dr William Moody, who had trained at the Maudsley Hospital where children had been seen and treated, although a separate department was not established until after World War II. Miller moved to the Tavistock Clinic in 1933 and founded its department for children and parents, pioneering the recognition of family influences on child psychopathology and the need to treat the whole family (Hersov, 1986).

Child guidance clinics spread rapidly and by 1948, when the National Health Service (NHS) came into being, there were services (often of a rudimentary kind) in most local authority districts, but there were only a few hospital-based child psychiatric clinics. By the end of the 1960s most child psychiatrists in the UK were employed by the NHS and were working in child guidance clinics with social workers, educational psychologists and a few child psychotherapists and remedial teachers. The premises were usually owned by local education authorities, who provided administrative services. Occasionally there was joint provision with the NHS.

The geographical isolation of the clinics from other health facilities led to the alienation of child psychiatrists from their roots in biology, medicine and general psychiatry. The educational psychologists were divorced from colleagues in academic and clinical psychology, and social workers were separated from their colleagues in hospitals and local authorities, so that there was little cross-fertilisation of ideas; the volume of work left little time or energy for teaching, research or the development of the political expertise necessary to enable effective expansion to take place. The lack of trainees, especially in child psychiatry, to challenge established dogma led to the entrenchment of outdated and ineffective practices in some clinics. There was little incentive to examine the best way of using scarce resources, to develop preventive services or to attend to research and the acquisition of new skills (Black, 1987). Classification was rudimentary, the aetiology and treatment of most disorders was ill-understood, and there had been almost no research on the therapies being used.

Furthermore we were reaching only the tip of the iceberg. Kolvin (1973) found that less than 1% of the child population were receiving help from child guidance clinics, yet 7–20% of children were identified as suffering from a definite and functionally handicapping child psychiatric disorder (Rutter *et al*, 1970).

Although academic departments of child and adolescent psychiatry were established earlier in the US than in Europe, the adherence there to psychoanalytic training for all child and adolescent psychiatrists led to many talented academics using their skills on relatively few patients. Psychoanalytic treatment is intensive and lengthy and often precludes its practitioners from conducting research. Research in the US moved more slowly into social and biological spheres than it did in the UK.

The first academic department of child psychiatry to open in England, in 1972, headed by Professor Michael Rutter at the Maudsley Hospital, enabled child psychiatric research to become established, although the growth of academic departments was slow. Kanner's delineation of the new syndrome of infantile autism (1943), Robertson's films on children in hospital (1952, 1958), Bowlby's seminal ideas on attachment and loss (Bowlby, 1969, 1973, 1980), Winnicott's concept of 'good-enough' mothering and his attention to mother–child relationships (1965), Robins' long-term follow-up of child guidance patients (1966), Rutter's work on epidemiology (Rutter *et al*, 1970), and Kolvin's careful assessment of treatment strategies (Kolvin *et al*, 1981) are landmarks in the recent history of child psychiatry.

Therapeutic techniques have also developed over the last 60 years. Early treatments were based on psychoanalytic theory and technique as applied to children by Anna Freud (1928) and Klein (1932), and play therapy as described by Lowenfeld (1935) with concurrent guidance for the mother (rarely was the father included) by psychiatric social workers trained at first in the US and then at the Child Guidance Training Centre and the Maudsley Hospital in the UK. Specific in-patient units for children and adolescents were largely a post-war development, although therapeutic schools run by charismatic pioneers developed earlier (Wardle, 1991*b*).

Other therapies such as behaviour therapy (developed mainly by clinical psychologists), family therapy, group therapy and drug therapies have been integrated into eclectic practice over the last 20 or so years (see Chapter 10).

Training for child psychiatry

A famous debate on training took place in the 1960s between Dr Donald Winnicott of Paddington Green Hospital and Professor Aubrey Lewis of the Maudsley Hospital (Lewis, 1963; Winnicott, 1963), with Winnicott advocating the route for training child psychiatrists through paediatrics and Lewis through general psychiatry. Although today's child and adolescent psychiatrists should have a sound basic training in both disciplines, before starting higher child psychiatric training (after passing the membership examination of the Royal College of Psychiatrists) many have had little or no experience of paediatrics. During the next four years, time spent in clinical training should be supplemented by a period spent in conducting research under supervision and acquiring diagnostic skills and a wide range of therapeutic skills. But clinical and research skills are not enough; child psychiatrists in the 21st century will require management and budgeting expertise, and leadership skills of a high order if they are going to serve the troubled children of the future.

Organisation of services

A series of studies and reports in the 1970s and 1980s (Brunel Institute, 1976; Royal College of Psychiatrists, 1978, 1986; Interdisciplinary Standing Committee, 1981) exposed the difficulties of the traditional way of organising child guidance services. The lack of clearly defined leadership and the muddled management structure led to intractable problems in some clinics, although Graham, in his review of trends in the practice of child psychiatry, saw the profession as a healthy one (Graham, 1976) and Rutter (1986) echoed that belief. This may have been more a reflection of the efforts which had been made over the years to maintain good relationships in the multidisciplinary team, often at the expense of efficiency and good practice. Traditionally the members were from psychiatry, social work and educational psychology, and child guidance work fossilised the historical triumvirate while lack of funding and inflexibility prevented new professions from being added. Modern practice has to be more flexible, and child psychiatrists and their colleagues should be able to call upon the services of clinical psychologists, psychiatric nurses, child psychotherapists, teachers, dieticians, occupational, art and music therapists, physiotherapists, pathologists, paediatricians, general psychiatrists, neuropsychologists, radiologists, neurologists, and others as needed.

The NHS reforms and funding constraints are bringing about changes in the way that child psychiatric services are delivered. Clinical directors and budgeting control, as well as better ways of measuring performance, will enable more flexibility in the staffing structure of child psychiatry departments and child guidance clinics which will be to the benefit of patients.

References

Black, D. (1987) The future of child guidance. In *Progress in Child Health*, vol. 3 (ed. J. A. Macfarlane). Edinburgh: Churchill Livingstone.

Bowlby, J. (1969, 1973, 1980) *Attachment and Loss* (3 volumes). London: Hogarth Press.

Brunel Institute of Organisation and Social Studies (1976) *Working Paper HS1. Future Organisation in Child Guidance and Allied Work*. Uxbridge: Brunel University.

Freud, A. (1928) *Introduction to the Technique of Child Analysis*. New York: Nervous and Mental Disease Publishing.

Graham, P. (1976) Management in child psychiatry: recent trends. *British Journal of Psychiatry*, **129**, 97–108.

Hersov, L. (1986) Child psychiatry in Britain – the last 30 years. *Journal of Child Psychology and Psychiatry*, **27**, 781–802.

Interdisciplinary Standing Committee (1981) *Interdisciplinary Work in Child Guidance*. London: Child Guidance Trust.

Kanner, L. (1943) Autistic disturbance of affective contact. *Nervous Child*, **2**, 217–250.

Klein, M. (1932) *The Psychoanalysis of Children*. London: Hogarth Press.

Kolvin, I. (1973) Evaluation of psychiatric services for children in England and Wales. In *Roots of Evaluation* (eds J. K. Wing & J. Hafner). Oxford: Oxford University Press.

——, Garside, R. F., Nicol, A. R., *et al* (1981) *Help Starts Here: The Maladjusted Child in the Ordinary School*. London: Tavistock.

Lewis, A. (1963) Symposium: Training for child psychiatry. *Journal of Child Psychology and Psychiatry*, **4**, 75–84.

Lowenfeld, M. (1935) *Play in Childhood*. London: Gollancz.

Renton, G. (1978) The East London Child Guidance Clinic. *Journal of Child Psychology and Psychiatry*, **19**, 309–312.

Robertson, J. (1952) *A Two Year Old Goes to Hospital* (film). Ipswich: Concord Films Council.

—— (1958) *Going to Hospital with Mother* (film). Ipswich: Concord Films Council.

Robins, L. (1966) *Deviant Children Grown Up*. Baltimore: Williams and Wilkins.

Royal College of Psychiatrists (1978) The role, responsibilities and work of the child and adolescent psychiatrist. *Bulletin of the Royal College of Psychiatrists*, **2**, 127.

—— (1986) The role, responsibilities and work of the child and adolescent psychiatrists. *Bulletin of the Royal College of Psychiatrists*, **10**, 202–206.

Rutter, M. (1986) Child psychiatry: looking 30 years ahead. *Journal of Child Psychology and Psychiatry*, **27**, 803–841.

——, Tizard J. & Whitmore, K. (1970) *Education, Health and Behaviour*. London: Longman.

Wardle, C. (1991*a*) Historical influences on services for children and adolescents before 1900. In *150 Years of British Psychiatry, 1841–1991* (eds G. E. Berrios & H. Freeman). London: Gaskell.

—— (1991*b*) Twentieth-century influences on the development in Britain of services for child and adolescent psychiatry. *British Journal of Psychiatry*, **159**, 53-68.

Winnicott, D. (1963) Symposium: Training for child psychiatry. *Journal of Child Psychology and Psychiatry*, **4**, 85-91.

—— (1965) *The Family and Individual Development*. London: Tavistock.

Further reading

Parry-Jones, W. L. (1989) Annotation. The history of child and adolescent psychiatry: its present day relevance. *Journal of Child Psychology and Psychiatry*, **30**, 3-11.

2 Normal development and specific developmental delays
Latha Hackett

Normal child development ● *Specific developmental delays* ● *Some theories of development*

Development, or the expectation of orderly change, is the backdrop against which all child psychiatry is practised. It is arguable that all psychiatric disorders in children represent deviations or delays of development. An understanding of development and the theories and evidence about what carries it forward, holds it up or deviates it from the expected path, is important because it affects our judgement of what is normal, it informs our clinical method, and it governs the framework in which we formulate cases and plan treatment.

Box 2.1 ICD-10 developmental disorders

The disorders have two features in common: an impairment or delay in the development of functions that are strongly related to biological maturation of the central nervous system; and a steady course that does not involve the remissions and relapses that tend to be characteristic of many mental disorders.

Specific developmental disorders of speech and language
   Specific speech articulation disorder
   Expressive language disorder
   Receptive language disorder
   Acquired aphasia with epilepsy (Landau – Kleffner syndrome)
   Other developmental disorders of speech and language
   Developmental disorder of speech and language, unspecified
Specific developmental disorders of scholastic skills
   Specific reading disorder
   Specific spelling disorder
   Specific disorder of arithmetical skills
   Mixed disorder of scholastic skills
   Other developmental disorders of scholastic skills
   Developmental disorder of scholastic skills, unspecified
Specific developmental disorder of motor function
Mixed specific developmental disorders
Pervasive developmental disorders
   See Chapters 7-9.
Other disorders of psychological development
Unspecified disorder of psychological development

Development is a lifelong process. It involves a continuous interaction between heredity and environment. Genetic determinants express themselves through the process of maturation. Motor development is largely a maturational process as normal children acquire skills like crawling, standing and walking in the same orderly sequence roughly at the same age. Development in other areas such as language, intelligence and personality may be permanently affected by early experience.

This chapter describes, briefly, normal development and some specific delays in development. Global developmental delay is described in a separate book in the series. Liaison with district handicap teams is described in Chapter 13. Box 2.1 gives a summary of the developmental disorders according to ICD-10 (World Health Organization, 1992).

The range of normal development is wide and merges with the abnormal. Table 2.1 describes the main features of development at different ages. For a detailed description see Illingworth (1990).

Normal child development

Motor development

Of all mammals, human infants are the most immature at birth and require the longest period of development before they are capable of all the skills characteristic of their species. The sequence of development is the same in all normal children, although some infants reach each stage ahead of others. Motor development is in the cephalocaudal direction, head control preceding hand control, which precedes walking.

Normal feeding

The feeding relationship between the newborn infant and mother in the first few days of life is largely dependent on instinctively determined behaviour based on physiological mechanisms. It also depends though on whether it is mutually enjoyable or not. The secretion of breast milk is a neurohumoral response; the infant's sucking triggers the milk letdown reflex. After a few days a rhythm is usually established between the baby's need and milk production. Similarly, in bottle-fed babies a pattern of feeding is established, with gradual lengthening of the period between late-night and morning feeds.

Newborn infants usually cannot place their lips tightly round the areola of the breast or the teat of the bottle, so milk leaks out at the corner of the mouth. As they mature, they are able to do so. They are able to drink out of a cup at four to five months, to chew at six months, and like to hold a bottle. At 15 months they are able to manage a cup without dropping it. They can manage a knife and fork by the age of two to three years.

Both the child and mother influence early feeding. The child should have an intact gastrointestinal system and a normal mouth. Premature infants or those who experienced perinatal trauma, or have cerebral palsy and other

Table 2.1 Developmental milestones

Age	Motor development	Speech	Vision and hearing	Social development
4–6 weeks				Smiles at mother
6–8 weeks		Vocalises		
3 months	Prone: head held up for prolonged period. No grasp reflex	Talks a great deal	Follows dangling toy from side to side. Turns head to sound	Squeals with pleasure appropriately; discriminate smile
5 months	Holds head steady. Goes for objects and gets them. Objects taken to mouth	Enjoys vocal play		Smiles at mirror image
6 months	Transfers objects from one hand to the other. Pulls self to sit and sits erect with supports. Rolls over prone to supine. Palmar grasp of cube	Double syllable sounds like mumum, dada	Localises sound 18 inches lateral to either ear	May show 'stranger shyness'
9–10 months	Wriggles and crawls. Sits unsupported. Picks up objects with pincer grasp	Babbles tunefully	Looks for toys dropped	Apprehensive of strangers
1 year	Stands holding furniture. Stands alone for a second or two then collapses with a bump. Lets go of objects	Babbles 2 or 3 words repeatedly	Drops toys and watches where they go	Cooperates with dressing, waves goodbye, understands simple commands

Continued

Table 2.1 *Continued*

Age	Motor development	Speech	Vision and hearing	Social development
18 months	Can walk alone, picks up a toy without falling over, gets up stairs and down stairs holding on to rail. Begins to jump with both feet. Can build a tower of 3 or 4 cubes, and throw a ball	'Jargon'. Many intelligible words		Demands constant mothering. Drinks from cup with both hands. Feeds self with a spoon
2 years	Able to run, walks up and down stairs 2 feet per step. Builds tower of 6 cubes	Joins 2–3 words in sentences		Parallel play. Dry by day
3 years	Goes upstairs one foot per step and downstairs 2 feet per step. Copies circle, imitates cross and draws man on request. Builds tower of 9 cubes	Constantly asks questions. Speaks in sentences		Cooperative play. Undresses with assistance. Imaginary companions
4 years	Goes downstairs 1 foot per step, skips on 1 foot. Imitates gate with cubes. Copies a cross	Questioning at its height. Many infantile substitutions in speech		Dresses and undresses with assistance. Attends to own toilet need
5 years	Skips on both feet, hops. Draws a man. Copies a triangle. Gives age	Fluent speech. Few infantile substitutions		Dresses and undresses alone
6 years	Copies a diamond. Knows right from left and number of fingers	Fluent speech		

forms of brain damage and infants with a cleft palate or lip could have difficulty in feeding. Medication used in the intrapartum period may impair the baby's ability to suck. Some babies can be difficult temperamentally, and this will affect their feeding (Thomas & Chess, 1977).

Early feeding is commonly affected by the emotional state of the mother, especially depression or anxiety. Mothers may be generally anxious or anxious specifically about feeding. A young inexperienced mother with little social and family support may have particular difficulties. The supply of breast milk may be affected by local problems affecting the nipple or breast or impairment of general physical health.

There is no evidence that whether a child is breast- or bottle-fed influences the later development of behavioural or emotional problems of the child (Orlansky, 1949; Sewell & Mussen, 1952).

Sleep

Newborn babies tend to alternate frequently between waking and sleeping. The total sleeping time drops from 16–17 hours a day to 13 hours per day within the first six months of the infant's life. A rhythm of two shorter naps during the day and a longer sleep at night is usually established. By six months over 80% babies sleep right through the night and only 10% at the age of one are still waking every night (Graham, 1986).

Environmental influences also affect the sleep patterns of infants during the first year of life. A change in the sleeping arrangements, an alteration in the bedtime ritual, or anxiety or depression in the mother may disturb the infant's sleep pattern. Difficulties in getting to sleep are common in two- and three-year-olds, and may be related to their limited capacity to retain an image in their minds of their parents. Inappropriate parental responses to the waking child may also reinforce night-time waking (see Chapter 7). 'Transitional objects' (Winnicott, 1958) like a teddy bear or a 'security blanket' may help some children to settle at night. Temperamentally difficult children commonly experience sleep problems.

Dreams

By the time children are three or four years old they are able to recognise dreams as such and to speak of them, although only one-fifth of children under five were able to describe traumatic dreams (Terr, 1987). Adults may infer that younger children dream as they vocalise or make movements in their sleep. Nightmares, troubled and frightening dreams associated with actual fears and traumas, which may occur at any age, must be distinguished from night terrors (pavor noctunus). These occur usually between three and four years of age, in stage 4 sleep, and are not associated with painful events, can be prevented by arousal of the child, are not remembered, and appear to be a maturational feature in some children.

Normal sleep in childhood and adolescence reflects the serenity and stability, or its reverse, of the life led by the sleeper. The content of dreams may be associated with the waking world through play, art, visualised memories and speech, which may allow access to traumatic memories. Sleep disturbances form one route to knowledge of the child's life events (Terr 1991).

Bowel and bladder control

In the newborn period micturition is reflex. Babies usually empty the bladder or bowels immediately after a meal; they can be conditioned at any age to pass urine when placed on a pot. Voluntary control does not begin until the age of 15 to 18 months, depending on maturation of the nervous system, which is influenced by genetic factors. Most children are reasonably dry by day at 18 months. By two years, 50% are dry at night; by three, 75%; and by five some 90% are dry.

For children to be continent, they need an intact nervous system supplying the bladder, no congenital malformation of the urinary system, physiological maturity, an understanding of what is required of them and the motivation to achieve this. In a child with generalised learning difficulties a delay in bowel and bladder control could be one aspect of general immaturity. If the family is under stress when the child is between the age of 18 months and 3 years he or she will achieve dryness more slowly. Parents who take a relaxed view of toilet training and start when the child is sufficiently mature, between the ages of 18 months to 2 years, and praise successful efforts, are likely to see their children gain control of their bowel and bladder with less effort. If bedwetting (enuresis) persists beyond the age of five, it is considered abnormal.

Bowel control is usually acquired before control of the bladder; faecal soiling (encopresis) beyond the age of four would be considered abnormal.

Sexual development

The process of sexual development enables the individual to conform to the gender-specific modes of behaviour and appearance expected by a society, form stable relationships with members of the opposite sex, and produce and rear children. Many areas of our lives are affected by our sex, from our choice of shoes to our choice of partner, from our chances of developing rheumatoid arthritis to our chances of ending up in prison. It is clear that sexual development covers an enormous area of change, ranging from universal aspects of physical development to relatively culture-specific aspects of social behaviour. It is conventional to divide this sweep of human development into its physiological aspects, which will be described first, gender identity, gender role, and finally sexual orientation.

Physical development

A happy sexual adjustment in adult life requires the necessary anatomical and physiological changes to have taken place. At about two months' gestation, the sex chromosomes cause the primitive, undifferentiated gonad to develop into either ovaries or testes. The ensuing phenotype depends on the secretion of foetal androgens, as without their masculinising influence female genitalia will result regardless of genotype.

The next decisive move towards a sexually adult body occurs some years before puberty. The maturing hypothalamus activates the pituitary gland, leading to increased release of luteinising hormone and follicular stimulating hormone. These in turn encourage the ovaries to secrete oestrogen (from about seven years) and the testes androgens, although the adrenals contribute to androgen output from the ninth year (adrenal puberty). Early on in puberty, before the final balance between oestrogen and androgens is established, temporary anomalies such as transient gynaecomastia in boys can commonly be observed.

The development of genitalia and secondary sexual characteristics starts earlier and proceeds faster in girls than boys, menarche occurring between the ages of 10 and 16, and the equivalent event – the capacity to ejaculate semen – happening between the ages of 13 and 17 years. The neural substrate of sexual activity responsible for erection, pelvic movements and ejaculation is present from an early age in the spinal cord, although pathways mediating the latter two functions require an appropriate hormonal input.

Human sexual behaviour and its development is influenced strongly by culture. Every society places some restrictions on sexual behaviour, and incest is prohibited by almost all cultures. By about three or four years of age, most children can identify correctly their own sex as well as that of other children.

Gender identity

This is the degree to which children regard themselves as male or female, and is usually well established by the age of four years. Transsexualism, which usually starts with cross-dressing and feminine behaviour (in the case of boys) in early or middle childhood, represents an extreme aberration of gender identity. Studies have suggested that an indulgent maternal attitude to the child's preference for behaving and dressing like a member of the opposite sex, and disinterest and failure to act as a role model on the part of the father, may contribute to gender identity problems (Green, 1985).

Though less extreme than the complete reversal of gender identity described above, insecurity of sexual identity can complicate late physical maturation, especially in boys. Such boys have been shown to feel dominated by their better developed peers and have a poorer self-concept of themselves as males.

Gender role

This refers to the ability of an individual to carry out the repertoire of behaviours, considered socially appropriate for his or her sex. By three years children show a preference for particular activities (e.g. boys for rough and tumble play) and sex-appropriate toys. Throughout childhood and adolescence many of these differences become accentuated. Processes by which the array of behaviours that constitute sex role are acquired include selective reinforcement by parents and identification.

Sexual orientation

This refers to an individual's choice of sexual stimulus and outlet. There is evidence of a genetic contribution to sexual orientation, particularly in homosexuals (Heston & Shields, 1968). In addition, the prenatal hormonal environment has been shown to play a part (Money & Ehrhardt, 1972). Sexual orientation represents a continuum from exclusive heterosexuality to exclusive homosexuality; only about 4% of men and 1–2% women become exclusively homosexual (Kinsey *et al*, 1948, 1953).

The wish to achieve sexual pleasure by stimulation of the genitalia is present from birth. This sexual drive persists throughout childhood and increases in early adolescence to peak in late adolescence and early adulthood. Masturbation is common in both boys and girls between the ages of two and five; sex play involving undressing and sexual exploration and interest in the genitalia of siblings and playmates is common and normal during this period.

It is only around puberty that the three components of sexuality – gender identity, gender role, and sexual orientation – become incorporated into the formation and maintenance of emotional dyadic relationships and our sexual orientation becomes organised and relatively fixed.

Infants develop their first feelings of affection and trust through a warm, loving, nurturant relationship with the mother. This is a prerequisite for a satisfactory interaction and affectionate relationships with youngsters of both sexes and for intimacy of later sexual relationship among young adults.

Language development

Infants have their own methods of communication. The first step towards communication is orientation towards the mother as a prelude to establishing eye contact. As she speaks, the child first smiles and then starts to vocalise. Communication occurs in other non-verbal modalities such as clinging, frowning, kissing, pushing her away, turning the head away, and later holding the mother's hand and leading her to something the child wants. From the first few weeks of life, babies and mothers can be observed to take turns when they interact, demonstrating a pattern of alternating responses that persists throughout life.

At four to six weeks infants smile in response to their mother's overtures. At eight weeks they smile and vocalise when talked to. At 12–16 weeks they hold long 'conversations' with their mothers and begin to babble. They squeal with delight at four months and laugh aloud. At seven months they combine consonants to say 'mumum' and 'dadada'. At 10 months they may say one word and at 12 months imitate dogs, cows and cats, and may say two or three words. At 15–18 months a child speaks in an expressive language of his or her own which is unintelligible ('jargon' speech). The average child begins to join words by 21–24 months and by the age of three is speaking in sentences.

The development of speech depends on the interaction of genetic, auditory, environmental, and intellectual factors. There are wide variations in the development of speech in normal children. Girls speak earlier than boys.

Play

Play is the work through which children learn about themselves, others, and the world in which they live. The earliest play, from a few weeks old, is social; smiling and moving the head to catch the eye of another soon lead to peep-bo, then the copying of other movements and attempts to copy sounds and rhythms (see also the account of attachment theory below) (Bowlby, 1977).

By the end of the first year children are learning to clap, smile, hide and seek, and to look for approval of shared jokes, tasks and movements.

Rhythm, rhymes, stories, songs, dancing, imitation of adults at work, giving and receiving, the potential, during the second and third years, for the development of cooperative play with other children, solving puzzles, building, drawing, modelling, all become available as activities for the maturing child. And play should not be an end in itself; children require opportunities to contribute to the life around them, by succeeding at household tasks, helping to care for siblings, preparing food, running errands, and so on. For children, there is no clear line between work and play; the need is for a valued role in family and community life.

The provision of such rich experience is as important for the psychosocial well-being of the child, the adolescent in transition, and the adult he or she will become as is the care of bodily needs and the acquisition of language.

Indeed, language, play and social learning are intertwined and all are essential for the development of autonomy, reciprocity, ethical awareness, creativity and resilience in adult life and for the availability of adults to each new generation of children.

Specific developmental delays

Specific motor retardation (clumsiness)

The main feature of this disorder is a serious impairment in the development of motor coordination with normal intelligence. The clumsiness is commonly associated with perceptual difficulties. Though language development is normal, clumsy children are somewhat slow to walk, and late in developing motor skills such as dressing, feeding, and walking. They have difficulty in writing, drawing and copying. They perform badly at ball games, are poor in handicrafts and tend to break crockery. Children with this disorder have been mistaken for being lazy or having generalised learning difficulties. They may develop secondary educational problems, their self-esteem may suffer, and they may present to the psychiatric department with emotional or behaviour problems.

A careful history confirmed by asking the child to draw, hop and catch a ball can clinch the diagnosis of a clumsy child. Formal testing can be done by administering the Wechsler Intelligence Scale for Children (WISC), which reveals a much lower performance than verbal IQ.

Once the diagnosis is confirmed, the treatment depends on the severity. It may be sufficient to explain to the parents and teacher that the child is not lazy but has a specific difficulty. Clumsy children can be helped to increase their confidence by enlisting the help of physiotherapists, speech therapists and occupational therapists with a special interest in this condition.

Specific delay in language development

Possible reasons for delay in speech acquisition include the following.

(1) Defects of hearing   If the child has severe hearing difficulty from birth he or she will not develop effective speech and will need special speech tuition. In general, the later the onset of deafness, the less seriously speech is affected.

(2) Delayed maturation   Comprehension long precedes the ability to articulate in normal children. It is thought that the rate of maturation of the central nervous system is a limiting factor in the acquisition of speech. No amount of practice can make a child speak before the nervous system is ready for it and mental handicap will therefore delay the acquisition of speech.

(3) Familial factors   If the child has normal hearing and intelligence and has no neurological disability like cerebral palsy, it is common to find that there is a history of delayed speech in the family, particularly in one of the parents, suggesting a familial pattern of delay in the maturation of speech areas of the central nervous system.

(4) The social environment   Language development is frequently delayed in children brought up in institutions. Children reared in large families or slums are usually slower to speak, as are twins compared with singletons. Children of higher social class are more advanced in their speech. Late speech development is commonly found in abused children.

The relation between handedness and speech acquisition is controversial, but left-handedness is commoner in children with generalised learning difficulties, for unknown reasons.

Language which is *deviant* (e.g. echolalia, pronominal reversal) as well as delayed is a feature of infantile autism (see Chapters 7, 8, 9).

Elective mutism is characterised by speech limited to a few people in familiar situations (see Chapter 8).

Specific delay in reading and writing

Writing and reading are complex acquired skills. Normal cognitive and language development are necessary for the acquisition of reading. Most children are able to read single short words by the age of 6–7 years, and by 10–12 years have acquired sufficient reading ability to cope with everyday tasks such as reading a newspaper.

General reading backwardness

This refers to reading that is poor in relation to the average attainment for that age regardless of intelligence. Many of these are children with mild mental handicap.

Specific reading retardation (SRR)

This syndrome (sometimes known as dyslexia) is defined in terms of a discrepancy between attainment and reading age as predicted on the basis of age and IQ. It is said to exist when a child is reading at a level (usually 1.5 or 2 standard deviations) below that expected from his or her non-verbal ability.

Severe reading difficulties are handicapping and are frequently associated with psychiatric symptoms. In the Isle of Wight study (Rutter *et al*, 1970), the prevalence of specific reading retardation was 4% of 9–10-year-olds; this increased to 10% in the London study (Berger *et al*, 1975).

The rate is higher in boys (3:1) and children from working-class families. It is associated with:

(1) delay in acquiring speech
(2) family history of reading difficulty
(3) conduct disorder
(4) brain injury
(5) confusion between left and right, and poor visuospatial ability
(6) large families, and overcrowding
(7) temperamental attributes such as impulsiveness and poor concentration
(8) episodic hearing impairment (usually due to recurrent ear infection), and visual defects such as uncorrected errors of refraction
(9) low birth weight (a weak association only).

Clinical presentation   Although the majority present because they cannot read, or because of their slow progress, some may present with somatic complaints like headaches or abdominal pain because of anxiety, or more commonly because of antisocial behaviour. SRR should always be looked for in children with a conduct disorder and those refusing to attend school. Roughly one-third of 10-year-old children with reading retardation were diagnosed as conduct disordered in the Isle of Wight survey (Rutter *et al*, 1970), and one-third of conduct disordered children had SRR.

Management Management of SRR is mainly the provision of appropriate remedial teaching. Any associated psychiatric disorder should of course be treated (see Chapter 10).

One important aim of parents and professionals dealing with children with SRR is to minimise secondary handicaps: these children should be helped to develop self-esteem by encouraging them to engage in activities in which verbal ability is not of prime importance.

Outcome Children over the age of 10 with SRR make very slow progress despite remedial help and most will continue to have reading and spelling difficulties in adolescence and adulthood. High IQ and socio-economic status predict better outcome. Final outcome may be related as much to associated conduct disorder as to SRR. Adolescents become vulnerable to conduct disorder and have poor employment prospects and limited acquisition of social skills.

Spelling difficulties

Spelling difficulties commonly accompany reading retardation. Frith (1978) has used the term 'dyslexic' to describe children with both reading and spelling difficulties, and 'dysgraphic' for those children whose reading is normal but their spelling is poor. Much less is known about this condition. It is thought to be due to either a failure of the internal lexicon or an inability to carry out phonological analysis, or both.

Specific arithmetic retardation

Arithmetic and mathematical difficulties in general have been little studied. Specific arithmetic retardation is a serious impairment in the development of arithmetic skills which is not explicable in terms of general intellectual retardation or inadequate schooling.

Rourke & Strang (1983) described two broad groups of children with arithmetic difficulties:

(1) those whose arithmetic is better than their reading and spelling, and
(2) those whose arithmetic is weak but reading and spelling is normal.

The first group perform well on visuospatial skills but have a general language disorder, while the second group have normal verbal skills but poor visuospatial skills. Classically these children misread signs or set out work incorrectly. They have particular problems with fractions or manipulations involving the moving of numbers around on the page. Arithmetic difficulties are less handicapping than reading disorder, although in a numerate society they may lead to emotional disturbance.

Some theories of development: a brief introduction

These theories are summarised in Table 2.2, except for Bowlby's, which does not lend itself to tabular presentation.

Table 2.2   Stages in psychosocial development

	Freud	Erikson	Piaget	Kohlberg
1st year	Oral stage	Trust versus mistrust	Sensorimotor (0–2 years)	Preconventional morality Level I
2nd year	Anal stage	Autonomy versus shame and doubt		
3rd to 5th year	Phallic stage	Initiative versus guilt	Preoperational (2–7 years)	(0–7 years)
6th year to puberty	Latency period	Industry versus inferiority	Concrete operational (7–12 years)	Conventional morality, level II
Adolescence	Genital stage	Identity versus confusion	Formal operational (over 12 years)	Post conventional morality, level III
Early adulthood		Intimacy versus isolation		
Middle adulthood		Generativity versus self-absorption		
Ageing years		Integrity versus despair		

Bowlby's descriptions of psychosocial development are not easily tabulated – see text.

Freud: psychoanalytic theory

The psychoanalytic theory of Sigmund Freud (1856-1939) described a predictable sequence of qualitatively distinct stages through which children pass, each differing as to the physical function that is invested with pleasure (Freud, 1905).

Freud stated that the personality was composed of three major structures – the id, the ego, and the superego – each having its own function but interacting to govern behaviour. The id, being the most primitive part of the personality, is present in the newborn infant, and from it the ego and superego later develop. The id mediates basic biological impulses such as feeding, drinking, eliminating, avoiding pain, and gaining sexual pleasures. It seeks immediate gratification and is said to operate on the pleasure principle.

Children soon learn that their impulses cannot be gratified immediately: hunger will have to wait until somebody provides food; relieving bladder or bowel pressure until a suitable place is available and certain other impulses like hitting another child may be punished. Ego develops as a consequence, as the young child learns to consider the demands of reality. The ego obeys the reality principle.

The superego is the internalised representation of the values of society as taught to the child by the parents and others. The superego develops in response to parental rewards and punishment. It strives for perfection.

Freud believed that the conflict between the id impulses and the restraining influences of the ego and superego constitutes the motivation for most behaviour. This conflict may give rise to much anxiety and the defence mechanisms are used to protect oneself against this anxiety.

The development of superego can be viewed as the equivalent of conscience; normal children internalise their parents' values because they want to be like their parents and fear that in not doing so might endanger their parents' affection for them. A child realises that certain actions are right and certain others wrong, and thus feels guilty when he or she commits a wrong action. A child who receives no affection from either parent may not fear the loss of their love and may not internalise parental values. Like children who are brought up in large institutions with impersonal carers, they may also develop poorly the capacity to feel guilt and the development of conscience may also be impaired, with progressive psychosocial disability in adolescence and adult life.

Piaget: cognitive development

Jean Piaget (1896-1980) was a Swiss psychologist who derived his theory of cognitive development from the observation of children: his own, those attending a nursery and, subsequently, school children (Piaget, 1932, 1951, 1952; Piaget & Inhelder, 1969). As well as describing a stage theory of development, he identified four necessary factors that brought this development about:

(1) maturation – physical development of the nervous system governed by inherent factors
(2) interactions with inanimate objects – learning as an ongoing experiment in the world of objects and physical forces
(3) opportunities for social interactions – learning derived from contact with other people, including imitation as well as formal teaching
(4) the ability to construct an internal representation of the world.

He described four stages through which children's cognitive development passes.

(1) Sensorimotor stage (0–2 years)

By encountering objects and people around them, infants acquire the ability to distinguish between self and other. Maturing infants' natural activity leads them to discover the properties of objects in their environment. Through physically acting on the world by reaching for a desired object they discover distance. By handling cloth or a plastic cup they discover texture and weight. Learning proceeds as an inevitable consequence of the infant's innate ability to act and perceive. At first an object removed from view is not searched for, at about 10 months it is searched for only where it was last seen, then finally the infant extensively searches. Piaget took this to indicate the infant's dawning sense of the permanence of objects.

(2) Pre-operational stage (2–7 years)

Having acquired familiarity with the properties of objects and the ability to retain a stable, internalised representation of them, the child learns that they can be represented by symbols, particularly words. This stage has four characteristics: egocentrism, animism, pre-causal logic, and an authoritarian morality.

Children in this stage are egocentric – they cannot imagine another person's viewpoint and see themselves as at the centre of their own universe. Children talk in each other's company but each child talks only about his or her own concerns; Piaget described this as the 'collective monologue'. Everything is seen to have life, feelings and thought; explanations are animistic. Most events are thought to happen by chance. Reasoning is non-scientific (pre-causal). In play a stick can symbolise a horse, and be ridden, despite its dissimilarity. The child is not yet able to see beyond the most superficial property of an object such as its height. If this changes, such as when water is poured from a tall thin glass to a short fat one, the child will insist that the actual amount of water has changed. Similarly, a child at this stage will insist that 10 sweets strung out in a long line are more than 10 sweets in a short, bunched-up line. The child has yet to appreciate the property of conservation of volume or number.

Children's authoritarian morality can be observed in their ideas about the rules of games. They are believed to be sacrosanct though understanding of them is limited. They also believe that bad events like illness or loss are punishments, that punishment should fit the crime, and that bad deeds are followed by retribution. This is also the stage of the development of conscience and guilt and a sense of obligation. Childhood phobias and fears are common in this animistic stage. Children misconstrue their ailments and the treatments they are getting. They have unrealistic fantasies about illness which is explained in moralistic terms. Painful procedures are seen as punishment and arouse guilt and anxiety, more so than at any later stage of development.

(3) Stage of concrete operations (7–12 years)

Children lose their egocentrism, animism and authoritarian morality during this stage. Children start to use categories; they are able to abstract from a number of objects a common property that allows them to be classified together. In a similar way, a child of nine years is able to ignore superficial differences such as the height of the column of water, while attending to its more essential characteristic, its volume. Conservation of number occurs at the age of six years, followed by conservation of weight at seven years on average. Children are now able to engage in cooperative activities with others. Justice is more a central concept than obedience.

(4) Formal operations (12 years onward)

By this stage children can entertain novel constructions and possibilities, completely divorced from objects around them. In addition they can anticipate consequences by manipulating mental constructions. Essentially, they can now hypothesise. This ability allows them to imagine the world from the point of view of others, an essential, albeit not always achieved, task of adolescence.

Piaget's work has had major effects on primary-school education and research into cognitive development of childhood. His theories have brought about a transformation from rote learning to learning by practical experimentation in primary schools. Piaget's findings have been largely confirmed, but he has been proved wrong on two issues. The development of intelligence in children is now known to be more complicated than he had suggested, and some of the apparent immaturities of children in the pre-operational stage are due to misunderstanding rather than faulty logic (Donaldson, 1978). On closer examination children's speech in the pre-operational stage reveals shared topics despite a superficial lack of relationship in their utterances, and Bower (1979) regards the 'collective monologue' as an artefact of the observer's lack of understanding of children's tendency to omit important connections in their speech.

Plate I. A typical painting by a one- or two-year-old. Only one or two colours were used, and they were layered on thickly. The painting did not use all of the paper

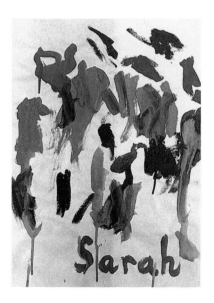

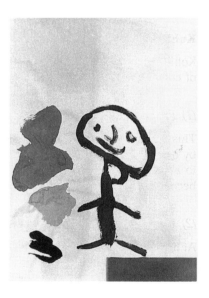

Plate II. A painting by a two-year-old. Lots of colours are used and the whole sheet of paper is employed

Plate III. A painting by a four-year-old. Note the large head and relative lack of other details, typical of paintings at this age

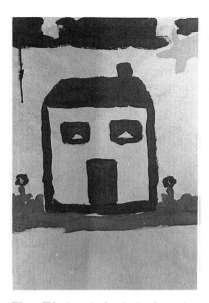

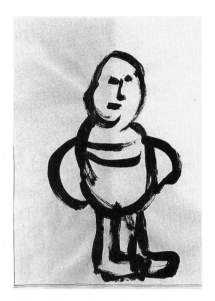

Plate IV. A typical painting by a six-year-old

Plate V. A painting by an eight-year-old. Although it is only a line painting, it shows a greater sense of proportion and more detail than the earlier paintings

Kohlberg: moral development

Kohlberg (1969, 1973) used Piaget's approach to account for the development of conscience and proposed three stages.

(1) Pre-conventional morality (level I)

This applies to children up to about seven years. Behaviour is guided entirely by external contingencies. Socially acceptable behaviour is exhibited purely to avoid punishment. Later on in this stage adherence to social rules also becomes driven by reward for conformity.

(2) Conventional morality (level II)

At first the child conforms to avoid the disapproval of others. This develops into a sense of an externally imposed obligation so that children will feel bad if they do not 'do their duty' (authority orientation).

(3) Post-conventional morality (level III)

Actions are guided by the principle of a social contract where one behaves towards others as one would wish them to behave to oneself. This finally evolves into 'ethical principle orientation', in which actions are determined according to abstract values such as justice and dignity, and are driven by the urge to avoid self-condemnation. According to Kohlberg many individuals never progress beyond level II. He sees the stages of moral development as parallel to Piaget's stages of cognitive development. By the age of 13-14 only those who have developed the capacity of abstract thought are able to function at this level. He also reports that only 10% of his subjects over the age of 16 were at the highest stage of moral development, the stage of 'ethical principle orientation'.

Bowlby: social and emotional development

Our knowledge of normal social development owes much to observational studies that have their roots in ethology. Indeed, man shares with most other higher species a propensity to associate and attach; in man this is experienced as affection. Studies have shown social development to be an interaction between an innate process of unfolding and a minimum necessary social environment. Bowlby (1977) combined theory and research from the fields of anthropology, ethology and psychoanalysis.

Within the first few weeks of life a baby's capacity for social behaviour shows itself by indiscriminant smiling and gurgling in response to attention from anyone. By two or three months babies preferentially respond to parents, and react most positively to a laugh or smile and least to an unresponsive, expressionless face. Even this early, the baby has the capacity to interact in the reciprocal 'turn-taking' manner so characteristic of all social interactions. Indeed, it would appear that in humans the readiness of an adult to engage with the baby in this way forms the basis for attachments; it is entirely analogous to the movement and visual salience of a hen that determines the chick's attachment to it.

By six to eight months these specific attachments or bonds have developed to an extent that if the particular adult leaves, the child protests (separation anxiety). Frightening situations lead the infant to seek proximity to the adult (the secure base) which, once achieved, gives the infant the confidence to move away and explore to an extent that increases with age. Conflicts between the child's increasing curiosity about the environment and the mother's concern for his or her safety can lead to temper tantrums, which are normally transient, ceasing by the age of five.

Concurrent with the development of specific attachment is an increasing wariness of strangers that develops into outright fear at 9 to 12 months, particularly if the encounter is unexpected and a parent is not present. The specific attachments of infants are often multiple but are hierarchical in preference. The intensity of these attachments peaks at 18 months, after which, in the preschool years, the child comes to tolerate the departure of attachment figures better, particularly if it is anticipated or explained, and clinging diminishes though it can reassert itself if the child is ill or tired.

Biological or social conditions can deviate or delay this orderly sequence of social development, with both immediate and delayed consequences. Temperament can render some children more prone to separation anxiety, as can the experience of a period apart from the mother, particularly if it carried with it the additional threat of family turmoil or illness, and was not mitigated by the presence of an alternative attachment figure such as a grandparent, or an assigned nurse if the child was admitted to hospital. Children denied the opportunity to form specific attachments through an upbringing in a poor institution can manifest an abnormality of social development characterised by numerous superficial attachments in which they respond indiscriminately to strangers.

Early social development encompasses the child's fantasy life as well as the concrete world. During the preschool years children often entertain elaborate fantasies involving imaginary friends or roles such as teacher/pupil or doctor/patient. This rehearsal serves to reduce anxiety and allows children to explore the world gradually and distort it to meet their current emotional needs. Though often appearing to be engrossed in fantasy, the child never loses the ability to distinguish between imagination and reality. At school this florid fantasy life should become less prominent.

The later consequences of aberrant social development include an inability to form stable relationships with sexual partners and any ensuing children, often perpetuating the cycle of emotional damage. Attachments broken by loss or separation in childhood expose individuals to the risk of depressive illness and self-harm in later life. In addition it is clear that the infant's ability to incorporate acceptable norms of behaviour successfully depends on a background of stable attachments in early life. Absence of these attachments may lead to delinquency and criminality in later life and in extreme cases to affectionless psychopathy.

Erikson: social development

Social development involves a broadening of the social domain from the dyadic mother–child relationship to incorporating siblings and then more distant relatives into the social world. The start of school involves integration into an even broader domain, with new opportunities to form friendships and enmities, as well as the first exposure to external authority figures such as teachers. During late childhood and adolescence the peer group starts to compete with the family for a child's allegiance. The increasing importance of the peer group reduces the prominence of the family in teenagers' social life, and though they may adopt, to the annoyance of their parents, the appearance and tastes of their peers, they still adhere to their family's social values and maintain a harmonious relationship with them.

Erikson (1968) proposed a series of eight psychosocial stages to describe development from cradle to grave, based on the individual's ability to resolve a series of psychosocial crises and to establish appropriate social relations at each of these life stages (Table 2.2).

Acknowledgement

Thanks are due to Jean Harris Hendriks for help in the preparation of some of this chapter.

References

Berger, M., Yule, W. & Rutter, M. (1975) Attainment and adjustment in two geographical areas. II. The prevalence of specific reading retardation. *British Journal of Psychiatry*, **126**, 510–519.

Bower, T. G. R. (1979) *Human Development*. San Francisco: W. H. Freeman.

Bowlby, J. (1977) The making and breaking of affectional bonds. *British Journal of Psychiatry*, **130**, 201–210, 421–431.

Donaldson, M. (1978) *Children's Minds*. Glasgow: Fontana/Collins.

Erikson, E. (1968) *Identity, Youth and Crisis*. London: Faber.

Freud, S. (1905) *Three Essays on the Theory of Sexuality*, standard edition, vol. 7. London: Hogarth Press.

Frith, U. (1978) Spelling difficulties. *Journal of Child Psychology and Psychiatry*, **19**, 279–285.

Graham, P. (1986) *Child Psychiatry: A Developmental Approach*. Oxford: Oxford University Press.

Green, R. (1985) Atypical sexual development. In *Child & Adolescent Psychiatry: Modern Approaches* (2nd edn) (eds M. Rutter & L. Hersov). Oxford: Blackwell Scientific.

Heston, L. L. & Shields, J. (1968) Homosexuality in twins: a family study and a register study. *Archives of General Psychiatry*, **18**, 149–160.

Illingworth, R. S. (1990) *The Development of the Infant and Young Child, Normal and Abnormal*. Edinburgh: Churchill Livingstone.

Kinsey, A. C., Pomeroy, W. B., Martin, C. E., *et al* (1948) *Sexual Behaviour in the Human Male*. Philadelphia: Saunders.

——, ——, ——, *et al* (1953) *Sexual Behaviour in the Human Female*. Philadelphia: Saunders.

Kohlberg, L. (1969) Stage and sequence: the cognitive developmental approach to socialisation. In *Handbook of Socialisation Theory and Research* (ed. D. A. Goslin). Chicago: Rand McNally.

—— (1973) Implications of developmental psychology for education: examples from moral development. *Educational Psychologist*, **10**, 2–14.

Money, J. & Ehrhardt, A. A. (1972) *Man and Woman, Boy and Girl: Differentiation and Dimorphism of Gender Identity from Conception to Maturity*. Baltimore: Johns Hopkins University Press.

Orlansky, H. (1949) Infant care and personality. *Psychological Bulletin*, **46**, 1–48.

Piaget, J. (1932) *The Moral Judgement of a Child*. London: Routledge & Kegan Paul.

—— (1951) *The Child's Conception of the World*. London: Routledge & Kegan Paul.

—— (1952) *The Language and Thought of the Child*. London: Routledge & Kegan Paul.

—— & Inhelder, B. (1969) *The Psychology of the Child*. London: Routledge & Kegan Paul.

Rourke, B. P. & Strang, J. D. (1983) Subtypes of reading and arithmetic disabilities: a neuropsychological analysis. In *Developmental Neuropsychiatry* (ed. M. Rutter). New York: Guilford Press.

Rutter, M., Tizard, J. & Whitmore, K. (1970) *Education, Health and Behaviour*. London: Longman.

Sewell, W. H. & Mussen, P. H. (1952) The effect of feeding, weaning and scheduling procedures on childhood adjustment and the formation of oral symptoms. *Child Development* **23**, 185-191.

Terr, L. C. (1987) Children's nightmares. In *Sleep and its Disorders in Children* (ed. C. Guilleminault). New York: Raven Press.

—— (1991) Childhood traumas: an outline and overview. *American Journal of Psychiatry*, **148**, 10-20.

Thomas, A. & Chess, S. (1977) *Temperament and Development*. New York: Brunner/Mazel.

Winnicott, D. W. (1958) Transitional objects and transitional phenomena. In *Collected Papers: Through Paediatrics to Psychoanalysis*. London: Tavistock. (Reprinted (1975) as *Through Paediatrics to Psycho-analysis*. London: Hogarth Press.)

World Health Organization (1992) *The ICD-10 Classification of Mental and Behavioural Disorders*. Geneva: WHO.

Further reading

Atkinson, R. L., Atkinson, R. C. & Hilgard, E. R. (1983) *Introduction to Psychology*. New York: Harcourt Brace Jovanovich.

Illingworth, R. S. (1990) *The Development of the Infant and Young Child, Normal and Abnormal*. Edinburgh: Churchill Livingstone.

Rutter, M. & Hersov, L. (1985) *Child and Adolescent Psychiatry: Modern Approaches*. Oxford: Blackwell Scientific.

3 Causes of disorder, I. Theoretical perspectives

Dora Black

Learning theories ● *Cognitive theory* ● *Developmental theories* ●
Psychodynamic theories ● *Systems theory* ● *The biological theories* ●
An attempted integration of theories

There is as yet no unifying theory of the causes of psychiatric disorder in childhood, nor is there likely to be until much more is known about the development and functioning of the brain, how the brain influences behaviour and how constitution and environment interact. Yet in the same way that infants become unbearably anxious or switch off completely in sleep, faced with the "blooming buzzing confusion" of the sensory input which assails them and which they cannot organise and integrate because of lack of knowledge and experience, so a practitioner, faced with the reality of troubled or troubling children, and complex family interactions, as well as the many, often conflicting, theories put forward to explain these phenomena, needs to develop a working hypothesis in order not to become unbearably anxious or switch off completely.

The theories which are set out below are those which currently seem to account for some of the observations made in the course of our work. The novice child psychiatrist could be forgiven for thinking that they are very much akin to the descriptions of an elephant made by blind men – each of them feeling a different part and each believing himself to be possessed of the whole truth. In practice, it is helpful to have a working knowledge of these organising concepts and to maintain a healthy scepticism towards those who claim that their theories embody the whole truth.

We do need to have an eclectic approach to childhood psychiatric disorders and yet practitioners need to develop a way of conceptualising the material they are presented with so that they can make enough sense of it to be able to offer help to their patients. This conceptual understanding will be increasingly based on the results of research. As the practitioner's curiosity becomes stimulated by the variety of problems they face daily in clinical practice and their compassion is aroused by the pain their patients and families suffer, it is to be hoped that they will become interested in adding to that body of knowledge themselves.

It is beyond the scope of this book to attempt to describe in detail all the theories and the research that underpins some of them. The reader is referred to Rutter & Hersov (1985) for a fuller exposition. A useful source is Tyrer & Steinberg's (1987) *Models of Mental Disorder*, which describes four conceptual models used in psychiatry, the behavioural, the disease, the psychodynamic and the social, and illustrates their advantages and limitations as well as describing how to use them in practice.

Learning theories

Human learning is an immensely complex phenomenon; most theories tend to oversimplify and do not account for all the observed data. Early theorists did not consider developmental changes or biological differences or processes.

Learning theory as expounded by Skinner and other behaviourists (see Berger, 1985, for a summary) postulates that all human and animal behaviour is learned by conditioning, either classic Pavlovian or operant conditioning (see Chapter 10, pp. 183-191). Deviant behaviour in children, therefore, is due to faulty conditioning (by parents or teachers) or relative inability to learn because of low intelligence or disorders affecting memory, perception, attention and concentration, or specific learning disabilities in the child. The early learning theorists postulated the idea of the infant as a *tabula rasa* - a blank slate on which could be written the adult prescription of behaviour and knowledge.

The work of the developmental and cognitive psychologists and particularly the direct observation of infants made this idea untenable. It was recognised that the infant came into the world with a repertoire of behaviours or potential behaviours which was genetically programmed and which unfolded as development proceeded. One did not teach children to talk or to control their bowels. One might teach them to deposit faeces in a particular place when they were able developmentally to control their anal sphincter but one could not, by conditioning, speed up development, although one could slow it by producing fear of the toilet by coercion to sit on it and punishment if children soiled their pants.

Similarly, children develop language by hearing others speak to them and begin to imitate speech as their speech apparatus develops sufficiently. Again, they can be prevented from speaking by lack of experience of hearing speech (if they are deaf, or if no one speaks to them, or if there are deviant communications from a psychotic parent, or if speaking is punished consistently) but they cannot be taught to speak like they are taught to read.

Strict learning theorists base their work on observed behaviour and do not recognise internal mental processes which cannot be measured or observed. Learning theory helps us to understand many childhood psychiatric disorders, particularly phobias, encopresis, some conduct disorders, and some cases of substance abuse.

Such theories do not account for much observed behaviour, for example attachment to an abusing parent, emotions such as joy and sorrow, many emotional disorders, and much else.

By paying attention only to what is measurable, learning theorists deny the complexity of much human experience and behaviour. Their theories are most useful in changing behaviour that is maladaptive, and are the basis of behaviour therapy (see Chapter 10).

Case example

A boy, aged seven years, refuses to go to school and wishes to stay home, becoming anxious, aggressive, or developing somatic symptoms when pressed to attend (school refusal). Learning theorists would explain the phenomenology by suggesting that the child had learned that it was safer or more advantageous to remain at home than go to school, and that this behaviour was reinforced by his parents. They might deal with it by a behavioural technique, flooding, in which the child would be forced to return, and supported through the panic attack that would follow.

Cognitive theory

This is an extension of learning theory and is based on the idea that patients who are anxious or depressed have distorted cognitions. The immediate appraisal of a situation, the perception of long-term consequences, or other associations may be distorted. Anxiety, in this model, is maintained by mistaken or dysfunctional appraisal (Beck & Emery, 1985). It has given rise to a treatment, cognitive therapy, which has been shown to be effective in adults but has not been evaluated in children as yet.

Case example

Our school refuser may believe that at school he will be ridiculed and that he cannot deal with this. Such a cognition may be based on one or more experiences when he became emotionally aroused, for example being teased at school, and experienced the feelings as life-threatening. A cognitive therapist would spend time elucidating the precise nature of the distorted cognitions and systematically, in a therapeutic relationship, attempt to restructure such cognitions (see Chapter 10).

Developmental theories

The observations by ethologists and developmental psychologists (e.g. Richards, 1974; Stern, 1977; Shaffer & Dunn, 1979) of biologically based innate behaviour present at birth or soon after and the work of Piaget (1955) on the development of the child's understanding, both empirically based, made the integration of learning theories easier to achieve. It could be understood for example that a child's reflex grimace could be conditioned by selective reinforcement. The newborn might grimace randomly or reflexly at birth, but within the course of the first month of life would produce a smile when he saw a human face, presumably because the appearance of the human meant a reduction in distress or because the human, delighted to see the smile (a social behaviour which is rewarding to the parent) would selectively reinforce its appearance by rewarding the child with sounds, touch and play. The child had therefore learned by conditioning (and so had the parent!) to produce the smile in response to rewards. However, the original behaviour, the unconditioned smile, was biologically produced, not taught, and there is an interaction (the delight of the parent, as well as possible innate social instincts of the child) to complicate and influence the final behaviour – the social smile.

The work of developmental psychologists, also experimentally based, has contributed greatly to an understanding of the way in which behaviour develops and changes as the individual matures (see Bentovim, 1979*a*, for a summary). The study of attachment (Bowlby, 1969) is of particular importance in the understanding of psychopathology. Put at its simplest, the types of behaviour called attachment behaviour are now seen to be adaptive, in that they keep immature and defenseless infants in proximity to their carer and thus protect them.

Attachment behaviour is at its height at about three years of age and then diminishes progressively and changes in nature. It becomes reactivated in a different form and with a different purpose in late adolescence in order to form procreational bonds. In early childhood the threat of bond disruption evokes separation anxiety, which is considered normal and is adaptive behaviour. However, similar behaviour in a 13-year-old would be viewed as maladaptive and pathological.

The attachment system is one of a series of behaviour patterns which is thought to have evolved by natural selection, and has the function of making it more likely that an infant will survive to adulthood and thus reproduce. While separation anxiety is seen as normal in a two-year-old, there are forms of attachment pathology which can be identified in children as young as one year, such as anxious attachment. These are different from the ways attachment pathology can be manifested in a seven-year-old (e.g. school refusal) or in a 19-year-old (e.g. difficulties in leaving home).

Case example
The developmental psychologists would view our school refuser as having an attachment pathology. He might be changing schools and finding such change difficult because he became insecurely attached to his mother in early childhood, perhaps as a result of premature separation.

Psychodynamic theories

These theories were the first to be applied to childhood psychiatric disorders, and for many years most child psychiatrists were psychoanalysts or analytically orientated. Although Sigmund Freud, who developed psychoanalysis from which all psychodynamic theories are derived, did not see any child patients himself, his daughter Anna and his pupil Melanie Klein both applied his technique of analysis to child patients, developing new ways of observing and interpreting children's non-verbal communications. Both of them came to England in the 1930s and pursued their work here, founding to some extent competing schools. Influential psychodynamic theoreticians included Erikson, Winnicott and Bowlby, who was trained as an analyst and never dissociated himself from the analytic movement, although his work is more akin to developmental psychology.

Many of the ideas and insights which originated with Freud and his followers have become so much part of our culture and in particular a clinician's stock-in-trade that it may be difficult to disentangle them. They are attractive because they are the only theories that attempt to describe and explain all the mental phenomena experienced by patients as well as those we can observe in their behaviour. These subjective experiences are not always what they seem, and psychoanalysts try to understand the meaning of communications, both verbal and non-verbal, according to a complex model of the mind. This model is a developmental one, but it is not easily verified by experimental means although attempts have been made to do so. It is largely derived from clinical work with patients, although observation of well children is increasingly used. A good summary of the ideas of the main theorists is given by Dare (1985).

The infantile psychological state is dominated by affects, of which anxiety and pleasure are the most important. At first these were seen as not under the infant's control but the current view is that there is an increasing integration over the first six months, aided by intuitive and sensitive mothering and the baby's attachment to her. Winnicott (1960) and Bowlby (1958) see the infant from birth as a responsive interactive being who actively structures the environment.

The importance of the traditional Freudian view of psychosexual develop-ment (the 'oral' first stage, the 'anal' second stage, and the 'genital' third stage, with a 'latency' period in later childhood before the development of adult sexuality) is accorded less importance in modern psychoanalytic thinking, although the Oedipus complex, the conflict in a child's mind between his love for his mother and his love for, rivalry, and jealousy of and fear of retaliation from his father, is still thought to be important as a source of conflict and psychopathology, particularly castration anxiety.

The idea that children develop firstly by imitation and then internalise their parents by identifying with them fits in with the observations of the learning theorists. The development of superego or conscience is part of this process. The concept of defences against anxiety, developed by Anna Freud and by Klein, has become part of psychiatric thinking and forms the basis for our understanding of the development of neurosis. Erikson's concepts of children developing through stages, each of which imposes tasks on them, is an attractive one but has not contributed to a greater understanding of the causes of psychiatric disorder in this age group.

Psychoanalysis and related theories are basically attempts to understand emotional and mental development, and are particularly important in helping us to understand that all behaviour has meaning, and that the meaning may be obscured by unconscious mechanisms and may need to be patiently unravelled. It has given us a therapeutic technique, psychodynamic psychotherapy, which is undoubtedly a useful and effective way of helping some troubled children (Kolvin *et al*, 1988), particularly those with relationship and emotional difficulties which stem from idiosyncratic experiences. The techniques employed which produce change may have less to do with the theoretical model used by the therapist than with the therapist him- or herself (Truax & Carkhuff, 1967).

> **Case example**
> Our school refuser would be seen by psychoanalysts as having developed conflicting feelings of love and hate towards his mother (perhaps because of her ridicule of his childish fears) and needing to stay home to guard her from his destructive, murderous fantasies about her.

Systems theory

Whereas learning theory and psychodynamic theory are concerned with the individual (although they take account of relationships), a different view of disturbed behaviour is that it is a manifestation of group processes, and in the case of children the group with whom they are most involved is the family. In the thinking of the other theorists, there is an interactive component but systems theorists, basing their thinking on the work of cyberneticists (von Bertalanffy, 1968), see individual function and dysfunction as a resultant of complex family interaction.

This view of a symptom or disorder as being the resultant of a systems disorder is relatively recent. The idea of studying families and their functioning started in the 1960s with the Timberlawn studies (Lewis *et al*, 1976). Looking at well and poorly functioning families, they found that they differed in their organisation in terms of power structure (structured versus chaotic), differentiation (clear identity versus fusion), communication (open versus evasive and confused), relationships (affiliative versus oppositional), reality sense, affect (warm, empathic versus cynicism, hopelessness), and attitudes to change and loss (adaptation versus denial). Healthy families had a strong parental coalition, good and varied relationships outside the family, and a transcendent value system.

Systems theorists are particularly interested in observing patterns of communication and conflict resolution in families, how homeostasis is maintained, similar types of behaviour across generations, and the positive value of symptoms.

Dare (1979) has suggested that to understand family functioning we need to consider three frames:

(1) the lifecycle of the family (courtship and early marriage, pregnancy, and infancy, toddlerhood and school, adolescence and leaving home, post-parenting, grandparenting)

(2) the intergenerational, historical aspects of the family
(3) the interactional structure of the family.

Minuchin *et al*'s (1978) findings that families with children suffering from certain disorders, such as anorexia nervosa, were enmeshed, with poor differentiation, and that the patient was detouring marital conflict led to the use of family therapy to try to alter these patterns of functioning with some success.

The success of a therapy based on a theory does not mean that the theory is correct or that it is the only explanation for the phenomena observed or inferred. The systems theorists, however, have widened the focus and attempted to make sense of the influences on children's functioning from the social groups, especially the family, of which they are a part and, reciprocally, of the influences on the family exerted by the child.

Case example

The systems theorist would view school refusal for example as a solution to a problem which had become a problem in itself. By staying at home the child was able to watch over the mother who was depressed and provoke the peripheral father into taking more interest in him and his mother. But the child was influenced to stay home by a family pattern of response to stress which may have extended back several generations and be expected of him. Indeed, it may enable his other siblings to behave more normally and he may have been inducted into the role of protector of mother to enable them to escape. The family therapist would address herself to the task of changing the system which had produced the symptom, rather than focusing solely on the identified patient.

The biological theories

This is the traditional disease or medical model, which views the patient as a passive recipient of noxious influences, be they constitutional or environmental. Diseases or disorders are seen as the resultant of a complex interaction between genetic endowment and environmental forces such as structural damage, infection, noxious substances or experiences, deficiencies in the provision of nutrients or other essential substances or experiences. Some diseases are almost completely determined by inheritance and others almost entirely by the environment, with most lying somewhere between the two. Psychiatric disorder in children would be seen as related to genetic influences modified by the environment.

Anorexia nervosa would be seen as a specific phobia of weight in a pubertal girl whose perfectionistic personality (genetic constitution) cannot accommodate change, particularly if she has had a trauma of a sexual nature which makes her perceive change as dangerous.

It can be seen here that the concept of experience as a precipitator of pathology is congruent with learning theory, and the idea of trauma as leading to disorder is an early psychodynamic concept, although it was later given less prominence. Families in the biological model are seen as general protectors, providers or stressors but not as being part of the disorder. It is essentially then an individual model.

Case example

School refusal is seen as being caused by a strong genetic predisposition to anxiety, as evidenced by agoraphobic and depressive tendencies in several generations, with the symptoms precipitated by the experience of separation or threat of permanent separation increasing anxiety.

An attempted integration of theories

It can be seen that it is possible to view the causes of various child and adolescent psychiatric disorders in very different and almost mutually exclusive ways.

It may be helpful to consider that one can view the child and family at different levels, each of which are most easily explained by a different model (Bentovim, 1979*b*). Rather as one views bodily functioning at cellular, organ or system level or as whole-body functioning, one could view the individual at an intrapsychic, dyadic, triadic or group level. Or at an individual, family, community, national or international level. Psychoanalytic understanding is particularly appropriate for individual, intrapsychic phenomena, and has some value for dyadic relationships, but is less helpful for understanding more complex groups. Biological and learning theories are predominantly individually focused, and systems theory is family focused and can accommodate triadic and group phenomena.

An interesting example of the complexity of explanatory hypotheses which are elaborated in the absence of evidence of the pathological basis of a disorder is the recent discovery that eradicating the bacterium *Helicobacter pylori* from the stomach and duodenum will cure most peptic ulcers (Potter, 1991). Now it is likely that all the work that has been done in understanding the personality characteristics of ulcer-prone individuals will be redundant as medication will cure and even prevent this condition. Similarly with tuberculosis; the 19th-century and early 20th-century literature was replete with observations about the personalities of people who developed tuberculosis but the discovery of the organism and then of an effective antibiotic made such observations redundant.

The question is which of the disorders we recognise today will be explained in the next century by a different model from the current one? It is likely that psychotic disorders will be found to have an organic basis, as may depressive illnesses – even if they are precipitated by experiences such as loss, the mechanism is a biological one and may be susceptible to direct influence, although the treatment may be a psychological one. The hyperactive syndrome, autism, anorexia nervosa, and tics, are likely to have a biological explanation. Conduct disorders and many emotional disorders, the bulk of child psychiatric practice, are likely to be seen as more complex in aetiology, as are personality disorders, habit disorders and some learning disorders.

In our present state of knowledge, the model that best helps us to understand our patients and their predicaments, and helps us plan an effective intervention, is an eclectic one that draws something from all the theories outlined above. To understand each child and each disorder we need to draw on these theories to different degrees.

A formulation for each child which balances the contributions to the disorder of genetic constitution, temperament, family functioning, environmental insults and deficiencies, stage of development, intellectual ability, and the meaning the child and others attribute to these experiences will enable us to help best. Such a formulation will take into account at which phase of the life cycle each family member is, what influences have been brought to bear from the parents' own families of origin, the idiosyncratic experiences and perceptions of those experiences which the child has, his or her inner construction of reality, the strengths and weaknesses of the child, family, school and wider network. It will also need to take into account what is available in terms of therapists and other services, and will consider the effect of any planned interventions on the other members of the family and network. The following case study attempts to illustrate such an approach.

Case example

A seven-year-old boy, Freddie, is referred because of difficulties in concentration and aggressive behaviour at school. At home his behaviour has always been more difficult than his 13-year-old brother's but his parents had not felt that it was abnormal until he started school; they had always been able to cope by isolating him and not rewarding him by attending to his disruptiveness. They were critical of the young and inexperienced teacher's inability to cope but recognised that their son was a handful. Their concern was mainly that he was not progressing as well at school as his brother, or as they felt he should be. They were both university graduates, but he had not yet learned to read. The father was inclined to make light of the aggressive behaviour – "Boys will be boys".

It was learned on direct questioning that he had been born after a long labour and had had difficulty establishing a normal sleep pattern. He had always been a very active baby and as a toddler had had more than his share of accidents because he was fearless and adventurous. He had been excluded from nursery school because he was so aggressive but had enjoyed staying at home with his mother as she had enjoyed his being there, as the father and older son were away all day and she felt somewhat frustrated at not being able to follow her career.

The family history was unremarkable. The older boy was seen as normal and helpful but had a tendency to suffer from asthma. The parents' marriage was basically good but was suffering some stress from the mother's career frustration and their different views about the patient.

During an assessment of the whole family the boy was extremely active and disinhibited, and he tended to escalate his dangerous activities when his brother was being attended to. When that happened his father laughed but his mother became sad and subdued. Neither acted to stop his dangerous behaviour and the psychiatrist felt impelled to take control. Psychological assessment indicated that the boy was of superior intelligence but was of poor attainment in reading, spelling, and maths. This seemed to be associated with defects in attention and concentration. When seen alone it became clear that he had a poor self-image, believing that he was bad and that he could not be good. He had few friends at school and he felt everyone hated him. He was often bullied and teased, and he hated school.

The formulation was that the boy was suffering from attention deficit syndrome with hyperactivity. This was probably present from birth and may have been influenced by the long labour or have been genetically determined. The influence of allergic factors was considered in view of the family history of allergy. On the whole the family had managed to cope with his difficult behaviour because the parents were competent, the older boy posed no problems and there was a large gap between the two brothers. The parents had found by trial and error a way of dealing with Freddie which was successful. Nevertheless his behaviour had caused tensions within the family and the boy was now not coping either educationally or socially at school. Some of his behaviour was being reinforced by his father, who did not recognise the extent of the boy's suffering because of his social isolation and his low self-esteem. The mother's loneliness leading to her wanting a companion at home had prevented them from recognising the problem earlier.

This view of Freddie's condition recognises the constitutional origins, and the maintaining forces within the family, the exacerbating forces at school and the resultant psychologically determined sadness and low self-esteem of the child. The complex influences of the family on the child and vice versa, and the resultant family dysfunction as well as the escalating suffering and handicap of the boy required a multifaceted approach to management and treatment. Freddie was prescribed methylphenidate. The school was visited by the psychologist and informed of the diagnosis, of his underfunctioning and low self-esteem, and a behavioural and remedial education programme was instituted. The family were offered family therapy aimed at helping them to teach the boy how to cope with his disability and to change their characteristic ways of reacting. The older boy was given a specific helping role which he enjoyed. Attention was given to helping his mother develop her own career and the marital tensions were addressed. The effect of the medication was to improve his concentration and lessen his distractibility and he began to make progress at school. His teacher started to treat him differently and so did his peers as his hyperactivity lessened and this improved his self-concept and self-esteem. The school felt less hopeless about him as they had a clear behavioural programme to follow which seemed to be helpful and effective. The family found that they could make changes in their functioning which were rewarding.

Conclusion

This case illustrates the advantages of an eclectic approach using several theoretical models (biological, systems, psychodynamic, and learning) and combining therapies (drug, behavioural, family and remedial educational therapy).

References

Beck, A. T. & Emery, G. (1985) *Anxiety Disorders and Phobias*. New York: Basic Books.

Bentovim, A. (1979*a*) Child development research findings and psychoanalytic theory: an integrative critique. In *The First Year of Life* (eds D. Shaffer & J. Dunn). Chichester: Wiley.

—— (1979*b*) Theories of family interaction and techniques of intervention. *Journal of Family Therapy*, **1**, 321–345.

Berger, M. (1985) Learning theories, development and childhood disorders. In *Child and Adolescent Psychiatry: Modern Approaches* (2nd edn) (eds M. Rutter & L. Hersov). Oxford: Blackwell Scientific.

Bowlby, J. (1958) The nature of the child's tie to his mother. *International Journal of Psycho-Analysis*, **39**, 350–373.

—— (1969) *Attachment and Loss, Vol. 1 - Attachment*. London. Hogarth Press.

Dare, C. (1979) Psychoanalysis and systems in family therapy. *Journal of Family Therapy*, **1**, 137–151.

—— (1985) Psychoanalytic theories of development. In *Child and Adolescent Psychiatry: Modern Approaches* (2nd edn) (eds M. Rutter & L. Hersov). Oxford: Blackwell Scientific.

Kolvin, I., Macmillan, A., Nicol, A. R., *et al* (1988) Psychotherapy is effective. *Journal of the Royal Society of Medicine*, **18**, 261–266.

Lewis, J. M., Beavers, W. R., Gossett, J. T., *et al* (1976) *No Single Thread: Psychological Health in Family Systems*. New York: Bruner/Mazel.

Minuchin, A., Rosman, B. L. & Baker, L. (1978) *Psychosomatic Families - Anorexia Nervosa in Context*. Cambridge: Harvard University Press.

Piaget, J. (1955) *The Child's Construction of Reality*. London: Routledge & Kegan Paul.

Potter, A. R. (1991) Duodenal ulcer: the villain unmasked? *British Medical Journal*, **302**, 919–921.

Richards, M. P. M. (ed.) (1974) *The Integration of a Child into a Social World*. London: Cambridge University Press.

Rutter, M. & Hersov, L. (1985) *Child and Adolescent Psychiatry: Modern Approaches* (2nd edn). Oxford: Blackwell Scientific.

Shaffer, D. & Dunn, J. (1979) *The First Year of Life: Psychological and Medical Implications of Early Experience*. Chichester: Wiley.

Stern, D. (1977) *The First Relationship: Infant and Mother*. London: Fontana/Open Books.

Truax, C. B. & Carkhuff, R. R. (1967) *Towards Effective Counselling and Psychotherapy: Training and Practice*. Chicago: Aldin.

Tyrer, P. & Sternberg, D. (1987) *Models for Mental Disorder*. London: Wiley.

von Bertalanffy, L. (1968) *General System Theory*. New York: Braziller.

Winnicott, D. W. (1960) The theory of the parent–infant relationship. *International Journal of Psycho-Analysis*, **41**, 585–595.

4 Causes of disorder, II. A review of the research findings
David Cottrell

Individual factors ● *Influences of the immediate family* ● *Wider environmental influences* ● *Conclusion*

Causation in child and adolescent psychiatry is complex and multifactorial. In general medicine a diagnostic label carries information concerning underlying aetiology, mode of presentation and likely successful treatments. In child and adolescent psychiatry this is not yet the case, although much evidence exists concerning causes of disorder. What is less clear are the mechanisms by which known aetiological factors combine to produce symptoms and clinical syndromes. Two children from seemingly similar backgrounds and with similar aetiological factors operating may present in markedly different ways; indeed, one of them may not even have any signs of disorder. On the other hand, two children with identical signs and symptoms may be found to have completely different aetiological factors contributing to their condition.

In the face of this complexity it is helpful to consider the different ways in which aetiological factors may impinge on the child. *Predisposing* factors will make some children more vulnerable to disorder in the first place. These need to be distinguished from *precipitating* factors which may trigger the onset of disorders, and *perpetuating* factors which will maintain symptoms long after the precipitants have disappeared. Thus a child with neurological disorder may be predisposed to a psychiatric disorder, which is then precipitated by a stress such as the birth of a sibling, and perpetuated by family factors, such as maternal depression, which result in impaired parenting. Table 4.1 indicates these areas of influence on the expression of childhood psychiatric disorder.

Table 4.1 Causes of child psychiatric disorder

	Individual	Family	Wider environment
Predisposing factors			
Precipitating factors			
Perpetuating factors			

As aetiology is multifactorial, consideration of possible aetiological factors in each cell will reduce the chance of important causes being overlooked.

It is important to consider circular (e.g. self-maintaining feedback loops) as opposed to linear (past cause leading to current effect) models of causality. As well as looking for causes in the past it is vital to examine how such past experiences are affecting current interactions in a way which perpetuates a child's problems. In a family, an individual's actions will influence others and in turn be influenced by their responses. A depressed mother's apathetic and inconsistent behaviour may contribute to her child's conduct disorder which in turn will exacerbate the mother's depression. Maternal depression may in turn influence and be influenced by marital discord, to set up further self-maintaining cycles. When attempting to understand possible perpetuators of behaviour it is helpful to ask about the family's past and current attempts to solve the problem, as such failed solutions are often repeated and themselves exacerbate the problem. All concerned will attribute some *meaning* to the problem, and this needs to be asked about. For further discussion of these areas see Chapter 6.

A further helpful division of aetiological factors is into those connected with the individual child and those resulting from the child's environment. Environmental factors can be further subdivided into those concerned with the child's immediate family and those concerned with the child's wider environment (neighbourhood, school, etc.) (Box 4.1).

Box 4.1   Types of influences on the expression of mental ill health in children

Individual factors
  Genetics
  Gender
  Cognition
  Temperament
  Chronic illness and disability
Influence of the immediate family
  Early attachment
  Brief separations
  Divorce
  Life events
  Family structure
  Family size
  Ordinal position
  Parenting style
  Marital discord
  Parental mental illness
  Parental criminality
Wider environmental influences
  Neighbourhoods
  Social class and disadvantage
  Schools

Individual factors

Until relatively recently, children have been seen as 'blank slates' upon which environmental influences have worked to produce the adult. It is only in the last 10 to 20 years that researchers have come to realise the degree to which young children, by virtue of their own innate characteristics, can influence their environment and thus their own development. Characteristics of the newborn such as temperament, gender, IQ, and so on, will affect and determine the behaviour of significant others in the child's environment, setting up recurrent patterns of interaction which may affect later development. Physical characteristics such as perceptual deficit or physical handicap will directly affect the child's ability to interact with or even be aware of his or her physical environment.

Within this framework arguments about nature/nurture are unhelpful. Instead, it must be recognised that innate individual characteristics interact with environmental influences from the moment of birth (or more probably from before birth) to produce a particular pattern of development. Children in the same family experience different environments as a result of differing responses to their individual characteristics, and the same child put in a different family environment may develop very differently.

As the child grows older, observed individual differences are clearly a result of such interactions. This section focuses only on those individual differences which are apparent early on.

Genetics

In general, specific genetic influences do not play a major part in child and adolescent psychiatry and there is little good evidence for a genetic role in most such disorder. However, there is good evidence for genetic factors in some specific conditions.

Sibling and twin studies suggest the importance of genetic factors in infantile autism (Folstein & Rutter, 1977), although the exact mode of inheritance is unclear.

Familial loading has been noticed with Tourette's syndrome, and twin studies confirm the role of genetic factors. Of interest is the repeated finding that chronic tics and obsessive–compulsive symptoms also occur more commonly than would be expected in the families of children with Tourette's. A dominant autosomal gene seems the most likely explanation of the current data (Rutter *et al*, 1990).

There is clear evidence that when a major affective disorder arises in childhood there is likely to be a greater genetic component than when the disorder arises later in life. However, there is less evidence about the contribution of genetic factors to depression generally in childhood and adolescence (Rutter *et al*, 1990).

Schizophrenia is fortunately rare in children and young adolescents. The evidence for a major genetic contribution to its aetiology is well established and discussed in more detail in another volume in this series.

Family and twin studies show a large genetic component to nocturnal enuresis (Bakwin, 1973). It is thought that what is inherited is a delay in the neuromuscular development of the bladder.

There is little evidence of a genetic role in conduct disorder and, surprisingly in view of the contribution of genetic factors to adult criminality, little evidence for a role in juvenile delinquency. Rutter *et al* (1990) point out that this is probably because most juvenile crime does not persist into adult life. Children with conduct disorder and delinquency are more likely to come from families with a criminal parent, but twin and adoption studies indicate that environmental rather than genetic causes are responsible.

Although early research suggested a role for genetic factors in hyperkinetic syndrome, more recent concerns about the rigour of these studies make any definite conclusions impossible (Rutter *et al*, 1990). Increased rates of alcoholism and antisocial personality in male, and hysteria in female adult relatives of hyperkinetic children have been found, but the association is as likely to be for psychological reasons as for genetic. Recent twin studies suggest a significant but small genetic contribution (Goodman & Stevenson, 1989*a,b*).

Although mental handicap is not in itself a psychiatric disorder it is an important aetiological factor in the development of such disorders. Genetic factors are a significant cause of mental handicap, with fragile X syndrome alone accounting for up to 10% of males with handicap. (Mental handicap and generalised learning difficulties are dealt with in another volume in this series.)

Gender

Epidemiological studies have shown consistently that boys are more vulnerable to psychiatric disorder in general than girls, usually by a factor of 2 : 1. Within this general category, boys are much more likely to have conduct disorder (4 : 1) but prevalence rates are equal for boys and girls with respect to emotional disorder (Rutter *et al*, 1970*a*). As children grow older there are some changes and in adolescence girls have higher rates of emotional disorder. Anorexia nervosa and attempted suicide are also much more common in teenage girls than boys. The explanation for the overall excess of problems in younger boys is unclear but is likely to be at least partially due to the increased rate of developmental delays in boys.

Cognition

There is an inverse relationship between IQ and the prevalence of psychiatric disorder (Rutter *et al*, 1970*a*). There is no link with particular types of psychiatric disorder – rather there is an increase of all types. However, it should be noted that social disadvantage, which is associated with higher rates of psychiatric disorder, is also associated with lower IQ and may partially explain the above finding for children with mild to moderate generalised learning difficulties (mental handicap). The siblings of children with such generalised difficulties are also at greater risk of psychiatric disorder (Gath & Gumley, 1987). Children with specific learning difficulties, for example specific reading retardation, show higher rates of conduct disorder and antisocial behaviour (Rutter *et al*, 1970*a*).

Temperament

Temperament refers to individual differences in the style of behaviour. It concerns the way a child does something rather than what that child actually does. It is possible to identify temperamental characteristics in the first few weeks of life although these are of variable stability over time. A cluster of temperamental characteristics (biological irregularity, predominantly negative mood, slow adaptability to and withdrawal from new situations, and intense emotional reactions), controversially labelled 'difficult' temperament, has been shown to be associated with problems in mother–child interaction and behavioural difficulties in childhood (Thomas *et al*, 1968). A more recent follow-up study has shown a significant association of 'difficult' temperament between three and five years with adjustment problems in later life (Thomas & Chess, 1982).

Chronic illness and disability

Children with chronic illness and disability show rates of psychiatric disorder increased two- to threefold (Cadman *et al*, 1987; see also Chapter 5). In the families of these children there is evidence of increased rates of marital difficulties, behavioural and emotional disturbance in siblings, and general family dysfunction (Garrison & McQuiston, 1989).

If the chronic condition involves the central nervous system, the rate of psychiatric disorder increases by a factor of five, even in those children with average IQ scores (Rutter *et al*, 1970*b*). The precise mechanisms of this link between brain injury and psychiatric disorder are unclear. A combination of factors is likely to be involved. Such children may have generalised or specific learning difficulties, or both. Medical treatment may involve many hospital admissions, the use of drugs with psychological side-effects and other potentially harmful sequelae. Stigmatisation will create an abnormal social environment outside the home and parental and sibling difficulties in coming to terms with the diagnosis may result in similar difficulties inside the home. Children with brain injury are, in any case, more likely to come from socially disadvantaged homes, which in itself is associated with psychiatric disorder.

Children with perceptual difficulties also have higher rates of psychiatric disorder. Rates are increased by a factor of about three in deaf children and a factor of about five in blind children (Freeman, 1977).

Influences of the immediate family

Most people spend most of their lives within a family, first their family of origin then their family of procreation. Their closest relationships and most intense emotional experiences occur within a family setting. For small children their family *is* their environment. Clearly the family will have a major influence on development. What is often less clear are the precise mechanisms of this effect. Teasing out the different contributions of different aspects of family life is made harder by the fact that dysfunctional families usually function badly in several different ways. Thus in a poorly functioning family there may be marital discord, parental mental illness, bond disruption, neglect and other examples of poor parenting. Indeed, these factors in combination may interact to further impair parenting. There is clear evidence that such dysfunctional families are likely to contain children with psychiatric disorder. Exactly what factor or factors produce which symptoms in the child, and how, is less well understood. This section reviews the evidence that is available concerning family function.

Early attachment

Small babies are able to recognise their mothers (by smell and by the sound of their voice) within days of birth. Within the first few months infants will be smiling differentially at familiar figures and at about the age of six to seven months infants start to make selective attachments as evidenced by an active striving towards an attachment figure, usually the mother, and anxiety when separated from that figure. Attachment behaviour is characterised by this proximity seeking; by a predictable sequence of *protest*, followed by *despair*, followed by *detachment* and an apparent contentment in the continued absence of the attachment figure with initial rejection when that figure returns; and by the 'secure base effect', whereby the presence of the attachment figure promotes exploration and reduces distress in strange situations. Infants usually form more than one attachment, although the first and most powerful is usually to their principal carer, usually the mother (Schaffer & Emerson, 1964).

Attachment behaviour is seen as the outward manifestation of a need to be near to a specific individual. Bonding implies a selective 'internal' attachment which persists over time and continues in the absence of the attachment figure. A securely attached child no longer needs to cling and can tolerate brief separations in the confident expectation that the attachment figure will return. Insecurely attached children (who usually become so as a result of inconsistent or anxious parenting) continue to be clinging and anxious at threatened or actual separations and may initially reject the attachment figure on their return. (For further information see Bretherton & Waters, 1985.)

Securely attached infants are more competent in peer relationships, have higher self-esteem, and are more sociable with adults. Children who have been brought up in environments which prevent the formation of lasting attachments have often been deprived in many other ways. However, some studies do allow conclusions to be drawn about the effect of a lack of early attachments.

Children reared in children's homes and residential nurseries 20 to 30 years ago were given adequate physical care and stimulation but little opportunity for lasting attachments because of high staff turnover and the deliberate discouragement of attachments between children and staff. Follow-up studies have shown that children who experienced such conditions for at least the first two years of their lives grew up to have social and emotional difficulties. At eight years they were clinging, over-friendly with strangers, and attention seeking. At school they were restless, disobedient and unpopular (Tizard & Hodges, 1978). As teenagers, problems persisted, with more behavioural and emotional difficulties than a control group and more difficulties with peer relationships (Hodges & Tizard, 1989a,b). One group of children have been followed up into adult life. The women in this group had an increased rate of psychosocial problems and performed significantly less competently as parents as measured by hard data such as the number of times their own children were removed into care (Quinton *et al*, 1984). Interestingly some of these ex-institutional mothers were able to parent as competently as controls despite their adverse early experiences. When this was examined further it became clear that those mothers with a supportive spouse were competent parents as often as mothers in the control group and much more commonly than ex-institutional mothers without a supportive partner.

Thus although an absence of early lasting attachment affects later functioning, positive change is possible if the right environmental supports are available.

Brief separations

The effects of separation on the child cannot be divorced from the reasons for the separation and the environment the child enters following separation. Thus research has shown that children have more problems following separation from a family with chronic difficulties than from a healthy family. Similarly, research into fostering and adoption indicates that separation and change of family environment *per se* is less important than whether there is a change in quality of parenting. Thus children who receive better parenting following a separation do well despite the change of family (Yarrow & Klein, 1980).

Hospital admission is one variety of brief separation which has been much researched. There is good evidence that a single brief hospital admission carries little long-term psychosocial risk. Children who experience multiple admissions are at a greater risk for later conduct disorder (Quinton & Rutter, 1976). This finding is complicated by the fact that children who experience multiple admissions are more likely to come from socially disadvantaged families who are themselves more at risk of psychiatric disorder.

Divorce

The caveats concerning separation, cited above, are equally applicable with regard to parental divorce. The effects on children are not just due to the separation but also the events leading up to the separation and its consequences. Children will usually have been exposed to considerable marital discord, which will not necessarily decline after divorce. In addition, children not only have to cope with much less contact with one parent – the parent with whom they live is likely to be experiencing considerable emotional distress and may therefore be less available for them at a time when they need more parental support.

It is not surprising then that children show a marked increase in emotional and conduct disorders in the aftermath of divorce. Boys exhibit more problems than girls, who, by two years, are no more likely than controls to have psychiatric disorder (Hetherington *et al*, 1982). There is evidence that children in well functioning single-parent families may do better than those in conflictual two-parent families in the first one to two years after a divorce. Parents who rate highly on warmth and communication but also on control do not let themselves become trapped in coercive cycles with their children, who do just as well after a divorce as controls. Thus, as with other family influences presented in this section, it is the quality of relationships between family members not the structure of the family which is of most importance.

Life events

Stresses arising from chronic adverse events such as disrupted early attachments, parental divorce, and parental mental illness and criminality are well recognised associations of psychiatric disorder in childhood. Less is known concerning the effect of recent acute life events. Douglas (1973) has found that experiencing four or more stressful life events between the ages of three and four years doubles the chance of enuresis. Goodyer *et al* (1985) found an excess of recent distressing life events in the 12 months before onset of psychiatric disorder in a group of out-patients.

Family structure

There is little evidence that any family structure *per se* is associated with a greater incidence of child psychiatric disorder. Children in one-parent families do have higher rates of conduct and emotional disorder but this can largely be explained by the greater social and economic hardship which such families experience. Teenage mothers have been shown to be as competent as older controls at parenting when receiving adequate emotional support themselves (Kruk & Wolkind, 1982).

Other studies looking at different family structures have indicated that children can do well when raised by single fathers, multi-family communes, and reverse-role nuclear families. Research has also indicated that children reared by lesbian couples show normal psychosexual development (Golombok *et al*, 1983). Although measurement of developmental progress and 'normal' relationships is not an exact science, these findings tend to confirm the view that it is the quality of relationships which is of most importance, not the organisational structure of the family.

Family size

Children who come from large families (four or more children) are twice as likely to develop conduct disorder (Rutter *et al*, 1970*a*). Presumably supervision and monitoring become harder for parents as numbers in the family rise and this in turn will make effective discipline harder. A further explanation may be that large families are more likely to be socio-economically disadvantaged.

Children from large families also have slightly lower intelligence and lower levels of reading attainment (Davie *et al*, 1972).

Ordinal position

Despite much research there are few clear findings in this area. Eldest children and only children tend to do better at school and work. Youngest children may be at a slightly greater risk of developing school refusal.

Parents will spend more time with their first children and provide more in the way of interaction and stimulation in the early years before the arrival of the second child, which may explain the first finding. The second finding may be partly explained by a family crisis when the last child starts school: mothers who have been at home for many years looking after preschool children have considerable adjustments to make at this time.

Although parents often ask about 'middle child syndrome', there is little evidence that middle children are at any disadvantage in families by virtue of their ordinal position.

Parenting style

Numerous classifications of child-rearing style have been advanced, with none seeming completely satisfactory. Parents who are warm, nurturant and supportive but who are also able to exert control over their children and have high expectations of them tend to have the best-adjusted children. Other studies suggest that a parental style of clear rule setting and enforcement coupled with an involvement of children in decision making is also associated with well adjusted children.

There is also evidence that a disorganised approach to discipline leads to conduct disorder and aggression (Patterson, 1982). Such an approach is characterised by a lack of clear rules for and expectations of children. In addition, poor supervision means that parents are unaware when rules are broken and cannot follow through effectively. Attempts to enforce rules, when they do take place, are often inconsistent and ineffective. There is also evidence that the parents of aggressive, conduct-disturbed children engage in fewer positive social interactions with their children (Patterson, 1982).

Marital discord

Substantial evidence exists that being raised in a family where there is frequent discord between parents puts children, especially boys, at risk of developing conduct disorder and delinquency (Emery, 1982). Despite this, marital discord in isolation is a relatively weak risk factor. What appears to be most damaging is the combination of a number of different varieties of family dysfunction.

Mechanisms are as usual complex, but presumably discordant parents, as well as providing poor role models and lacking warmth, will also find it difficult to agree clear and consistent limits for their children and then monitor and implement these effectively. A number of studies have highlighted a close association between family discord and poor discipline.

Parental mental illness

Many studies have shown strong links between parental psychiatric illness and child psychiatric disorder. Genetic factors have been discussed elsewhere in this chapter; here we are concerned with those non-genetic influences that having a mentally ill parent brings about. The key factor seems to be the general level of functioning of the parents, and therefore it is with long-standing and recurrent conditions such as alcoholism, personality disorder, chronic depression and other chronic emotional difficulties that the risk to children is greatest (Rutter, 1966). Risk is heightened if the parental illness leads to discord in the parental relationship and hostility towards the child. There is evidence that children of parents with non-psychotic mental illness may be at greater risk than those of psychotic parents. This is presumably because psychotic parents, if treated effectively, may have substantial periods of good functioning between episodes of illness, whereas children of the parents described above will be exposed to continuous parental dysfunction.

Most of the evidence concerns psychiatric morbidity in mothers, which has been related to child psychiatric disorder generally, conduct disorder in older children, and general competence and performance. Richman *et al* (1982) found that having a depressed mother doubled the likelihood of psychiatric disorder in three-year-old children. Discord has been shown to be an important mechanism linking maternal depression and conduct problems in children, but depressed mothers are also likely to be inconsistent, less stimulating, and more irritable with their children.

Postnatal mental illness

With respect to postnatal *psychosis*, the evidence suggests that children do well in the long term irrespective of mental state post-partum, duration of illness and mother–child interaction while ill. Chronic psychiatric and social problems before childbirth are much better predictors of eventual outcome (Oates, 1984). However, there is increasing evidence that depressive disorder during some or all of the first year post-partum adversely affects the infant's cognitive (Cogill *et al*, 1986) and emotional (Stein *et al*, 1991) development.

Parental criminality

Parental criminality is associated with a two- to threefold increase in child psychiatric disorder (West & Farrington, 1973). This risk is further increased if both parents are criminal and more so still if siblings are also delinquent. These findings persist after socio-economic status and the possibility of selective prosecution have been taken into account.

West & Farrington (1973) showed that criminal parents provided poor supervision of their children and that this was likely, at least partially, to explain these findings.

Wider environmental influences

Neighbourhoods

Numerous studies have found marked differences in prevalence rates for child and adolescent psychiatric disorder in different areas (see also Chapter 5). Rates tend to be highest in run-down areas of inner cities. All types of disorder are increased; there are no psychiatric conditions unique to inner cities. These differences are unlikely to be due to 'drift' of dysfunctional families into such areas as they remain when just those children born in the area are examined (Rutter *et al*, 1975*a*). Confirming this view are the results of another study into delinquency in boys which found that rates fell when the boys moved out of London (West, 1982).

One of the best-designed studies compared rates in the Isle of Wight and an inner-London borough (Rutter *et al*, 1975*b*). In both areas rates of psychiatric disorder were associated with factors such as marital discord, family disruption, parental mental illness and criminality, and socio-economic disadvantage. In the inner-London borough there were much higher rates of these family and social factors and that accounted for the higher rates of psychiatric disorder. It seems likely that the effects of inner cities are mediated via the family rather than acting directly on young people themselves.

Why it is that these families are more common in inner cities is difficult to answer. Poor housing conditions may provide part of the answer. At least one study has suggested that living above the fourth floor in a tower block is associated with psychiatric disorder in preschool children (Richman *et al*, 1982). Other studies have provided conflicting evidence, but this may be because it is a family's perception of their housing rather than any objective measure of housing quality that is important. Thus families who are dissatisfied with their housing will be operating under stress whether their housing is inferior to their neighbours' or not.

There is some evidence for the idea that some aspects of the design of housing (e.g. housing estates with large areas of semi-public space for which no resident feels responsible) may contribute to increased rates of delinquency (Wilson, 1978). A lack of safe outdoor play areas is a further handicap to mothers in inner cities. Overcrowding may be especially important where it leads to competition for scarce resources, for example, many parents competing for scarce places at a day nursery.

Social class and disadvantage

Although there is clear evidence that working-class mothers interact differently with their children, for example they talk less and smack more when disciplining their children (Newson & Newson, 1968), there is only a weak association of social class with psychiatric disorder in children and adolescents.

Mild generalised learning difficulties are strongly associated with children from working-class families (Craft, 1985).

While social class may not be associated with psychiatric disorder there is clear evidence that social adversity is. Poor housing, lack of play space and overcrowding have been mentioned above. There is also evidence for financial hardship (Richman *et al*, 1982) and unemployment (Banks & Jackson, 1982; Warr & Jackson, 1985) being linked with psychiatric disorder in children and their parents.

Schools

Children spend large amounts of their time in school. Research has shown that schools influence their pupils' social and behavioural development as well as their academic attainments (Rutter *et al*, 1979). Thus it has been demonstrated that schools with pupils from similar backgrounds at intake may have markedly different rates of conduct and behavioural problems and levels of absenteeism.

It has been suggested that these differences can best be accounted for by differing qualities in the school ethos. In many ways the desirable factors in schools are similar to those outlined above in the section on parenting styles. Thus children do best in schools where staff have clear expectations, consistent methods of disciplining children and work together as a group supporting each other. Teachers must be firm but show respect for the child and involve the child in decision making whenever appropriate. Encouragement and praise get better results than regimes based on punishment. Research also indicates the importance of staff having similar standards for their own behaviour as they do for the pupils'. Finally, the evidence indicates that pupils do worse in schools where there is a high proportion of other children with behavioural difficulties.

Conclusion

It is clear that much is known about the causes of childhood psychiatric disorder. It is also clear that much more needs to be known. Current research tends to throw light first on one particular area of the child's experience and then on another. What is missing are plausible explanations for how the many different causes that may be identified in any one child link together to produce that child's disorder and why it is that one child develops a phobia and another child, in seemingly similar circumstances, a conduct disorder. Only further research, looking at the underlying mechanisms and looking at the children and families that flourish in adversity, as well as those who do badly, can answer these questions.

References

Bakwin, H. (1973) The genetics of bed wetting. In *Bladder Control and Enuresis* (eds I. R. MacKeith & R. S. Meadow). Clinics in Developmental Medicine, nos 48/49. London: Heinemann/Spastics International Medical Publications.

Banks, M. & Jackson, P. (1982) Unemployment and risk of minor psychiatric disorder in young people: cross sectional and longitudinal evidence. *Psychological Medicine*, **12**, 789-798.

Bretherton, I. & Waters, E. (1985) Growing points of attachment theory and research. *Monographs of the Society for Research in Child Development*, serial no. 209, vol. 50, nos. 1-2.

Cadman, D., Boyle, M., Szatmari, P., *et al* (1987) Chronic illness, disability and mental and social well-being: findings of the Ontario child health study. *Pediatrics*, **79**, 805-813.

Cogill, S., Caplan, H., Alexandra, H., *et al* (1986) Impact of postnatal depression on cognitive development in young children. *British Medical Journal*, **292**, 1165-1167.

Craft, M. (1985) Classification, criteria, epidemiology and causation. In *Mental Handicap. A Multidisciplinary Approach* (eds M. Craft, J. Bicknell & S. Hollins). London: Baillière Tindall.

Davie, R., Butler, N. & Goldstein, H. (1972) *From Birth to Seven: A Report of the National Child Development Study*. London: Longman.

Douglas, J. (1973) Early disturbing events and later enuresis. In *Bladder Control and Enuresis* (eds I. Kolvin, R. MacKeith & R. S. Meadow). Clinics in Developmental Medicine, nos. 48/49. London: Heinemann/Spastics International Medical Publications.

Emery, R. E. (1982) Interparental conflict and the children of discord and divorce. *Psychological Bulletin*, **92**, 310-330.

Folstein, S. & Rutter, M. (1977) Infantile autism: a genetic study of 21 twin pairs. *Journal of Child Psychology and Psychiatry*, **18**, 297-321.

Freeman, R. D. (1977) Psychiatric aspects of sensory disorders and intervention. In *Epidemiological Approaches in Child Psychiatry* (ed. P. Graham). London: Academic Press.

Garrison, W. & McQuiston, S. (1989) *Chronic Illness During Childhood and Adolescence: Psychological Aspects*. Newbury Park: Sage.

Gath, A. & Gumley, D. (1987) Retarded children and their siblings. *Journal of Child Psychology and Psychiatry*, **28**, 715-730.

Golombok, S., Spencer, A. & Rutter, M. (1983) Children in lesbian and single parent households: psychosexual and psychiatric appraisal. *Journal of Child Psychology and Psychiatry*, **24**, 551-572.

Goodman, R. & Stevenson, J. (1989*a*) A twin study of hyperactivity - I. An examination of hyperactivity scores and categories derived from Rutter teacher and parent questionnaires. *Journal of Child Psychology and Psychiatry*, **30**, 671-689.

——— & ——— (1989*b*) A twin study of hyperactivity - II. The aetiological role of genes, family relationships and perinatal adversity. *Journal of Child Psychology and Psychiatry*, **30**, 691-709.

Goodyer, I., Kolvin, I. & Gatzanis, S. (1985) Recent undesirable life events and psychiatric disorder in childhood and adolescence. *British Journal of Psychiatry*, **147**, 517-723.

Hetherington, E. M., Cox, M. & Cox, R. (1982) Effects of divorce on parents and children. In *Non-traditional Families* (ed. M. E. Lamb). New Jersey: Lawrence Erlbaum.

Hodges, J. & Tizard, B. (1989*a*) IQ and behavioural adjustment of ex-institutional adolescents. *Journal of Child Psychology and Psychiatry*, **30**, 53-75.

——— & ——— (1989*b*) Social and family relationships of ex-institutional adolescents. *Journal of Child Psychology and Psychiatry*, **30**, 77-97.

Kruk, S. & Wolkind, S. (1982) A longitudinal study of single mothers and their children. In *Families at Risk* (ed. N. Madge). London: Heinemann Educational.

Newson, J. & Newson, E. (1968) *Four Years Old in an Urban Community*. London: Allen & Unwin.

Oates, M. (1984) Assessing fitness to parent. In *Taking a Stand: Child Psychiatrists in Custody, Access and Disputed Adoption Cases*. London: British Agencies for Adoption and Fostering.

Patterson, G. (1982) *Coercive Family Process*. Oregon: Castalia.

Quinton, D. & Rutter, M. (1976) Early hospital admissions and later disturbances of behaviour: an attempted replication of Douglas's findings. *Developmental Medicine and Child Neurology*, **18**, 447-459.

———, ——— & Liddle, C. (1984) Institutional rearing, parenting difficulties and marital support. *Psychological Medicine*, **14**, 107-124.

Richman, N., Stevenson, J. & Graham, P. (1982) *Pre-school to School: A Behavioural Study*. London: Academic Press.

Rutter, M. (1966) *Children of Sick Parents: An Environmental and Psychiatric Study*. Institute of Psychiatry, Maudsley Monograph no. 16. London: Oxford University Press.

———, Tizard, J. & Whitmore, K. (eds) (1970*a*) *Education, Health and Behaviour*. London: Longman.

———, Graham, P. & Yule, W. (1970*b*) *A Neuropsychiatric Study in Childhood*. Clinics in Developmental Medicine, nos 35/36. London: Heinemann/Spastics International Medical Publications.

———, Yule, B., Quinton, D., *et al* (1975*a*) Attainment and adjustment in two geographical areas. III. Some factors accounting for area differences. *British Journal of Psychiatry*, **126**, 520-533.

———, Cox, A., Tupling, C., *et al* (1975*b*) Attainment and adjustment in two geographical areas. I. The prevalence of psychiatric disorder. *British Journal of Psychiatry*, **126**, 493-509.

———, Maughan, B., Mortimore, P., *et al* (1979) *Fifteen Thousand Hours: Secondary Schools and their Effects on Children*. London: Open Books.

———, MacDonald, H., Le Couteur, A., *et al* (1990) Genetic factors in child psychiatric disorders – II. Empirical findings. *Journal of Child Psychology and Psychiatry*, **31**, 39–83.

Schaffer, H. R. & Emerson, P. E. (1964) The development of social attachments in infancy. *Monographs of the Society of Research in Child Development*, **29**, 1–77.

Stein, A., Gath, D. H., Bucher, J., *et al* (1991) The relationship between post-natal depression and mother–child interaction. *British Journal of Psychiatry*, **158**, 46–52.

Thomas A., Chess S. & Birch, H. G. (1968) *Temperament and Behaviour Disorders in Children*. London: University of London Press.

——— & ——— (1982) Temperament and follow up to adulthood. In *Temperamental Differences in Infants and Young Children* (eds R. Porter & G. M. Collins). London: Pitman.

Tizard B. & Hodges, J. (1978) The effect of early institutional rearing on the development of eight year old children. *Journal of Child Psychology and Psychiatry*, **19**, 99–118.

Warr, P. & Jackson, P. (1985) Factors influencing the psychological impact of prolonged unemployment and of re-employment. *Psychological Medicine*, **15**, 795–807.

West, D. (1982) *Delinquency: Its Roots, Careers and Prospects*. London: Heinemann Educational.

——— & Farrington, D. (1973) *Who Becomes Delinquent?* London: Heinemann Educational.

Wilson, S. (1978) Vandalism and 'defensible space' on London housing estates. In *Tackling Vandalism. Home Office Research Study No. 47* (ed. R. Clarke). London: HMSO.

Yarrow, L. J. & Klein, R. P. (1980) Environmental discontinuity associated with transition from foster to adoptive homes. *International Journal of Behavioural Development*, **3**, 311–322.

5 Classification and epidemiology
Michael Wieselberg

The need for classification ● Criteria for classification ● Disadvantages of diagnosis ● Categorical versus dimensional classification ● Multi-axial framework ● Prevalence rates of psychiatric disorder

---

The need for classification

In making sense of the varied ways in which child and adolescent psychiatric disorder presents, ordering information and setting it in the context of what is known about normal development is a central task. Classification is a means for grouping phenomena into categories based on shared characteristics. This is a necessary precursor to the exploration of relationships between entities and events. It also functions as a language for communication between professionals in writing clinical reports, applying research findings, and in the preparation of statistics.

A classification system for general use must satisfy several criteria if it is to be acceptable to professionals who may have different theoretical views. Diagnosis involves selecting key features of a disorder and assigning them to one or more predetermined categories which are meaningful not only through identifiable symptoms, but which also carry some implications for aetiology, course, prognosis and treatment. Rather than specifying unique features about the individual bearing the disorder, the process abstracts certain characteristics which he or she has in common with others bearing the same condition.

The diagnosis of a mental disorder does not imply the existence of an organic disease state. A commonly accepted definition of psychiatric disorder in young people is the presence of abnormalities of behaviour, emotions or relationships which are developmentally inappropriate and of sufficient severity and duration as to cause persistent suffering or handicap in the child, or distress or disturbance in the family or community (Rutter *et al*, 1970).

Criteria for classification

It is disorders that are classified, not people. The diagnosis does not take account of many other qualities of the individual. Nor is a diagnosis lifelong. It concerns disturbance at a particular point in the individual's life and does not necessarily predict the form of disorder at earlier or later stages, although the diagnosis may have prognostic value. Children are developing, and a classification system needs to take this into account, for example by allowing for conditions which manifest themselves in particular ways during childhood, without the requirement of a separate classification at different ages.

The system must be practicable, set out in a clear, unambiguous, convenient form, using information which is routinely available. It needs to be reliable, that is it should be used similarly by clinicians in varying settings, and there needs to be adequate differentiation between disorders, giving minimal overlap. It should encompass all the important conditions known to professionals. The classification needs to be clinically relevant, identifying conditions which warrant clinical attention, and aiding decision making.

Diagnoses need to be valid, that is differing in terms of variables other than those which are used initially to define them, such as aetiology, course, and response to treatment. Some logical consistency and conceptual coherence is necessary, although the present state of knowledge best suits a descriptive approach involving a minimal amount of inference on the part of the observer.

Disadvantages of diagnosis

Objections are sometimes raised against the labelling involved in the diagnostic process. It has been claimed that the process obscures individual differences and hinders a detailed understanding of disordered mental function. Moreover, it has been held responsible for producing social stigma and social deprivation. The implication of deviance can lead to an altered view of oneself, and hence to a self-fulfilling prophecy. It may lead to a change in the way others act towards the individual, even to the extent of justifying inappropriate social control.

Sometimes the expectations of others can be altered by a process of labelling, with increased likelihood of a poor outcome for the child, for example, with regard to teacher expectations of low achievers, and court appearance of teenage boys.

If diagnosis is to be justified, its clinical value must be demonstrated. It should help clarify thinking about the nature of the child's disturbance. It should improve therapeutic responses and facilitate the delivery of services.

The classification reflects problems of adjustment, not qualities of individuals. A classification of people is not only morally offensive in regarding people as vehicles of problems, but can convey an assumption of persistence which is often incorrect. Furthermore, diagnosis does not necessarily imply the need for psychiatric treatment or some other form of administrative action. These may depend on many other factors such as social impairment, the persistence of disorder, the availability of resources, and the readiness of the social and professional network to accept the need for intervention. The harmful effects of labelling are therefore to be found in the misuse of the diagnostic process, rather than the process itself. Importantly, informal and sometimes much more harmful labelling has often already taken place in the network of the suffering child long before mental health professionals become involved. Correcting misperceptions is often an important part of the assessment.

Categorical versus dimensional classification

Historically, there have been a number of approaches to classification in child psychiatry which have not met the criteria outlined above. Modern approaches fall into two groups, the categorical and the dimensional. Both the *International Classification of Diseases* (ICD-10) of the World Health Organization (Rutter, 1989*b*) and the *Diagnostic and Statistical Manual* (DSM-III-R) of the American Psychiatric Association (1987) use categorical systems, requiring the clinician to make a selection from a list of diagnoses, each consisting of identifiable behavioural symptoms. Ultimately, these categories are based upon clinically derived syndromes through professional consensus. Inclusion and exclusion criteria encourage a qualitative forced choice.

By contrast, the dimensional approach to classification derives from the use of multivariate statistical techniques to measure the tendency of specific types of behaviour to occur together in characteristic patterns (e.g. Achenbach & Edelbrock, 1978). Such definitions tend to be tied to specific scores on assessment instruments. Once dimensions of disturbance are identified, for example, by factor analysis, techniques such as cluster analysis or principal-components analysis can be used to assign symptoms to mutually exclusive diagnostic groups. The method is therefore more empirical than the categorical approach, produces groups which have greater reliability and homogeneity, and is linked to standard assessment tools. Variation is quantitatively ordered, so that there is no need for an index of severity to define 'caseness'.

There are a number of problems with the latter approach. Although the main dimensions of disturbance derived from non-clinical and clinical populations are quite comparable, they depend upon the population studied, and rare conditions may be omitted. With the dimensional approach, different solutions may also emerge from the same data set using different mathematical models. Moreover, statistically significant dimensions may not be clinically or conceptually meaningful. Furthermore, such a system tends to be cumbersome. Nevertheless, both the categorical and dimensional approach may have separate usefulness in exploring the factors associated with disturbance, and ultimately a classification may emerge which combines the strengths of both.

Multi-axial framework

The ICD system is the classification used by most countries (World Health Organization, 1992; Rutter *et al*, 1975*b*), DSM-III-R being used in the USA, Canada and Australia. ICD-10 is now available (Rutter 1989*b*; van Goor-Lambo

Table 5.1 Axes on ICD–10 and DSM–III–R

Axis no.	ICD–10	DSM–III–R
I	Clinical psychiatric syndrome	Clinical syndromes
II	Development disorders	Developmental disorders, mental retardation and personality disorders
III	Intellectual level	Physical disorders and conditions
IV	Medical conditions	Severity of psychosocial stressors
V	Associated abnormal psycho-social situations	Global assessment of functioning

et al, 1990). DSM–III–R has been in use since 1987 and DSM–IV is in preparation (Shaffer *et al*, 1989). Both systems are regularly updated, and by influencing each other's development, have been coming closer over the past 20 years. No single diagnostic category can sufficiently convey the complexity of an individual child's disorder. For this reason both systems have developed five separate axes along which different components of a child's disorder can be recorded without overlapping (see Table 5.1). Clinicians are required to make judgements on each axis.

Psychiatric syndromes axis

Both ICD–10 and DSM–III–R follow similar basic principles. They use a categorical rather than dimensional approach, based upon non-theoretical phenomenological principles (see Table 5.2). Clinical psychiatric syndromes on axis I are divided into similar major groupings comprising hyperkinetic and attentional deficit disorders, conduct disorders, and emotional/anxiety disorders arising in childhood or adolescence. These major divisions also emerge from dimensional studies of childhood disorder and have the greatest degree of empirical validation. Disorders which can arise at any age are not separately designated in the children's section, but DSM–III–R sometimes gives additional guidelines for children, for example with depressive disorders. ICD–10 is anomalous in placing anorexia nervosa and gender identity disorders within the adult section, although they normally have their onset rather earlier.

Both classifications carry detailed glossaries giving specific criteria for each diagnosis, although neither is truly operational in the sense of defining how the diagnostic information is to be gathered. ICD–10 differs in specifying a concept for each disorder detailing the knowledge upon which each category is based, and breaks new ground by suggesting more tightly designated criteria for research purposes.

Table 5.2 A comparison of ICD-10 and DSM-III-R

ICD-10	DSM-III-R

Axis I

ICD-10	DSM-III-R
Behavioural and emotional disorders with onset usually in childhood or adolescence	Disorders usually first evident in infancy, childhood or adolescence
F90 Hyperkinetic disorder	Disruptive behaviour disorders
.0 Disorder of activity and attention	Attention-deficit hyperactivity disorder (314.01)
.1 Hyperkinetic conduct disorder	Undifferentiated attention deficit disorder (314.00)
F91 Conduct disorders	Conduct disorder
.0 Conduct disorder confined to family context	
.1 Unsocialised conduct disorder	Solitary aggressive type (312.00)
.2 Socialised conduct disorder	Group type (312.20)
.3 Oppositional defiant disorder	Oppositional defiant disorder (313.81)
F92 Mixed disorders of conduct and emotions	
.0 Depressive conduct disorder	
F93 Emotional disorders with onset specific to childhood	Anxiety disorders of childhood or adolescence
.0 Separation anxiety disorder	Separation anxiety disorder (309.21)
.1 Phobic disorder of childhood	Avoidant disorder of childhood or adolescence (313.00)
.2 Social sensitivity disorder	Overanxious disorder (313.21)
.3 Sibling rivalry disorder	
F94 Disorders of social functioning with onset specific to childhood or adolescence	
.0 Elective mutism	Elective mutism (303.23)
.1 Reactive attachment disorder of childhood	Reactive attachment disorder of infancy or early childhood (313.89)
.2 Disinhibition attachment disorder of childhood	
F95 Tic disorders	Tic disorders (307.20-23)
F98 Other emotional and behavioural disorders with onset usually occurring during childhood	Elimination disorders
.0 Enuresis	Functional enuresis (307.60)
.1 Encopresis	Functional encopresis (307.70)

Continued

Table 5.2 *Continued*

ICD–10	DSM–III–R
.2 Feeding disorder of infancy or childhood (Anorexia nervosa and bulimia nervosa are in the adult section)	Eating disorders Anorexia nervosa (307.10) Bulimia nervosa (307.51)
.3 Pica	Pica (307.52) Rumination disorder of infancy (307.53) Other eating disorders (307.50)
.4 Stereotyped movement disorder	Stereotyped habit disorder (307.30)
.5 Stuttering	Stuttering (307.00) Identity disorder (313.82)
(Gender identity disorder is in the adult section)	Gender identity disorders (202.60, 50, 85)

Mental and behavioural disorders not classified by age in both classifications

Organic mental disorders, psychoactive substance disorders, psychotic disorders, affective disorders, neurotic disorders, sexual disorders, sleep disorders, adjustment disorders, psychological factors affecting physical condition

Axis II

Developmental disorders	*Specific developmental disorders (315)*
F80 Specific developmental disorders of speech and language	Language and speech disorders
F81 Specific developmental disorders of scholastic skills	Academic skills disorders
F82 Specific developmental disorders of motor function	Motor skills disorders
F83 Mixed specific developmental disorder	
F84 Pervasive developmental disorders	Pervasive developmental disorders (299)
.0 Childhood autism	Autistic disorder
.1 Atypical autism	Pervasive developmental disorder
.2 Rett syndrome	
.3 Other childhood disintegrative disorders	
.4 Overactive disorder associated with mental retardation and stereotyped movements	
.5 Asperger syndrome	

Axis III

Mental retardation (F70–79)	*Mental retardation (317–319)*

The two systems deal with the problem of overlap rather differently. ICD-10 generally assumes that a child has a single disorder and the clinician is expected to choose according to the predominant picture, accepting that the underlying disorder may express itself differently at another time. On the whole, clinical guidelines are more flexible than in DSM-III-R. The problem of comorbidity is recognised by a small number of combination categories, notably the association of conduct disorder with either depressive disorder or hyperkinetic disorder, because this may significantly alter the prognosis. By contrast, DSM-III-R has tighter definitions and allows multiple diagnoses. A particular child might meet the criteria for a depressive disorder, conduct disorder, and attention deficit hyperactivity disorder. Care is needed in avoiding conceptual confusion around individual cases. Usually there are duration and exclusion criteria, and sometimes a specified severity rating. The problem of rating symptoms is addressed by listing items in descending order of discriminating power based on data from field trials.

Hyperkinetic syndrome

The two classifications differ over some diagnoses (Table 5.2). Hyperkinetic syndrome within ICD-10 has a much more empirical base than in ICD-9 or DSM-III-R. It requires early onset and emphasises pervasiveness and persistence of activity across situations, with a disorganised and poorly regulated style, reckless impulsiveness, social disinhibition and problematic peer relationships. DSM-III-R offers a rather wider and less specific definition, requiring 8 out of 14 characteristics to have been present for more than 6 months since before the age of 7 years. Defining characteristics include "has difficulty playing quietly" and "often does not seem to listen to what is being said to him or her", which must be rather doubtful discriminants. However, there is an acceptance that hyperactivity is a vital part of this syndrome, and that the earlier DSM-III conception of an underlying deficit in selective attention has not been supported by empirical evidence.

Conduct disorder

The traditional distinction between socialised and unsocialised conduct disorder has been preserved in both systems, despite limited validation. DSM-III-R makes the distinction rely upon offences that are carried out with peers, rather than whether the youngster has adequate peer relationships *per se*. Predicting poor outcome may depend more upon general competence in peer relationships. DSM-III-R relies on selecting 3 out of 13 items. Despite the length of the list, the scope is narrow, consisting mainly of types of behaviour which are severe enough to reflect illegal activities such as fire setting, stealing, and forcing sexual activity.

Both systems now carry an oppositional defiant disorder category which does not include delinquent activity or extreme aggressiveness, but occupies an uncertain territory between unacceptable misbehaviour and conduct disorder.

Emotional disorder

Although the superordinant category of emotional disorder is a reliable and valid diagnosis in children, its subclassification does not yet have a firm empirical basis and reliability between clinicians has been rather low in studies using both systems (Rutter *et al*, 1988). ICD-10 makes it easier to distinguish between anxiety disorders of childhood and neurotic disorders of adults than does DSM-III-R by introducing developmental appropriateness of the form of disorder as a key defining criterion. For example separation anxiety as defined would be normal in a five-year-old but not in a 15-year-old. Subcategories in both systems are very different, apart from separation anxiety disorder, and both lack validation in terms of associated phenomena, course and treatment response.

Affective disorders

Affective disorders in both systems are now classified in the adult section. DSM-III-R does include some criteria for childhood diagnosis, going beyond the research data so far available. ICD-10 only makes specific reference to this by including a special subcategory of depressive conduct disorder, which is emerging as an association carrying increased prognostic risk.

Attachment disorder

ICD-10 introduces a new major category of "disordered social function" which focuses mainly upon disorders of attachment. A distinction is made between *reactive* attachment disorder, with markedly insecure selective attachments, and contradictory social responses in the presence of associated emotional disturbance, and *disinhibition* attachment disorder, manifest in infancy by clinging and diffuse non-selectively focused attachment behaviour, and in middle childhood by attention-seeking and indiscriminately friendly behaviour accompanied by diffuse attachments. In contrast, DSM-III-R has a single category of reactive attachment disorder which also requires for its definition a history of gross abnormalities in the provision of care, limiting the opportunity for investigating the connections between clinical presentation and presumed aetiology.

Developmental disorders axis

In both systems developmental disorders are classified on a separate axis because they often coexist with psychiatric disorder, and one or other important condition may be omitted if they were placed in the same list. Developmental disorders are included in the psychiatric classification because they are commonly associated with reduced social skills, lowered self-esteem and problematic peer relationships which may not merit a clinical psychiatric diagnosis but might nevertheless warrant intervention.

ICD-10 is rather more demanding in distinguishing them from normal variations by specifying severity (e.g. for language disorders, scoring more than two standard deviations below the mean on standardised testing), requiring a prior history of severe delay, even if the problem is less marked on presentation, needing deviance in function as well as delay, and associated abnormalities in socio-emotional functioning or scholastic attainment. The categories and definitions are similar under DSM-III-R but looser. For example the definition of language disorder requires only a score "substantially below" that expected on a standardised measure, but there is a requirement for significant impairment in daily living or academic function.

Differences in boundary definition also characterise the pervasive developmental disorders. DSM-III-R now has only two categories: autism, and a residual group. The diagnosis of autism is considerably broader than in DSM-III or ICD-10, for example not including a language comprehension criterion, and the requirement for a markedly restricted repertoire of activities can be met merely by the presence of head banging. There may also be difficulties distinguishing a residual category from severe developmental receptive language disorder.

Mental retardation axis

ICD-10 carries a separate axis for mental retardation, now more usually called non-specific or generalised learning disability. This is separately coded because it carries significant prognostic information quite separately from axis I disorders. DSM-III-R keeps it on axis II, partly to avoid a proliferation of axes, partly for conceptual reasons. This does not mean that it cannot be coded alongside other axis II diagnoses, but there is no requirement that it should be. Intellectual level is one of the most reliable and valid of all categories, being tied to standard accepted measures.

Medical axis

The separate medical axis allows codings of medical conditions, such as fragile X syndrome, which may or may not prove to have aetiological significance in psychiatric disturbances.

Psychosocial axis

The psychosocial axis lists a range of stressors for the separate coding of factors which are relevant to aetiology, but also may help with prognosis and therapeutic planning. Unfortunately, field trials of both DSM-III and ICD-10 gave relatively low inter-clinician reliabilities for these ratings. This is partly because clinicians differ in their interpretation of causal events, partly because there is often no empirical way of weighting the contribution of a particular cause of a particular disorder.

ICD-10 therefore codes psychosocial factors according to whether specified criteria are present, irrespective of whether they may be considered a direct cause. A total of 39 stressors are listed under nine main headings, half of which describe abnormal or unusual family environments. Stressors which result from the child's own disorder, such as reception into care because of antisocial behaviour, are rated separately from those which are more independent, such as reception into care following death of a parent. This still does not remove conceptual confusion, for example, the circularity between separation anxiety disorder and parental overprotection. ICD-10 rates items over the six months before assessment.

DSM-III-R definitions are less tied to specified criteria. Heterogeneous stressors are pooled, and the clinician is asked to rate severity "as experienced by an average person", rather than by this particular individual. Severity is rated on a six-point scale, and involves problematic judgements. For example, the birth of a sibling and chronic parental discord score similarly, though the latter has far greater empirical status as an aetiological and prognostic factor. Stressors are rated over the year before assessment, and there is a subdivision between acute and enduring factors, with a six-month cut-off. There are difficulties here too; for example, parental divorce is coded as an acute event, but the impact may depend more upon the long-term changes in family life than upon the event itself.

It is perhaps inevitable that the complex multifactorial aetiology of child and adolescent psychiatric disorders can be squeezed only with great difficulty into a tight classification system, but research in this area is still at an early stage, perhaps comparable with that of axis I some 30 years ago.

Global assessment axis

DSM-III-R carries an additional axis for global assessment of personal functioning on a hypothetical continuum of mental health-illness. Unlike psychosocial stressors, it does not have a separate scale for children and adolescents, though one has been piloted in this age range (Shaffer *et al*, 1983). Psychological, social, school and leisure functioning are combined on a composite scale ranging from superior to grossly impaired, with separate ratings for current level, and highest level in the past year. It is intended for this measure to be of prognostic value, partly acting as a measure of premorbid state. Although it may have some value for adult disorder, it is a relatively crude measure and there are problems with its reliability.

Prevalence rates of psychiatric disorder

Since 1970, a number of rigorous epidemiological surveys of prevalence rates of psychiatric symptoms and of disorder have been published in the developed world. Differing purposes, target populations, methods and completeness of data sets have understandably led to different findings. Illustrative prevalence rates are given below, but more detailed reviews have appeared (e.g. Rutter, 1989*a*; Brandenberg *et al*, 1990).

Preschool period

Emotional and behavioural problems at this age consist of symptoms varying in number and severity, most of which do not appear to fall into clearly differentiated categories permitting classification.

Richman *et al* (1975) interviewed more than 800 mothers of randomly selected three-year-old children in Waltham Forest, an outer-London borough with a social class distribution similar to that in the country as a whole. They used a behaviour screening questionnaire of tested reliability, and interviewed mothers of about 100 high-scoring children and 100 controls matched for gender and social class. The commonest individual items of difficult behaviour in the whole population were bedwetting (37%), daytime wetting (17%), poor appetite (17%), night waking at least three times weekly (14%), difficulty settling at night, soiling, fears and overactivity (13% each).

Taking the clinical picture as a whole, 7% had moderate to severe behaviour problems, and another 15% had mild behaviour problems. Overall rates for boys and girls were roughly similar. The most frequent clinical picture was of a child who was restless, attention seeking and difficult to manage, but not particularly anxious or unhappy. A strong link between language and behaviour disorders emerged. For example, of children with expressive language disorder, 59% had a behaviour disorder compared with 14% in the general population.

The study revealed a high rate of maternal depression in both groups (39% of problem children, 26% of control children), but there was a strong interaction with the quality of the parental marriage (Richman *et al*, 1982). Other studies in south and east London confirm these findings. Follow-up not only showed strong continuities both for behaviour and language disorder after one year, but behaviour disorder persisted in two-thirds of the preschool sample when they were eight years old, indicating that preschool behaviour disorder is common, and can be both handicapping and persistent (Stevenson *et al*, 1985).

Psychosocial adversity played an important role. For example, maternal depression or family discord at three years predicted the development of child behaviour disorder by eight years even in children who did not show disturbance at three years. Speech and language delay at three years was a similarly powerful predictor.

Middle childhood

The classic study was carried out in the 1960s on the total 10- and 11-year-old population of the Isle of Wight, chosen because it was an easily defined stable geographical and administrative unit, socially representative of England as a whole. Standardised measures of physical health, intelligence, educational and psychological status were obtained on 2334 children, over 90% of the total (Rutter *et al*, 1970). Parent and teacher screening questionnaires identified similar proportions of children with deviant behavioural scores, but only 19 out of 271 were identified by both, emphasising that multiple sources of information are essential in epidemiological studies. Other studies bear this out (e.g. Sandberg *et al*, 1980). Stage 2 of this study involved interviewing the parents and diagnostic examination of children having deviant scores, with an additional random sample to estimate cases missed by the screening, to reduce interview bias, and provide normative data. Of the children screened, 5.7% had a psychiatric disorder, corrected to 6.8% for the missed cases. Boys were affected more often than girls (1.9:1). In most cases disorder had been present for at least three years. Only 10% were attending a psychiatric clinic.

The survey was designed to estimate possible service need, and used a broad concept of handicap as meaning a disability which interferes with development or adjustment to daily life. On the Wechsler Intelligence Scale for Children, 2.5% had IQs below 70, but half of these children were attending ordinary day schools. Three per 1000 had severe learning disability (IQ < 50). Reading backwardness, defined as more than 28 months (2 standard deviations) below the age mean on a standardised test, affected 6.6%. Controlling for IQ as well as age, 3.7% suffered from specific reading retardation. Physical disorders involving handicap present for at least a year affected 5.7% of children, asthma being the commonest. Overall, 12% of 9–11-year-olds had one handicap, 3% had two, and 0.8% had three, giving a rural population total of 16% with at least one significantly handicapping condition.

Offord *et al* (1987) examined the six-month prevalence rates for disorder among 1400 4–11-year-olds in Ontario. They used a standardised screening questionnaire for parents which yielded four main DSM-III diagnoses, with thresholds validated against psychiatric interview of a subsample, and estimated that 19.5% of boys and 13.5% of girls had a conduct, emotional, somatisation or attention deficit with hyperactivity disorder, or combined diagnoses. Only 16% of boys and 9% of girls with disorder in the total survey from age 4 to 16 had used mental health or social services in the preceding six months, though about half had consulted a physician during that time.

Adolescence

Prevalence rates of psychiatric disorder among adolescents in the general community vary between 10% and 20%, depending upon the method used and population. All studies identify larger numbers of disturbed adolescents from individual interview than from data given by parents and teachers.

Leslie (1974) screened over 1000 13–14-year-olds in Blackburn, a northern English industrial town, with a parental questionnaire and interviewed high-scoring adolescents and their parents. Randomly selected controls were also interviewed. In all, 17.4% had moderate disturbance (equivalent to appropriate psychiatric clinic referrals) or severe disturbance (long-standing, with several very abnormal traits). The boy:girl ratio was 1.5:1. Only 65% of their parents regarded their child's behaviour as abnormal, and only 1 in 20 were receiving psychiatric treatment at the time of the survey.

Rutter *et al* (1976) screened all the 2300 14–15-year-olds on the Isle of Wight with parent and teacher questionnaires of tested reliability and validity, four years after the original survey. On teacher questionnaires, 7% had deviant scores, similar to rates for 10–11-year-olds. Interviewers, who were blind to the selection process, saw high-scoring adolescents and randomly selected controls, their parents and teachers. Diagnosis based on corroborating sources of information gave an 8% prevalence rate for psychiatric disorder, rising to 13% based solely on the parental interview, but this rose to 21% on taking account of individuals not picked up by screening. Many adolescents expressed considerable anxiety or misery not evident to their parents or teachers. Persistence of corroborated disorder since the earlier survey accounted for two-fifths of the cases, and was strongly associated with educational disadvantage, maternal psychiatric disorder, family discord and separation (as was the presence of disorder at age 10) but these associations were much weaker or absent with newly arising disorders, except for marital disharmony.

Among 1200 12–16-year-olds in the Ontario study mentioned above, 19% of boys and 22% of girls were estimated to have a psychiatric disorder (Offord *et al*, 1987).

McGee *et al* (1990) have been following a cohort of 1000 children born in Dunedin, New Zealand, in 1972–73. At age 15, 943 adolescents were given a modified version of a standardised interview (Diagnostic Interview Schedule for Children) from which DSM–III diagnoses were derived, and their parents given a standardised questionnaire. Of the 22% who had a psychiatric disorder, one in four received more than one diagnosis, most commonly depression. (Nearly half had some form of anxiety disorder, and a similar number had a conduct/oppositional disorder; half of the latter reported police contact.) The boy:girl ratio was 1:1.4. Parental interview only identified half the adolescents who had a disorder, and these cases were no more or less severe than the rest. Of the 10% with parent-corroborated disorder, half had sought professional help. The Dunedin sample is somewhat advantaged in socio-economic terms relative to the rest of New Zealand.

Major differences between studies in criteria and populations make it difficult to be clear whether there are changes in overall prevalence rates with age during the course of adolescence. However, both the Isle of Wight and Dunedin studies following up the same cohort with the same measures have shown an increase in prevalence between 11 and 15 years.

Prevalence rates of individual disorders

Table 5.3 gives illustrative rates of specific psychiatric disorders from epidemiological surveys. Rates may vary considerably. This may reflect true differences across age and populations, or methodological differences and limitations. Explanatory details will be found in other chapters. Male:female ratios are given where studies show marked differences.

Prevalence rates in primary care

Work with children is estimated to occupy 25–33% of a general practitioner's time. Although most children present with physical ailments, 'behaviour disorder' was found in one study to be the third commonest reason for presentation to a general practice after acute otitis media and bronchitis (Campion & Gabriel, 1984). Garralda & Bailey (1986), using Rutter A (Parent) questionnaires and psychiatric interview found that 23% of 7–12-year-old children attending general practices in the north of England had psychiatric disorder. Costello *et al* (1988) found that 22% (±3.4%) of 7–11-year-olds visiting their primary-care paediatrician in the US had a DSM–III child psychiatric disorder.

Physical illness

Chronic physical illness of any kind is a potent vulnerability factor for psychiatric disorder. The Isle of Wight study identified 5.7% of 10–12-year-olds as having a chronic physical disorder (2.3% asthma, 0.9% epilepsy, 0.3% cerebral palsy). Illnesses not involving the central nervous system were associated with double the base rate of psychiatric disorder. Idiopathic epilepsy was associated with a tripling of the base rate, but where epilepsy and other unequivocal evidence of brain damage were present together, the rate of psychiatric disorder in 10–11-year-olds rose to nearly 40%. This rise was non-specific in terms of the type of psychiatric disorder, and family/social/educational factors were also commoner here than in the general child population (Rutter *et al*, 1970). These rates show that pathology of brain function adds significantly to the less specific stress factors present with physical illness *per se*.

The increased vulnerability of chronically ill children is also reflected in the Ontario study (Cadman *et al*, 1987) showing a doubling of the general risk for psychiatric disorder. Disability on top of chronic illness raised the risk further to 3.4 times base rate. For the population as a whole, chronic physical disorder was responsible for 9% of total child psychiatric morbidity.

Physical symptoms, mostly without diagnosed illness, are much commoner. For example, Faull & Nicol (1986) found that 25% of 5–6-year-old children had recurrent abdominal pain, defined as at least three episodes of pain over at least three months in the preceding year leading to the child missing normal activities.

Table 5.3 Prevalence rates of individual disorders

Clinical syndrome	Reference	Age of subjects	Prevalence
Anorexia nervosa (DSM-III)	Whitaker et al (1990)	14–17	3 per 1000 girls, 0 boys
(ICD-9)	Szmuckler (1985)		0.37–4.6 per 100 000
Clinical eating disorder	Johnson-Sabine et al (1988)	14–16	1% of female sample
Autism			
nuclear/Kanner type	Steffenburg & Gillberg (1986)	2–9	4 per 10 000 (4M:1F)
partial/autism spectrum	Wing & Gould (1979)	2–15	20 per 10 000 (3M:1F)
	Gillberg et al (1986a)	13–17	20 per 10 000 (2M:1F)
Bulimia nervosa (DSM-III)	Whitaker et al (1990)	14–17	2.5% (1M:20F)
Conduct disorder	Offord et al (1987)	4–11	8.3% (3.5M:1F)
		12–16	14% (2.5M:1F)
	Rutter et al (1970)	10–11	4% (3M:1F)
Delinquency (accumulated conviction rate)	Rutter & Giller (1983)	10–16	14% (5M:1F)
Depressive disorder	Fleming & Offord (1990)	6–11	0.4–2.5%
		12–19	0.4–6.4%
Elective mutism	Fundudis et al (1979)	7	0.8 per 1000
Emotional disorder	Rutter et al (1970)	10–11	2.5% (1M:1.5F)
	Offord et al (1987)	4–16	10% (1M:1.5F)
Enuresis	Butler & Golding (1985)	5	10.5% (4M:3F)
	Rutter et al (1973)	7	5% (2M:1F)
		10	2.5% (1.5M:1F)
		14	0.75% (2M:1F)
Encopresis	Bellman (1966)	7–8	1.5% (3M:1F)
	Rutter et al (1970)	10–11	0.8% (4M:1F)
Foetal alcohol syndrome	Abel & Sokol (1987)	0	0.6–2.6 per 1000 live births

Disorder	Reference	Age	Prevalence
Hyperkinetic syndrome (ICD-9)	Taylor et al (1991)	7–8	1.7% male sample
Attention deficit disorder with hyperactivity (DSM-III)	Taylor et al (1991)	7–8	16% male sample
Mental retardation	Offord et al (1987)	4–16	6% (3.5M:1F)
severe (IQ<50)	Rutter et al (1970)	9–10	0.3%
	Myers (1981)		0.3%
Non-organic growth retardation	Dowdney et al (1987)	3	2%
Obsessive–compulsive disorder	Flament et al (1988)	14–17	1%
–mixed obsessional anxiety	Rutter et al (1970)	10–11	0.3%
Oppositional disorder	Anderson et al (1987)	11	2.2% (2M:1F)
Overanxious disorder	Bowen et al (1990)	12–16	3.6% (4M:1F)
	Anderson et al (1987)	11	2.9% (1.7M:1F)
Separation anxiety disorder	Bowen et al (1990)	12–16	2.4% (6M:1F)
	Anderson et al (1987)	11	3.5% (1M:2.5F)
	Anderson et al (1987)	11	2.4% (1M:2F)
Phobias – single	Gillberg et al (1986b)	13–19	0.5%
Psychoses	Faull & Nicol (1986)	5–6	23%
Recurrent abdominal pain	Welte & Barnes (1987)	11–15	25% (1M:1.7F)
Smoking	Rutter et al (1970)	9–10	3.7% (3M:1F)
Specific reading retardation	Andrews & Harris (1964)	4–16	1% (4M:1F)
Stammering (persistent)	Swadi (1988)	11	2%
Substance abuse (i.e. regular use of solvents/ illicit drugs)		16	16%
Suicidal attempts	Hawton & Goldacre (1982)	12–15	1% 12 years (1M:1F) 14 years (1M:6F)
Suicide	McClure (1988)	10–14	1 per 1 000 000
	McClure (1986)	15–19	54 per 1 000 000 (3M:1F)
Tics (handicapping)	Rutter et al (1970)	10–11	0.1%

Urban-rural differences

Within the preschool period, there are few comparative studies. Earls (1980) replicated Richman's study in rural Massachusetts, a cohesive community of low population density, and found the same prevalence rates for moderate and severe behaviour problems. There too, rates were unaffected by gender and social class.

Further support for a lack of an urban-rural difference in prevalence of behaviour disorder in young children comes from a study comparing six-year-old Danish children from Aarhus (population 250 000) and a rural island (Kastrup, 1977).

Ten-year-olds in an inner-London borough were compared with those living on the Isle of Wight after screening with a teacher questionnaire and using a similar two-stage method (Rutter *et al*, 1975*a*). Excluding immigrants, rates of behavioural deviance (on questionnaire), psychiatric disorder and specific reading retardation were all twice as high in London. Association with background factors were similar in both settings. The differential rates were largely accounted for by much higher levels of family disadvantage as measured by family discord and breakdown, parental mental disorder and criminal history, family size, overcrowding, lack of home ownership, receptions into care, and greater school disadvantage as measured by high teacher and pupil turnover, pupil absenteeism, and a high proportion of children then receiving free school meals. It was the stress of urban living reflected in family and school efficacy rather than migration or differential school entry which underlay the differences.

An adolescent urban-rural comparison was undertaken by Lavik (1977), who found a 20% rate of psychiatric disorder among 15-year-olds in a suburb of Oslo, and an 8% rate in a rural Norwegian valley 200 miles away. Cases were equivalent to those seen in adolescent psychiatric clinics. The bulk of the difference was due to conduct problems. A much higher rate of family breakdown in Oslo was the most striking demographic contrast. Contrary to Rutter's research, class was lower in the rural sample, but the cumulative effect of other urban factors made the impact of low social class, family breakdown and poor scholastic performance more deleterious in Oslo than outside it.

Prevalence rates in ethnic minority groups

There has been little systematic study of prevalence rates within the UK of psychiatric disorder among children from ethnic minorities, although there are several clinical and anecdotal accounts. In the Waltham Forest preschool study, a 7% subsample of three-year-old chilren whose mothers were born in the West Indies showed the same prevalence rate of overall disorder as did indigenous children (Earls & Richman, 1980). They also scored similarly on the Vineland scale of social maturity. There were some differences in the pattern of symptoms. West Indian children were more faddy eaters, more difficult to settle at night, more fearful and had more articulation problems. Indigenous children were more likely to soil, wet the bed, and have tempers. These differences may reflect contrasting child-rearing practices, but not necessarily so. West Indian mothers were more likely to have been educated beyond the age of 16, and to work longer hours. Among other disadvantages, their children were more poorly housed and had experienced more separations from their parents.

A national cohort of 13 000 children born in one week in 1970 was followed using questionnaires administered by health visitors (Butler & Golding, 1986). At five years of age, a subsample of 174 ethnic West Indian children, compared with the whole sample, were more likely to have had tantrums and speech problems. The excess risk for these symptoms disappeared with adjustment for social disadvantage, but higher rates of bedwetting and feeding problems did not. In both this and the Waltham Forest study, West Indian children suffered on a wide range of social indices; they were more likely to live in a single-parent family, with more siblings, more overcrowding, and lower social class. A subsample of 257 five-year-old children whose parents were of Indian, Bangladeshi or Pakistani origin showed fewer behaviour problems than the indigenous population even after controlling for social class and maternal age. There were fewer sleeping problems and accidents. Increased rates of tempers and headaches disappeared after controlling for social class. They too lived in larger families, with overcrowding, lower income and social class.

Hackett *et al* (1991), using Rutter parental questionnaires, compared community samples of 4–7-year-old Gujerati and indigenous English children. The immigrant children had only a quarter (5%) of the rate of disorder of the English sample (21%), and this difference related to family structure (especially single parenthood) and child-rearing patterns.

Rutter *et al* (1974), in their survey of 10-year-olds in inner London, found that children of West Indian parents did not show more disorder on parent interview than indigenous children (18% v. 25%), but did show higher rates of disorder on teacher interview (38% v. 28%). The difference was largely due to higher rates of conduct problems. There were also higher rates of restlessness and poor concentration, but not of non-sanctioned school absence, which was higher in indigenous pupils. Rutter concluded that two probable explanations were racial discrimination (not necessarily by teachers) and the educational retardation of West Indian compared with indigenous pupils. Girls of West Indian origin differed from indigenous girls in having rates of disorder closer to that of boys, and for the disorder to be antisocial rather than emotional. Nicol (1971) reported similar findings in a child guidance clinic study.

Such studies open new routes to understanding clinic referral patterns and their relation to adult expectations, but also will make it possible to explore which aspects and associations of psychopathology are relatively culture-bound, and which may have universal application.

References

Abel, E. & Sokol, R. (1987) Incidence of foetal alcohol syndrome and the economic impact of FAS-related anomalies. *Drug and Alcohol Dependence*, **19**, 51-79.

Achenbach, T. & Edelbrock, C. (1978) The classification of child psychopathology: a review and analysis of empirical efforts. *Psychological Bulletin*, **85**, 1275-1301.

American Psychiatric Association (1987) *Diagnostic and Statistical Manual of Mental Disorders* (3rd edn, revised) (DSM-III-R). Washington, DC: APA.

Anderson, J., Williams, S., McGee, R., *et al* (1987) DSM-III disorders in pre-adolescent children. *Archives of General Psychiatry*, **44**, 69-76.

Andrews, G. & Harris, M. (1964) *The Syndrome of Stuttering*. London: Heinemann.

Bellman, M. (1966) Studies on encopresis. *Acta Paediatrica Scandinavica* (suppl. 170).

Bowen, R., Offord, D. & Boyle, M. (1990) The prevalence of overanxious disorder and separation anxiety disorder: results from the Ontario child health study. *Journal of the American Academy of Child and Adolescent Psychiatry*, **29**, 753-758.

Brandenberg, N., Friedman, R. & Silver, S. (1990) The epidemiology of childhood psychiatric disorders: prevalence findings from recent studies. *Journal of the American Academy of Child and Adolescent Psychiatry*, **29**, 76-83.

Butler, N. & Golding, J. (1986) *From Birth to Five: A Study of the Health and Behaviour of Britain's 5 Year Olds*. Oxford: Pergamon.

Cadman, D., Boyle, M., Szatmari, P., *et al* (1987) Chronic illness disability and mental and social well-being: findings of the Ontario child health study. *Paediatrics*, **79**, 805-813.

Campion, P. & Gabriel, J. (1984) Child consultation patterns in general practice comparing 'high' and 'low' consulting families. *British Medical Journal*, **288**, 1426-1428.

Costello, E., Costello, A., Edelbrock, C., *et al* (1988) Psychiatric disorders in pediatric primary care. *Archives of General Psychiatry*, **45**, 1107-1116.

Dowdney, L., Skuse, D., Heptinstall, E., *et al* (1987) Growth retardation and developmental delay amongst inner-city children. *Journal of Child Psychology and Psychiatry*, **28**, 529-541.

Earls, F. (1980) Prevalence of behaviour problems in 3 year old children: a cross national replication. *Archives of General Psychiatry*, **37**, 1153-1157.

—— & Richman, N. (1980) The prevalence of behaviour problems in three year old children of West Indian parents. *Journal of Child Psychology and Psychiatry*, **21**, 99-106.

Faull, C. & Nicol, A. (1986) Abdominal pain in six year olds: an epidemiological study in a new town. *Journal of Child Psychology and Psychiatry*, **27**, 251-260.

Flament, M., Whitaker, A., Rapoport, J., *et al* (1988) Obsessive compulsive disorder in adolescence: an epidemiological study. *Journal of the American Academy of Child and Adolescent Psychiatry*, **27**, 764-771.

Fleming, J. & Offord, D. (1990) Epidemiology of childhood depressive disorders: a critical review. *Journal of the American Academy of Child Psychiatry*, **29**, 571-580.

Fundudis, T., Kolvin, I. & Garside, R. (1979) *Speech Retarded and Deaf Children; Their Psychological Development*. London: Academic Press.

Garralda, M. & Bailey, D. (1986) Children with psychiatric disorders in primary care. *Journal of Child Psychology and Psychiatry*, **27**, 611-624.

Gillberg, C., Persson, E., Grufman, M., *et al* (1986*a*) Psychiatric disorders in mildly and severely mentally retarded urban children and adolescents. *British Journal of Psychiatry*, **149**, 68-74.

——, Wahlstrom, A., Forsman, A., *et al* (1986*b*) Teenage psychoses – epidemiology, classification and reduced optimality in the pre-, peri- and neonatal periods. *Journal of Child Psychology and Psychiatry*, **27**, 87–98.

Hackett, L., Hackett, R. & Taylor, D. (1991) Psychological disturbance and its associations in the children of the Gujerati community. *Journal of Child Psychology and Psychiatry*, **32**, 851–856.

Hawton, K. & Goldacre, M. (1982) Hospital admissions for adverse effects of medicinal agents (mainly self-poisoning) among adolescents in the Oxford region. *British Journal of Psychiatry*, **141**, 166–170.

Johnson-Sabine, E., Wood, K., Patton, G., *et al* (1988) Abnormal eating attitudes in London schoolgirls – a prospective epidemiological study: factors associated with abnormal response on screening questionnaires. *Psychological Medicine*, **18**, 615–622.

Kastrup, M. (1977) Urban–rural differences in 6 year olds. In *Epidemiological Approaches in Child Psychiatry* (ed. P. Graham). London: Academic Press.

Lavik, N. (1977) Urban–rural differences in rates of disorder. A comparative psychiatric population study of Norwegian adolescents. In *Epidemiological Approaches in Child Psychiatry* (ed. P. Graham). London: Academic Press.

Leslie, S. (1974) Psychiatric disorder in the young adolescents of an industrial town. *British Journal of Psychiatry*, **125**, 113–124.

McClure, G. (1986) Recent changes in suicide among adolescents in England and Wales. *Journal of Adolescence*, **9**, 135–143.

—— (1988) Suicide in children in England and Wales. *Journal of Child Psychology and Psychiatry*, **29**, 345–349.

McGee, R., Feehan, M., Williams, S., *et al* (1990) DSM-III disorders in a large sample of adolescents. *Journal of the American Academy of Child and Adolescent Psychiatry*, **29**, 611–619.

Myers, A. (1981) First seven years of a new NHS mental handicap service, 1974–81. *British Medical Journal*, **285**, 269–273.

Nicol, R. (1971) Psychiatric disorder in the children of Caribbean immigrants. *Journal of Child Psychology and Psychiatry*, **12**, 233–281.

Offord, D., Boyle, M., Szatmari, P., *et al* (1987) Ontario child health study II. Six month prevalence of disorder and rates of service utilisation. *Archives of General Psychiatry*, **44**, 832–836.

Richman, N., Stevenson, J. & Graham, P. (1975) Prevalence of behaviour problems in 3 year old children: an epidemiological study in a London borough. *Journal of Child Psychology and Psychiatry*, **16**, 277–287.

——, —— & —— (1982) *Preschool to School: A Behavioural Study*. London: Academic Press.

Rutter, M. (1989*a*) Isle of Wight revisited: twenty-five years of child psychiatric epidemiology. *Journal of the American Academy of Child and Adolescent Psychiatry*, **28**, 633–653.

—— (1989*b*) Child psychiatric disorders in ICD-10. *Journal of Child Psychology and Psychiatry*, **30**, 499–513.

——, Tizard, J. & Whitmore, K. (eds) (1970) *Education, Health and Behaviour*. London: Longman.

——, Yule, W. & Graham, P. (1973) Enuresis and behavioural deviance: some epidemiological considerations. In *Bladder Control and Enuresis* (eds I. Kolvin, R. MacKeith & S. Meadow). London: Heinemann.

——, ——, Berger, M., *et al* (1974) Children of West Indian immigrants - I. Rates of behavioural deviance and of psychiatric disorder. *Journal of Child Psychology and Psychiatry*, **15**, 241–262.

——, Cox, A., Tupling, C., *et al* (1975*a*) Attainment and adjustment in two geographical areas - I. The prevalence of psychiatric disorder. *British Journal of Psychiatry*, **126**, 493–509.

——, Shaffer, D. & Shepherd, M. (1975*b*) *A Multiaxial Classification of Child Psychiatric Disorders*. Geneva: WHO.

——, Graham, P., Chadwick, O., *et al* (1976) Adolescent turmoil: fact or fiction? *Journal of Child Psychology and Psychiatry*, **17**, 35–56.

—— & Giller, H. (1983) *Juvenile Delinquency: Trends and Perspectives*. London: Penguin.

——, Tuma, A. & Lann, I. (1988) *Assessment and Diagnosis in Child Psychopathology*. London: Guilford.

Sandberg, S., Wieselberg, M. & Shaffer, D. (1980) Hyperkinetic and conduct problem children in a primary school population: some epidemiological considerations. *Journal of Child Psychology and Psychiatry*, **21**, 293–311.

Shaffer, D., Gould, M., Brasic, J., *et al* (1983) Children's global assessment scale. *Archives of General Psychiatry*, **40**, 1228–1231.

——, *et al* (1989) Child and adolescent psychiatric disorders in DSM IV: issues facing the working group. *Journal of the American Academy of Child and Adolescent Psychiatry*, **28**, 830–835.

Steffenburg, S. & Gillberg, C. (1986) Autism and autistic-like conditions in Swedish rural and urban areas; a population study. *British Journal of Psychiatry*, **149**, 81–87.

Stevenson, J., Richman, N. & Graham, P. (1985) Behaviour problems and language abilities at three years and behavioural deviance at eight years. *Journal of Child Psychology and Psychiatry*, **26**, 215–230.

Swadi, H. (1988) Drug and substance abuse among 3333 London adolescents. *British Journal of Addiction*, **83**, 935–942.

Szmuckler, G. (1985) Review: the epidemiology of anorexia nervosa and bulimia. *Journal of Psychiatric Research*, **19**, 143–153.

Taylor, E., Sandberg, S., Thorley, G., *et al* (1991) *The Epidemiology of Childhood Hyperactivity*. Institute of Psychiatry Maudsley Monographs. London: Oxford University Press.

van Goor-Lambo, G., Orley, J., Poustka, F., *et al* (1990) Classification of abnormal psychosocial situations: preliminary report of a revision of a WHO scheme. *Journal of Child Psychology and Psychiatry*, **31**, 229–241.

Welte, J. & Barnes, G. (1987) Youthful smoking: patterns and relationships to alcohol and other drug abuse. *Journal of Adolescence*, **10**, 327–340.

Whitaker, A., Johnson, J., Shaffer, D., *et al* (1990) Uncommon troubles in young people in prevalence of selected psychiatric disorders in a non-referred adolescent population. *Archives of General Psychiatry*, **47**, 487–496.

Wing, L. & Gould, J. (1979) Severe impairments of social interaction and associated abnormalities in children. *Journal of Autism and Developmental Disorders*, **9**, 11–30.

World Health Organization (1992) *The ICD-10 Classification of Mental and Behavioural Disorders. Clinical Descriptions and Diagnostic Guidelines*. Geneva: WHO.

6 Assessment in child and adolescent psychiatry

Mary Eminson

Considerations before the first interview ● *The structure of the assessment* ● *Parents' account* ● *The family interview* ● *Interview with the child* ● *Physical examination and investigations* ● *Psychometric testing* ● *Conclusion*

Assessment in child and adolescent psychiatry is among the most sophisticated and complex assessment tasks in psychiatry. There are several reasons for this. *First*, it is rarely a child who is making a complaint and usually adults (often parents) who are presenting their view of the problem. The interviewer is immediately faced with the need to examine carefully what is essentially an interpretation by parents of what they perceive as wrong, and also the need to engage these parents in this assessment process as they have the power to bring their child for further treatment if needed. The assessment involves enabling parents to describe in detail what they have observed and helping them to give an account of many areas – behaviour, feelings, communication – which will help the psychiatrist draw his or her own conclusions.

The child is often not making any complaint and this provides the *second* special challenge of child psychiatric assessment: the need to communicate with children, not only about 'the problem', but to gain access to their thinking and feelings and a view of their inner world. With the youngest and the most disturbed children, this access may be difficult and achieved only through play and non-verbal techniques.

In addition, throughout the assessment, the interviewer must have in mind normal developmental milestones for a child of this age. Thus the *third* special aspect of the assessment in child psychiatry is the emphasis on learning about the child's functioning from a variety of sources: the child him- or herself, parents and teachers being a conventional minimum. To these sources are added the observations of the child made during the consultation.

Finally, evidence from direct observation of interaction between family members is considered important. This is in contrast to many other areas of psychiatry, where interaction is studied only between an interviewer and a patient. Skills in structuring family interaction, organising one's observations and categorising them in a reliable way have often *not* been acquired at earlier stages in training; together with the need to learn to communicate with children, there is much that is novel.

Because of the complexity of these tasks and the many aspects of the child's and family's functioning to be examined, it is natural that professionals from several disciplines have contributions to make in the assessment. It is important to learn how best to use the skills of other professionals (nurses, social workers, psychologists, psychotherapists, occupational and art therapists and teachers) for both assessment and treatment. On the other hand, it is also vital that the psychiatrist is able to make at least a preliminary assessment of all aspects of a child and the family's problems, for those occasions when this is necessary (e.g. emergencies) or to prepare for working where there is no other professional support.

A further consideration, easily forgotten when the interviewer is grappling with many new aspects of history gathering, is that there is no arbitrary boundary between assessment and treatment. The therapeutic process begins, potentially at least, at the start of the assessment. In some cases it may be the *only* therapeutic opportunity. This chance can be lost by concentrating too narrowly on eliciting 'facts' alone, but balancing the demands of history gathering and therapeutic intervention is almost always a skill to be acquired, rather than one which comes naturally.

One consequence of the complexity of assessment is for novice practitioners to simplify the form of their interviews and perhaps to stick too rigidly to the first assessment format they learn. A useful way to counteract this is to observe as many different professionals as possible (who employ different styles) early in one's training. This also helps to establish how to dovetail the different aspects of assessment in multidisciplinary team work.

The Royal College of Psychiatrists has made it clear that trainees should acquire skills in all aspects of assessment and treatment: individual approaches (psychotherapeutic, cognitive and behavioural, neuropsychiatric, pharmacological) and family assessment and treatment (Joint Committee on Higher Psychiatric Training, 1990). This does not mean that all can necessarily be learnt simultaneously, but consideration should be given to an initial interview to examine all factors which have a bearing on the child's problems. The style in which the initial assessment is made makes a powerful impact on how the problem is conceptualised and the type of treatment the interviewer considers appropriate. It follows that an assessment where individual family members are seen both separately and together (if necessary over more than one session) helps the decision about treatment to be made in a balanced way.

Considerations before the first interview

Spending time thinking about the context of the referral will reduce non-attendance and may save time in the interview itself.

The referral letter or call

(1) Where did the impetus come from to bring about the referral (a desperate mother, or an aggrieved one where her child's school has told her 'something must be done', the harassed general practitioner, a social worker or paediatrician who wishes some respite from a troublesome problem?). Does it sound as if the referrer has met the child or adolescent, or just heard

a report and sent a letter? The parents or child could be quite hostile to the referral, which means special consideration must be given to engagement if any work is to be done.

Three further questions are posed as a result.

(2) Who should be invited to the first interview? In intact families, two parents and the child is a usual minimum, but should the whole family be invited? When should a non-custodial parent be included? Should other members of the 'network' be invited? The family's social worker, if they have initiated the referral, can give helpful information, or perhaps one should meet the social worker before the family attend?

(3) Which professionals should be involved from one's own service? Although all the professionals in the team are able to carry out assessments, the letter may suggest considerable attention needs to be given to the parents' own background, in which case a psychiatric social worker will be an invaluable help in assessment. Alternatively the description of the child's problem may suggest some form of psychometric assessment will be useful, in which case the psychologist might perform the assessment.

(4) What are the likely diagnoses? This question determines one's own preparation. It may seem premature to be thinking about this while considering the referral letter but a mental list of differential diagnoses will encourage reading beforehand and help to focus questioning to distinguish one diagnosis from another.

Practical matters

The waiting area

This needs to be of adequate size and comfort and equipped with suitable toys. An opportunity to observe briefly how the family behaves there will give a useful impression of their noise, chaos, physical closeness, seating arrangements and general affect. Children must be able to be supervised at times when their parents are being interviewed.

The consulting room

A common practice is to start the assessment interview with all who have attended, to explain the structure of the assessment and check the various agenda items with them. This means the room must be of an adequate size and temperature to accommodate all comfortably and with furniture which gives children an opportunity for quiet play (paper and crayons or pens will do at this stage). The impression must be created quickly that the environment is safe (both physically and emotionally). If using this room for longer interviews or with children alone, then further play materials should be easily available. These may include:

For younger children   There should be available posting and construction toys, plasticine, tea-set, small figures, cars (ambulances, fire engines, police cars), a doll's house, furniture and figures, a couple of toy telephones for 'messages', paper and crayons.

For older children   There is no need to hide away the toys mentioned above as the child may choose or need a toy associated with a younger age group; felt-tips and paper go a long way, but more complex construction toys, perhaps dolls, even simple board games should be available to facilitate interaction in a safe, undemanding way with a child who is anxious about either play or conversation.

The structure of the assessment

Introductions

These should include all who are present, including the youngest children and any trainees or students. Particular clarification of the role of social workers in the clinic may be needed so that the family does not assume they are being accused of abuse or inadequate parenting. The care taken in introduction gives, from the start, an important message of interest in the contributions each individual has to make; altering one's position for introduction to the small children shows one can 'get down to their level'.

Any technology to be employed (e.g. one-way screen, television link or video recording) is explained and consent acquired from all family members. There must be an explicit explanation of the use to which any video recording is to be put.

Preparing for the interview

Establish the source and purpose of the referral in language understandable by parents and children; explain the timing and structure of the assessment. A clear statement to young children (e.g. "I'm a doctor who sees children with upset feelings") or to older children who look particularly angry, anxious or disengaged (e.g. "I'm a doctor who often sees young people with problems like yours; I need to hear your point of view") may be needed.

After the introductions and explanation a decision must be made about when to separate parents and child and, for adolescents, a decision about whether to see adolescent or parents first. There is good evidence that even the most sensitive parents do not have complete knowledge of their child's feelings and experiences (Barrett *et al*, 1991) and some time should be spent with each separately. This also permits parents to tell secrets about their own experiences and history, or the parentage of the child, which they would be uncomfortable disclosing in front of him or her. On the other hand, it is also clear that information about family relationships is strengthened by direct observation of the family interactions, so both family and individual interviews are needed for a full assessment.

What follows assumes that, after introduction, parents are seen separately from their child; this is often easiest for a novice. Once a comfortable routine has been learnt, however, greater flexibility may be introduced. Large parts of the history and current complaints can be gathered in the family interview (see below), giving more opportunity to observe family interaction. If the interview is with parents and child together from the start, reassurance must be given that separate interviews will take place at some point and that 'secrets' need not be disclosed unwillingly in front of other family members.

Parents' account of present complaints and history

When parents are seen alone, the interview should begin by allowing them to describe the problems which are their current concern, elicited by open-ended questions. Their views (which are their interpretation) should be noted carefully; the interviewer's impression of their attitudes and feelings is as important as the facts recounted. After the initial complaint, the parents should be asked if there are other concerns and encouraged to offer worries about as many areas as they wish.

The next stage is to examine the parents' spontaneous concerns in more detail, and more closed questions will be required to elicit:

(1) the precise nature of the symptom
(2) a recent detailed example
(3) its onset (and any connections to other events at that time)
(4) its duration, effects and factors which exacerbate or ameliorate it
(5) the pervasiveness of the behaviour (home/others' homes/school), and
(6) an example of the antecedents and consequences on a particular occasion.

Enquiry is made about the parents' beliefs about causation and the strategies they have used in dealing with the symptom; their success or otherwise is detailed, as is the effect the symptom is having on *all* family members. Gathering information in such detail helps the professional to form an objective view of the severity of the problem.

The next symptom presented by the parents should be considered similarly, and so on down their list, until their current concerns have been thoroughly examined and the interviewer also has a good grasp of the parental attitudes, management style and feelings about their child's symptoms. Notes at this stage will consist largely of a verbatim account of how parents conceptualise the problems.

The other psychiatric symptoms which have *not* arisen in the spontaneous account are next examined: in broad terms, this involves enquiring about a

√

Box 6.1   Areas of current psychiatric symptoms to be enquired for: the young child

Anxiety (separation anxiety particularly), panic, fears, phobias
Misery, withdrawal
Changeability of mood, sensitivity, irritability
Sleep: difficulty in settling, sleeping alone, night terrors or nightmares
Eating problems: faddiness, reluctance, restriction, gorging or stealing
 food
Wetting, soiling
Obsessional traits, thoughts, ruminations, rituals, compulsions
Motor restlessness and level of activity
Poor attention, concentration or distractibility
Disobedience, non-compliance
Aggression, lying, stealing, fire setting
Physical and verbal temper tantrums, outbursts, destructiveness

---

wide range of possible emotional difficulties where only problem *behaviour* has been offered spontaneously, and checking for conduct issues where parents have focused on emotional symptoms. The range of these probes is informed by a knowledge of likely difficulties at this age and developmental stage, and by reading or experience of symptoms which cluster together (for example, following the description of florid symptoms of Tourette's syndrome, asking carefully about obsessions and compulsions would be crucial) (see Boxes 6.1–6.3).

The child's current functioning in other areas

The interview now moves from a focus almost exclusively upon the patient to a wider examination of his or her functioning in other areas.

(1) Current academic abilities and performance

Permission is sought to contact the child's school for a report; head teachers often like to be the point of entry for enquiries. Areas of functioning to ask about include any behavioural or emotional problems, the child's academic ability, attainment and any change in this, other interests and activities and relationships with peers and staff.

(2) Peer relationships

Are the child's current friendships with children of the same age, younger or older? How long do the friendships last and are they predominantly with children of the same or different sex? Has there been a change recently? Is the child constantly falling out with friends? Do other children call for them,

---

Box 6.2   Areas of current psychiatric symptoms to be enquired for: middle childhood

Anxiety, panic, fears, phobias
Obsessional traits, thoughts, ruminations, rituals, compulsions
Eating problems: special fads or restrictions
Sleep problems, night terrors, nightmares
Frequent changeability of mood, irritability
Marked or frequent low or high moods, withdrawal
Level of motor activity, degree of restlessness
Attention span, distractibility
Impulsiveness
Wetting, soiling
Self-harming urges, threats or actions (including running away)
Oppositional behaviour, temper tantrums
Conduct problems: lying, stealing, destructiveness, fire setting, aggression
School attendance problems: refusal, truancy, running out
Hallucinations

---

come to the house or contact them, or is all contact either at the instigation of this child or only achieved through some structured activity such as a club? For adolescents, sexual relationships need consideration.

Peer relationships must be considered in the context of the child's and family's general level of social integration; this is highly dependent on the family's culture, beliefs and geography, as well as the child's functioning. This area, like that of parental management techniques, is particularly prone to value judgement by the interviewer.

(3) Current relationships within the home

Do the parents see problems in the relationship between the child and either of them, the siblings or other family members? Non-verbal communication about relationships should be noted, together with the degree of hostility, scapegoating or idealisation of family members.

Personal history and development

The assessment is now broadened to include the child's functioning in the past. The amount of detail recorded in each area listed below will depend on the type of problem presented (for example, a referral of a possibly autistic child will require great detail about early physical and linguistic development).

(1) The history of the child's functioning before this current referral, not only in the areas of important symptoms but also generally. Contact with

---

**Box 6.3   Areas of current psychiatric symptoms to be
enquired for: adolescence**

Anxiety, panic, fears, phobias (especially social phobias)
Obsessional traits, thoughts, ruminations, rituals, compulsions
Eating and weight problems: comfort eating, anorexic or bulimic traits
Moods: severe or frequent low or high moods
Mood changeability, loss of interests, withdrawal
Suicidal or self-harming thoughts, threats or actions
Conduct problems at home: stealing, destructiveness, aggression
School attendance problems: reluctance, refusal, truancy
Substance abuse: solvents, drink, drugs
Antisocial and risk-taking activities outside home and school
Psychotic phenomena, delusional mood, hallucinations

---

any other agencies or specialists is recorded; what was help sought for and what was the effect? Permission to contact other agencies is sought.

(2) The child's personal development including the pregnancy and birth, and attainment of developmental milestones; his or her reactions to predictable developmental challenges such as attending nursery, play group, and school. Significant separations and disruptions should be recorded; the stage of pubertal development is established and whether the menarche has been reached.

(3) The child's temperament or personality: examples of how he or she reacts to strange situations, ways of showing feelings.

(4) The child's physical health throughout his or her life. In addition to a strictly factual record of sickness and hospital admissions, some idea of the meaning that these illnesses had for the parents and the way they viewed the child afterwards may help in an understanding of any overprotection and rejection within the parent–child relationships. Specific details of dates, consultants and hospitals attended may be essential if records have to be scrutinised subsequently. Particular care should be taken where neuro-psychiatric conditions are concerned.

(5) The personal and social histories of both parents. Particular reference needs to be made to any mental illness in family members, especially if any genetic component in the illness is suspected. Previous partners and a non-custodial parent need special and delicate enquiry so that one can acquire a view of the nature of the relationship. The practicalities surrounding the break-up of the relationships are considered, as is the likelihood that the child's feelings were considered at all. Feelings about current relationships with the non-custodial parent and about access arrangements may need exploration.

(6) The rest of the family: problems or strengths of other siblings, the quality of their relationship with the referred patient.

(7) Current or recent social stresses and supports, such as bereavements, changes in job, health and school must be examined. They may be forgotten by parents intent upon a history of the problem, particularly if they do not see a connection between the events and the child's symptoms.

(8) Finally, it is important to make a general enquiry about whether parents think that the interviewer has failed to ask about any other area which *they* think could have a bearing on what has taken place. In this fashion not only is unexpected information sometimes discovered, but also one has access to parental beliefs about the cause of the problem which they may have been uncertain about declaring earlier.

The family interview

At whatever stage of the assessment this takes place, some of the same rules apply: the interviewer needs to *engage* all family members by introduction, eye contact and a clear message that their contribution will be valued. It must be established that there will be an opportunity to speak to the psychiatrist separately if they wish; it is helpful to state clearly that only one person can 'hold the floor' at any time. Much of the information about family relationships, history and communication patterns can be gathered in a family interview with greater richness than in individual interviews.

Small children can be given permission to play quietly while listening; a low table with drawing materials in the centre of the room facilitates this. The interviewer should avoid hearing a long initial account from parents by showing quickly that he or she is interested in knowing all points of view and in how other family members felt and communicated about the issue.

Interaction should be encouraged between family members as well as with the interviewer. A good tactic is to check that children have understood what a parent has said and if not, to ask the parent to simplify it.

Texts on family assessment (e.g. Barker, 1986) give more details about the different dimensions of family functioning which can be examined, but even without this, psychiatrically trained interviewers should be able to look out for, and record their impressions of:

(1) the family's affect (tension, sadness, anger)
(2) their communication patterns (verbal and non-verbal)
(3) the degree of organisation and structure (can the parents help the children to play quietly in the session and control them effectively?)
(4) their responsiveness and sensitivity to different family members and the interviewer.

Although the order in which the history is gathered within the interview is up to the individual psychiatrist, it may be helpful to place the child within the family by constructing a genogram (family tree) with the family (Rogers & Durkin, 1984). This will often obviate the need for some detailed questioning in other areas mentioned. Gathering of family history and relationships using a family tree is enormously rewarding for those who incorporate it as a routine technique. Time and patience are required, and a sensitivity to hesitations and uncertainties in each parent's account which merit further gentle questioning to elicit painful issues from the past, or denote an area to leave for an individual interview. The family tree should cover at least three generations and personal preference will dictate whether one starts with a parent or the presented child. Children can be involved in the task by inviting them to help in drawing the tree and writing in names and birthdays.

When enquiring about the children in this sibship it is important to frame the question not as "Was Johnny your first child?" but "Was Johnny your first pregnancy?", which quickly reveals miscarriages, terminations or other children adopted away who might not have come to light in the narrative otherwise. The planning and welcome given to each pregnancy, the mother's and baby's health, the mode of birth and weight of the infant follow naturally in the sequence as each pregnancy is considered.

By making a start at patiently working through the current sibship and set of pregnancies, parents appreciate that they are telling their family story and it is easy to move back a generation in order to enquire how the couple met and made a relationship and then to look at each individual parent and the parenting they themselves received. They are placed within their own sibship and enquiries made of current family relationships and any problems of the parents, siblings or other relations which could be germane to the current difficulties (for example reading problems, physical stigmata or mental illness). From enquiries about the parents' own parenting a picture of the grandparental generation is built up which is led back to the current patient through enquiries about contact between grandparents and children.

Interview with the child

The tasks of the interview

These are:

(1) to assess whether the child has a psychiatric illness
(2) to examine the child's functioning in terms of motor skills, hearing and language (structure, articulation, expression), social relating and cognitive abilities; objective assessments of educational and cognitive attainments can be used
(3) to make an assessment of the child's emotional state, including affect, thoughts and experiences
(4) to carry out a physical examination if appropriate

(5) to give the child a sense of being accepted and understood by the interviewer, both to make this assessment a positive experience and to prepare the ground for future therapeutic endeavours.

General considerations

It has already been emphasised that children rarely present themselves at the clinic and their expectations need to be considered. An explanation should be offered of how the time will be spent (getting to know them, trying to understand what has been making them upset, playing or talking with them) and misapprehensions should be corrected (they will not be taken away, put in hospital, given an injection). With teenagers particularly, issues of confidentiality should be clarified. If an issue arises during the interview which must be discussed with parents or other agencies, explain this and the reasons explicitly to the child.

Consider carefully the place of any physical examination in relation to the interview with the child. Judgement is required to decide whether making a relationship with the child or adolescent first will ease their embarrassment or fears about an examination, or whether it is easier to complete the physical examination initially and then to carry out the interview. In some cases it may be felt advisable to ask a paediatric colleague to carry out the physical examination.

Children up to age five or six years

Generally speaking, the interview will be conducted through play and the child's account of his or her symptoms will form only a very peripheral part. Play materials must be readily accessible, clearly distinguished from any area of the room which is 'out of bounds', appropriate for the child's age, not broken, and chosen so that interaction is facilitated. If necessary, set the rules early on: toys cannot be taken home, a clear 'we don't do that here' to any behaviour which is dangerous or physically hurtful or damaging.

Initially one should notice how the child copes with the separation from parents (if protest is extreme, allow one parent to join the interview briefly and then slip out); allow the child to explore the toys before gently joining in the play. The task at this time is to consider the relationship made with the psychiatrist and to observe skills demonstrated spontaneously. After a period of play and exploration which is child led, it may be useful to initiate activities which will test the child's skills more directly.

Motor activity

Relate observations to both *gross* and *fine* movements (their extent and skill), and to laterality (and how well established). What is the level of motor restlessness, activity, and coordination; is there any clumsiness? If there are tics, which muscle groups are affected? Are there any stereotypies or mannerisms?

Speech and language

Is the child attentive/responsive to speech? Could hearing be impaired? The child's vocalisation is considered in terms of:

(1) amount (is the child mute or virtually so?)
(2) volume
(3) spontaneity, appropriate gestures, and any abnormality in articulation (stammering, odd intonation, dysarthria, or other defect of word or sound production)
(4) unusual features in expression: pronominal reversals, echoing, repeated stereotyped utterances
(5) complexity of speech in terms of vocabulary, grammar and ideas expressed in relation to age.

Social relating

(1) *Initial rapport.* Is the child appropriately cautious? How anxious, shy or disinhibited is he or she? Is there any eye contact initially; does the child seem aloof or avoidant?
(2) *The quality of relationship after the first few minutes.* Is the child responsive in conversation and play, allowing or inviting joint activities? Is there much reciprocity? Does he or she organise the interviewer's activities, or passively wait to be organised? Can the child initiate games; and can the topic be changed with ease or difficulty? Is he or she disinhibited, distractible, cheeky, intrusive? How satisfying did the interaction feel? What was the range and extent of emotional expression?

Children between five years and puberty

In interviewing children of five or six years onwards, it is increasingly important to make clear the purpose of the assessment and to clarify why the child thinks he or she has come. Strictly factual closed questions may be useful initially to help the child settle down and appreciate that the interviewer is interested: for example an enquiry about the journey to the clinic, the structure of the family, pets or hobbies. This general introduction will quickly give an impression of the child's level of verbal facility and current anxiety. As ever, it is crucial to match one's language and complexity of grammar to the child's understanding.

The first decision is how to start the interview: by simply talking with children about the difficulties that have brought them to the clinic, inviting them to play and then using this as an indirect method of understanding their difficulties, or by starting an activity such as drawing which will allow discussion of the problems alongside it? Obviously the child's ability to relate in straightforward conversation with a new adult will increase as adolescence approaches, but the decision about how much 'the problems' should be the focus of the discussion or how much is gathered by play is highly dependent on the rapport established, the child's cognitive abilities, how the assessment has progressed, and the philosophy and orientation of the psychiatrist.

Observations in the areas mentioned for a preschool child (motor, sensory, language, social relations) still apply. After the first few minutes open questions will be useful; sometimes offering a range of possible answers in 'multiple choice' fashion is a help. As children respond particularly to non-verbal communication, the interviewer's face and posture must express the appropriate emotion clearly. If talk is difficult (and this is quite likely when one is unused to interviewing children) long silences should be avoided by a move to play or drawing.

Taking notes at the interview is undesirable, but by the end the psychiatrist should have at least tentative answers to the following questions:

(1) What is the child's view of the problems that have brought them to the clinic and what do they think is the cause of these? (When conduct problems are present, how much do they acknowledge their own part in the activities, or are they all someone else's fault?)

(2) What are the child's feelings? It may be tempting to shy away from, or fail to explore, painful subjects so as to avoid upset, but an appraisal of distress cannot be made without consideration of sensitive areas. Children will not be damaged by evoking distress providing this is acknowledged with sympathy and sensitivity. How sad, miserable, guilty and responsible do they feel? How often do they have these feelings and what are they about? What type and range of affect is expressed about the parents? Great ease in talking about feelings should not be expected in children of this age, who are probably quite unused to such discussions. If the child is trying to identify feelings but having trouble in finding words, two alternatives may be offered (but this should be noted). A request for other examples of times when they have had these feelings may be helpful (it is always tempting to take agreement for understanding). Phrases such as 'I knew a boy once who . . .' or 'some children tell me . . .' allow children to explore difficult areas of feelings to which they might not admit directly.

(3) Are there difficulties which may be *secondary* to mood or emotional problems: for example problems with sleep (vivid or unpleasant dreams or nightmares, insomnia) or appetite and enjoyment of food?

(4) What kind of friendships does this child have? (See also section under "Parents' account", pp. 80–81.) Are these *confiding* friendships ("Could you tell him a secret or a worry if you had one?"); are they accompanied by hostility, falling out and name calling?

(5) How does the child view school – as a place of terror and humiliation, or success and stimulation?

Interviews with adolescents

Earlier conjoint parts of the interview will have given adolescents an idea about the level of interest in their point of view, but if conduct or antisocial activities form any part of the problem, they probably still assume the psychiatrist will take sides with the parents. A stance should be cultivated which is morally neutral towards the symptoms while still being very interested in the adolescent's concerns, point of view and feelings. This does not involve faking enormous enthusiasm for particular aspects of youth culture; this will unerringly be identified as phoney. It is often helpful to start with a sympathetic remark such as "It sounds as if this has been a pretty difficult time, why don't you tell me about it?" While this sounds banal, few adolescents disagree with it, whatever the disorder.

Because adolescents hate to lose face, they are unlikely to admit the interviewer's language is too complex for them. Young adolescents, those from non-verbal families or with cognitive limitations, may require considerable simplification of vocabulary and concepts.

Although the style and language of the assessment may differ from that used with adults, the content of the interview and mental state examination is very similar; questions about experiences and cognitions examine the same range of disorders. In addition the questions raised under the previous two headings remain valid. Long silences are generally experienced as persecutory and should be avoided.

Physical examination and investigations

The importance of a physical examination may vary with the history and type of disorder but it should always be considered; the inexperienced should learn to incorporate it as a routine. See under "General considerations" (p. 85) for timing.

Observation of the child's skill in dressing and undressing may alert one to the need for a neurological examination later by an appropriately skilled person. Plot the height, weight and head circumference on centile charts if this has not been done. Note the child's hand preference, the degree of clumsiness, incoordination or unsteadiness; look carefully for asymmetrical physical development, unusual facial appearance, any skin blemish (pigmented or depigmented patches, naevi, unusual nails or hair texture, bruising, scars, etc.).

Children generally find it entertaining to perform for 'Fog testing' (Fog & Fog, 1963) (walking in a straight line, heel–toe walking, and walking on tip toes, on heels, and on the outer edge of the foot); asymmetry in and extent of overflow movements are relatively easily seen. Coordination of hands and arms can be assessed by asking to see the child's handwriting, drawing and copying of figures; then, with the child standing, eyes shut, arms outstretched, watch for tremor or drifting of one arm. This may be followed by finger to nose with eyes still closed. Rapid finger–thumb opposition and tapping the back of the opposite hand complete a brief examination.

Even without postgraduate paediatric experience the psychiatrist has now considered basic biological growth and neurological integrity; the young child's developmental progress should be checked with a standard manual (e.g. Sheridan, 1980).

Findings in the history or examination may prompt a request for paediatric (or paediatric neurological) assessment. Details are beyond the scope of this chapter, but in addition to biochemical, haematological and urine tests, some special investigations are quite common. Neurological and neuropsychiatric disorders may require investigation by electroencephalography, brain scans, and blood investigations of drug levels. Genetic and chromosomal investigations may be required where there is developmental delay, a suspicion of a disintegrative condition, a significantly related condition in the family pedigree, or the child's appearance is unusual. Gene mapping is a possibility as advances in molecular genetics increase the chance of the discovery of disease-related genes in mental disorders; the laboratory should be consulted about conditions suspected in view of special techniques required (e.g. for fragile X chromosome testing).

Psychometric testing

The indication for psychometric assessment may have been evident at the referral stage, but the initial history and examination is often the place where it is clear that this should be considered, because of the suggestion of inconsistencies in the child's cognitive performance or the possibility of a learning disability. A discussion with a psychologist will clarify this. The three commonest indications in ordinary practice are when:

(1) Developmental delay, either specific or generalised, is suspected in young children who have not been assessed before. If this seems to be a specific language delay it would be reasonable to ask a speech therapist for an assessment.

(2) There are discrepancies in educational attainment: between the child's apparent potential and achievement, including the possibility of specific learning disorders. These discrepancies may operate in either direction; that is to say, the low attainment may in fact be because the child's potential is much less than expected, or greater than expected. If the difficulties are likely to result in 'statementing' procedures (see p. 265) under the Education Act 1981, or in the need for remedial intervention,

any testing should be carried out in active collaboration with psychologists responsible for educational provision.

(3) Neuropsychiatric deficits are suspected: large discrepancies between verbal and performance skills, problems with memory, visuospatial ability, speed in psychomotor tasks. When a deteriorating condition is under consideration, serial testing may be required.

Even when the child's primary difficulty is evident (e.g. severe attention deficit) it can be useful to see what can be achieved under optimal conditions.

In any of these circumstances, the report of the child's behaviour in the test is very useful in addition to test results. (The psychologist's experience in how children approach tests parallels the psychiatrist's in judging how children respond to an interview.) The degree of organisation, concentration and anxiety about tests, the extent of fear of failure, the type of problem-solving approach and response to difficult items all increase the understanding of the child's functioning and difficulties.

Commonly used tests

Berger (1985) provides a useful introduction to the psychological assessment and testing of children.

Griffiths Mental Development Scale, 0-8 years

The test has four subscales: locomotor, personal/social, hearing/speech, hand/eye coordination. It yields a quotient for each subscale and a general quotient which has a mean of 100 and standard deviation of 12. It has been standardised on a British population and is used quite often by medical personnel with appropriate training. It is used uncommonly in the upper age range except in the learning disabled.

Wechsler Intelligence Scale for Children (Revised) (WISC-R), 6-17 years

Verbal and performance subscales yield a verbal, performance, and full-scale IQ; there is a short form of four subtests. Probably still the most commonly used intelligence test, it is lengthy and was standardised on an American sample though a British version of the test is usually used. It is helpful as a first-line neuropsychiatric assessment to indicate the need for more specific tests.

Wechsler Preschool and Primary Scale of Intelligence (WPPSI), 4-6½ years

This version of the WISC for younger children also yields verbal, performance, and full-scale IQ.

British Ability Scales, 2½–17 years

Standardised on a British population, the scales were designed to assess a broader range of competencies than just IQ. Subscales are speed, reasoning, spatial imaging, perceptual matching, short-term memory, retrieval and application of knowledge. For each, a percentile rank is given and an overall IQ calculated.

Neale Analysis of Reading Ability, 6–12 years

This tests the rate of reading, accuracy of reading and comprehension, giving an overall reading age.

Schonell Graded Word Reading Tests and Spelling Tests, 6–12 years

These tests yield reading and spelling ages. Educational psychologists might wish to complement Schonell tests with further educational diagnostic assessments where specific difficulties are apparent.

Conclusion

Once the initial assessment interview is completed, the psychiatrist is in a position to decide whether or which further physical and psychometric investigations are necessary, together with any views or information to be acquired from schools, hospitals or other agencies (see also Box 6.4). Occupational, speech or physiotherapy assessment may be merited. Further psychiatric interviews may also be considered: a plan for a longer individual or family assessment perhaps.

The type of formulation again depends on orientation but consideration of the multi-axial framework is helpful (see Chapter 5). Thus at the end of the assessment the child has been evaluated in terms of the presence, or absence, and type of psychiatric disorder, with consideration of organic and dynamic components. The educational and cognitive deficits are labelled, albeit tentatively at this stage. Some measure of severity is usually included in both these areas. The context of the disorder has also been established, including the physical, psychiatric, social and developmental issues in child and family. The individual's or family's predicament has been examined, together with patterns of family interaction. Although this is rarely included in a formulation, the individual's and family's strengths have also been appraised: a vital issue if treatment is considered.

Another type of formulation outlines precipitating, aetiological and maintaining factors in any disorder, and this, too, is often helpful in identifying potential routes for intervention. Overall, an assessment places the parents and child's subjective account of difficulties in the context of the psychiatrist's knowledge of normal and psychopathological child and family development.

Box 6.4 The information the psychiatrist should have at the end of the psychiatric interview

Source and nature of referral
  Who made referral
  Who initiated referral
  Family attitudes to referral
Description of presenting complaints
  Onset, frequency, intensity, duration, location (home, school, etc.)
  Antecedents and consequences
  Ameliorating and exacerbating factors
  Specific examples
  Parental and family beliefs about causation
  Past attempts to solve problem
Description of child's current general functioning
  School – behaviour and emotions
          – academic performance
          – peer and staff relationships
  Peer relationships generally
  Family relationships
Personal/developmental history
  Pregnancy, labour, delivery
  Early developmental milestones
  Separations/disruptions
  Physical illnesses and their meaning for parents
  Reactions to school
  Puberty
  Temperamental style
Family history
  Personal and social histories of both parents
    especially – history of mental illness
                – their experience of being parented
  History of family development
    – how parents came together
    – history of pregnancies
    – separations and effects on children
  Who lives at home currently
  Strengths/weaknesses of all at home
  Current social stresses and supports
Information from observation of family interaction –
  structure, organisation, communication, sensitivity
Information from observation of child at interview –
  motor, sensory, speech, language, social relating skills
Mental state, concerns, and spontaneous account if age appropriate
Results of physical examination
Plan for future investigation and management

Concluding the interview

It is crucial that the assessment is drawn to a proper conclusion for the patient and family as well as the professionals. The family will have come with certain expectations which will need to be addressed at the end of the assessment. Both parents and child may have revealed a great deal about many aspects of their past and present lives; the process and content may have been emotionally highly charged for them. This interview with a family may or may not have been therapeutic in itself. It is not adequate to respond to one's encounter solely by informing the parents and child that "more information will be acquired from different sources".

The family should be given a version of the psychiatrist's diagnostic formulation, couched in appropriate terms. There should be a clear indication of what the next stages of either assessment or treatment will be, and the aims, form, and likely outcome of this. Even where no further meetings are anticipated, a summary of what understanding has been gained from the interview must be shared with the family and there must be an acknowledgement of the effort they have made in sharing their predicament.

Sample formulation

B is an 11-year-old Hindu Gujerati boy with Tourette's syndrome, characterised by involuntary use of English swear words together with facial grimacing and tics. The assessment was made of him with his 18-year-old sister and a family friend as interpreter.

These difficulties have been gradually worsening over the last two to three years and have resulted in considerable difficulty in school with teasing and bullying, where he has also been disruptive and silly in class. The information available at present does not lead to an additional diagnosis of conduct disorder and there is no evidence of secondary emotional disorder.

B has learning difficulties; his reading and writing were found in the clinic to be very poor for his age. He seemed emotionally somewhat immature. The referrer says the educational psychologist has been asked to see him, but he is in mainstream classes.

On physical examination, apart from the facial tics, there were no specific abnormalities, though both height and weight were between the 3rd and 10th centiles. He was poorly coordinated, with extensive overflow movements on Fogs testing, but there were no asymmetries to suggest a specific neurological lesion.

The family are members of the local Gujerati community and have been in Britain about 14 years; B is their only son. Neither parent speaks English; both work in a local garment factory. The family are deeply embarrassed by the symptoms and have been reluctant to seek professional help. There are three older sisters; the one who attended the interview seemed affectionate but irritated with B. She allowed the family friend to do much of the talking although he knew little detail; the family seem to have traditional ideas about sex roles.

Plan

The knowledge of his early history and development is inadequate because his parents did not accompany him and the family friend was acting as interpreter. On the next occasion, the parents have been asked to come and an independent Gujerati interpreter arranged.

The sister, friend, and B were told the diagnosis and given a brief explanation. Medication has not been started because of the language difficulties and the need to have a qualified interpreter when drug effects, side-effects and the outlook are explained. Because of the severity of the condition and the presence of language and communication difficulties, behavioural intervention was not considered appropriate alone.

Opening communication with education services is a priority to discover what assessments are planned and discuss placement possibilities and B's prognosis. B's sister has given consent for this.

References

Barker, P. (1986) *Basic Family Therapy* (2nd edn). Oxford: Blackwell Scientific.

Barrett, M. L., Berney, T. P., Bhate, S., *et al* (1991) Diagnosing childhood depression. Who should be interviewed – parent or child? The Newcastle Child Depression Project. *British Journal of Psychiatry*, **159** (suppl. 11), 22–27.

Berger, M. (1985) Psychological assessment and testing. In *Child and Adolescent Psychiatry: Modern Approaches* (eds M. Rutter & L. Hersov), pp. 264–279. Oxford: Blackwell Scientific.

Fog, E. & Fog, M. (1963) Cerebral inhibition examined by associated movements. In *Minimal Cerebral Dysfunction* (eds M. Box & R. MacKeith). Clinics in Developmental Medicine, no. 10. London: Spastics International Medical Publications/Heinemann Medical.

Joint Committee on Higher Psychiatric Training (1990) *JCHPT Handbook*. London: Royal College of Psychiatrists.

Rogers, J. & Durkin, M. (1984) The semi-structured genogram interview: I protocol, II evaluation. *Family Systems Medicine*, **2**, 176–185.

Sheridan, M. D. (1980) *From Birth to Five Years: Children's Developmental Progress*. Windsor: Nfer-Nelson.

7 Clinical syndromes in early childhood
Ann Le Couteur

*Classification and prevalence of significant disorder ● Temper tantrums ●
Sleep disorders ● Eating disorders ● Encopresis (faecal soiling) and
enuresis ● Attention deficit disorder (hyperkinetic syndrome) ● Specific
developmental disorders ● Pervasive developmental disorders ● Disorders
of social functioning ● Emotional disorders ● Conduct disorder ● Gender
identity disorders ● Summary and conclusions*

In the preschool period young children rapidly develop some independence
for motor and bodily functions, gain the ability to use language to communicate
and develop important selective social relationships, initially within the family
and then gradually with others.

When reviewing the clinical syndromes of this age group there are five points
to consider.

Firstly, a sound knowledge of the normal variations and variabilities in
development is needed (see Chapter 2). Performance in infancy and later
childhood is of limited predictive power (Kagan, 1979), and this needs to be
taken into account when assessing the significance of disturbance in such
young children.

Secondly, the skills and techniques required for the assessment of this age
group may be rather different and complementary to those necessary for
assessing older children (Chapter 6). The developmental stage of the young
child will influence the way in which they can use language and words
to communicate. For example, they may not be able to describe their
feelings and thoughts directly but indirectly through their behaviour, play and
other activities.

Thirdly, the young child's changing degree of dependence upon their
caring adults and the development of parent-child relationships form an
important part of the assessment of young children. Bowlby (1969) and
subsequent writers have highlighted the significance on later development
of the important early social relationships (see Chapter 3). Research has
focused not only on the nature of the good experience in the mother and
infant interaction, but also the crucial role that conflict and distress may
play in helping the infant develop a sense of competence and resilience
(Hinde, 1982). The complex interplay between the young child's early
relationships, developmental competence and environment in determining
the outcome and quality of infant-adult relationships is illustrated in the study
of infants raised in a very poor environment: Rutter (1980a) reported that such
young children can make very good progress providing their subsequent
rearing is adequate.

Fourthly, the effect of the complex interaction of individual characteristics (such as temperament) that young children and their parents bring to their relationships will change as young children rapidly pass through their developmental stages. For example, for some children and parents periods of rapid developmental change can provoke intense stress and anxiety. Language acquisition, or the gaining of bladder control or bowel function, may be accomplished by such tensions that their relationship is adversely affected.

Fifthly, for young children their nurturing environment also provides all their social experiences. This means that children of this age are especially susceptible and vulnerable to tensions and other stresses within the family. Indeed, it may be difficult or inappropriate to separate how much any presenting symptom may be a function of the child's individual difficulties or reflect wider issues for the family.

The considerations outlined above have led some professionals involved in the assessment, treatment and management of young children to encourage the development of the subspecialty of infant psychiatry (Minde & Minde, 1986).

All preschool children are referred for child psychiatric assessment because of the concerns of others. For most of these children their disorder or difficulties will be mainly behavioural, for example difficulties with eating or sleeping, problems with elimination, reactions to separation or illness. Many of these young children will have initially been seen by the health visitor or family general practitioner and then referred to a hospital-based or community-based consultant paediatrician. For other children and families, problems with managing behaviour might be referred to a local social services department. All or any of these professionals might then consider referral to a child psychiatric service, or indeed the parents or general practitioner might make a direct referral.

A number of features must be looked at when deciding whether a significant disorder exists. These will include the number, severity and persistence of the behavioural difficulties, together with evidence of disturbed relationships within the family and the consideration of whether the child's development is impaired or delayed.

During the later preschool years, the child may attend a play group or nursery group and in this setting, too, concerns will be mainly in terms of the child's behaviour, as gradually a greater emphasis will be placed on the young child's ability to relate socially outside the immediate family.

In addition to concerns about behaviour, emotions and quality of the child's relationships, all of which may be considered as extremes of normal behaviour, there are rare, severe disorders with a much worse prognosis. These include the pervasive developmental disorders such as infantile autism, Rett's syndrome and the disintegrative psychoses. These are also considered in more detail within this chapter.

Classification and prevalence of significant disorder

The majority of young children who are referred for assessment present with a mixture of symptoms or behaviour problems and as such the difficulties do not fall into clearly differentiated categories, and they are distinguished from other children in the general population by the severity and persistence of their difficulties. Some of the disorders discussed below are given in Box 7.1.

Among referrals to a community child guidance service or hospital-based child psychiatry service, approximately 30% are likely to be children under the age of five years. These will include children with autism and developmental problems – such as disorders of speech, language and late development – elimination disorders (enuresis and encopresis), overactive children and behaviour and management problems including temper tantrums and breath holding, sleeping and eating problems and difficulties involving the processes of developing relationships, such as disorders of attachment and separation anxiety.

Box 7.1　Some disorders of early childhood

Sleep disorders
　Wakefulness
　Night terrors
　Sleep walking
　Nightmares
Eating disorders
　Food refusal and faddiness
　Non-organic failure to thrive
　Pica
　Obesity
Pervasive developmental disorders
　Infantile autism
　Rett's syndrome
　Childhood disintegrative disorder (Heller's syndrome)
　Asperger's syndrome
Disorders of social functioning
　Reactive attachment disorder
　Social disinhibition syndrome (primary attachment disorder)
　Preschool behavioural adjustment disorders
Emotional disorders
　Separation anxiety disorder
　Phobic disorder of childhood
　Social sensitivity disorder
　Sibling rivalry disorder
　Depression

Temper tantrums

Modes of presentation

Temper tantrums involving screaming, kicking and thrashing the arms about are normal in toddlers and usually subside as the child learns to accept the behavioural limits imposed by parents or others. However, they may be a problem if they are persistent or severe and when parents find they are unable to deal with them.

Aetiological factors

Tantrums and severe behavioural disturbance seem to increase when, for whatever reason, the infant or young child receives attention or feels that somehow he or she has benefited from the behaviour. Young children whose behaviour gets 'out of control' because they feel they have been denied something they want will have further episodes of very disturbed behaviour if, through the behaviour or temper tantrum, they eventually see that they do get their own way.

Investigations and treatment

In common with many of the behavioural disorders of early childhood, the first step is to obtain a detailed account of the behaviour and their reaction to it from the parents. This can then form the basis of a programme to modify and curtail the tantrums. Wherever possible tantrums should be avoided. Parents can learn to anticipate situations and circumstances likely to lead to a tantrum and divert or distract their child, and so avoid confrontation. In addition, parents need to develop planned, predictable reactions to their child's behaviour which ensures that the child is safe but that the behaviour is ignored. This behavioural approach is often successful. Physical restraint should be necessary only when the child is at risk of harming him- or herself or others or is dangerous and destructive.

Firm, caring, limit setting, particularly if non-critical, increases the likelihood of (rapid) improvement. In contrast, in disorganised chaotic families, particularly when the parental reaction to both disciplining and the child's behaviour in general is inconsistent, there is an increased risk of persistent disturbance.

For this very common condition, the outcome is closely linked to the quality of the child–parent relationship – the more 'positive' and mutually rewarding their interaction, the better the outlook. The role of individual and family factors and how these may affect particular parent-child relationships and attachments is discussed in more detail in Chapter 4.

Sleep disorders

Wakefulness

Modes of presentation

Most infants and young children do develop a fairly regular, predictable sleeping pattern, such that by the age of six months 85% of babies sleep through the night and by one year most have established a regular pattern. However, there will still be approximately 10% who continue to wake every night. Wakefulness is the commonest presenting sleep difficulty, with a peak of incidence between 12 to 24 months of age (Richman, 1981). This type of behaviour difficulty seems to be related to temperamental characteristics of the child, family stress factors, and parental factors such as maternal depression. For most physically healthy children, the problem clears after a few weeks or months, and for many individual children with sleep problems none of these factors are present (Graham, 1986).

Case example

Jonathan, aged 17 months, was referred by his general practitioner because of his mother's concerns about his frequent waking at night. He had always been a very active baby and had been difficult to settle. Jonathan's early development was normal. He was described as an early walker and although he was said to miss father since his parents' divorce, he had a close relationship with his mother and enjoyed physical affection. Before referral he and his mother had experienced major upheavals, including a number of changes of accommodation and day care. His mother, when reassured about the wide range of normal sleeping patterns among young children, was able to acknowledge the stress and distress that her recent divorce had caused both herself and her son. Once they had moved to permanent accommodation and his mother to full-time employment, and regular day care for Jonathan had been organised, as well as contact with his father, his sleep gradually settled.

Investigations and treatment

For wakefulness and other sleep problems a detailed history of what actually happens during the night is necessary. In addition, it is important to identify what types of treatment the child has already received. Jonathan (above) had, before referral, been prescribed a sedative antihistamine. These have been shown not to be as effective as behavioural methods in re-establishing normal sleep patterns in infants and toddlers (Richman, 1985). Additional emotional, family and behavioural factors must also be considered, as illustrated above.

The treatment of choice is a behaviour management programme. Initially the parent(s)/carer(s) are asked to keep a careful diary over one to two weeks, detailing both the child's sleeping patterns and the parents' or carers' responses. They may then spontaneously perceive ways of altering the child's and their own response to the wakeful periods, or the therapist can help parents first clarify and then alter their behaviour to avoid inconsistency and inappropriate rewarding of their child for wakefulness. Chapter 10 deals with treatments used in child and adolescent psychiatry in more detail.

For older preschool children there may be other relevant factors; for example they may become frightened by real or imaginary worries or may wish to rejoin their parents later in the evening. The same strategy of charting the child's and parents' night-time behaviour and helping to devise a behavioural management programme is frequently successful. For some older preschool children, this approach could be used in conjunction with a star chart.

However, for families where, because of parental difficulties or social circumstances it is impossible to undertake a consistent programme, or when the sleep difficulties are associated with severe emotional problems, behavioural therapy alone is less likely to be successful. Sleep problems as part of a more widespread disturbance are considered under preschool behavioural adjustment disorders (p. 115).

Night terrors and sleep walking

Modes of presentation

Night terrors, as described in ICD–10 (World Health Organization, 1992), have a dramatic presentation which is frequently distressing for parents. They affect 3% of children, often occurring every night. The child will suddenly sit up during sleep, appear terrified and shout, scream or moan. On occasions they may try getting out of bed but cannot be comforted and have no memory of the event the next day.

Sleep walking, like night terrors, usually begins with a sleeping child sitting up in bed and then rather mechanically getting out of bed and walking, usually about the house. Although the child avoids objects, he or she is unresponsive and will usually return to bed if guided in that direction.

Both disorders are described in the older preschool child and may continue into early middle childhood.

Aetiological factors

Kales *et al* (1980) reported that approximately 50% of children with one or other of these disorders has a close family relative who has experienced a similar difficulty. It has, therefore, been suggested that there may be a genetic contribution. Night terrors are rarely evidence of an associated psychiatric disorder. They may occur following a stressful event but are not considered, in isolation, to be evidence of an emotional disorder. The attacks are thought to represent a fault in slow-wave sleep (Matthews & Oakley, 1986).

Treatment

These conditions usually resolve spontaneously within a few months. However, treatment is indicated for night terrors because of the extreme distress experienced by both parents and children. Lask (1988) reported a successful behavioural treatment programme. The success of the treatment seemed to depend on the alteration of faulty slow-wave sleep by interruption of the child's sleep pattern just before the onset of the symptoms. The author assumes that this then causes a reversion to a more normal sleep pattern. Drug treatment is not recommended.

Nightmares (frightening dreams)

The child may wake in terror or distress but is able to describe the content of the dream and be comforted. Nighmares are common, and the peak age is between five and six years.

Aetiology

These are often associated with physical disorder (such as acute febrile illness) or an emotional disorder such as anxiety. They are also a cardinal symptom of post-traumatic stress disorder (PTSD). In contrast, a much rarer cause of persistent and unusual nightmares is nocturnal epilepsy. This may be suspected if the episode includes stiffening or jerking movements or if the child wakes at the start of the nightmare and reports strange sensations. These experiences may be followed by impairment of consciousness. Such a history would require a further detailed assessment and investigations, including full electroencephalographic evaluation.

Treatment

Parents should be reassured that nightmares are common and can rapidly disappear, irrespective of their duration and severity. A cognitive–behavioural treatment initially developed with adults has now been used successfully with children (Matthews & Oakley, 1986). These techniques of 'rehearsal–relief' enable the child to face the feared experience and so habituate to it. In addition the child is encouraged to produce some different, triumphant endings to the dream – this will enhance his or her sense of mastery and control.

Eating disorders

ICD-10 states that minor difficulties in eating are sufficiently common during both infancy and early childhood that, of themselves, they should not be considered as indicative of disorder; rather the category of 'eating disorder' should be reserved for those children where the eating problem is qualitatively abnormal or sufficiently severe that the child fails to gain weight or loses weight and the severe symptoms have lasted for at least one month. In addition, a diagnosis of eating disorder should be made only once the possibilities of organic disease have been excluded and in the absence of some other psychiatric disorder such as a pervasive developmental disorder.

Food refusal and faddiness

Feeding, as well as being one of the first tasks that newborn infants master, represents for parents an early measure of their skill and competence. Gradually, the baby's instinctual behaviour will be modified by the interactions between baby and carer(s).

Problems with early feeding and later difficulties with faddiness, poor appetite and other food-related concerns are common in infants and young children: 12% of mothers report moderate or severe feeding problems (Richman *et al*, 1982). Excessive food faddiness is more common in children over one year of age. It is characterised by a child's refusal to eat a wide range of foods or demanding that the food be prepared or presented in specific ways. For example, the child may refuse to eat food of a particular colour or consistency, or refuse everything except one or two types of food (e.g. cereal or puddings). At the time of referral, the problem may be presented as a 'battle of wills'.

This confrontation emphasises, again, the need to consider the quality of child–parent relationships and the family's particular social circumstances.

Non-organic failure to thrive

Children who are consistently below the 3rd centile in weight or who have a reduction in growth velocity require detailed assessment and investigation. The causes of failure to thrive may be organic, non-organic, or a mixture of the two. Investigation will include assessment of the role of genetic, constitutional and organic factors as well as the family's social circumstances, parental and child difficulties. The role of environmental deprivation and child abuse or maltreatment is covered in Chapter 11.

A community survey (Dowdney *et al*, 1987) showed that approximately 2% of inner-city Caucasian children suffered from chronic, non-organic failure to thrive or 'growth retardation'. Skuse (1985) reported that for most cases of non-organic failure to thrive, inadequate food intake, as a consequence of the impaired mother–child interactions, seemed the most likely final common pathway.

Investigations and treatment

Assessment needs to include careful medical investigations to ensure that any underlying physical condition is diagnosed and treated appropriately. In addition, infants with a history of congenital abnormalities and other serious perinatal and neonatal disorders may be more at risk of later feeding difficulties. However, in many cases the organic factors are not sufficient to account for the picture. A detailed history of the young child's feeding behaviour needs to be taken, together with assessments of the parental behaviour and parent–child relationships. A detailed food diary and observation of a family meal will also be required.

Developmental counselling (Fraiberg, 1980; Minde & Minde, 1981) in conjunction with a behavioural management programme is successful for many infant eating disorders. However, for some families, the focus of treatment needs to take into account not only the parents' fears and anxieties about the child, but other psychosocial factors. These might include adverse living conditions, problems with social relationships such as the absence of a supporting and confiding relationship for the parent, or psychiatric illness. Maternal depression and emotional disorders are relatively common. Such families may require additional support, for example practical help and advice from their health visitor or counselling from a community child psychiatric nurse. Also the development of extra support from within the family or in the local community through local support groups for mothers may allow some sharing of the responsibilities for child care (Cox *et al*, 1991). In more extreme situations, a parent (usually mother) may require referral for psychiatric assessment. Finally it may also be necessary to involve local social services departments to consider the use of respite care, shared care with experienced foster parents, or day nursery placement.

Case example

Judith, aged four years, was referred by a consultant paediatrician because of a long history of poor eating and extreme faddiness with her foods. She was the youngest of three children born three weeks pre-term following an unplanned pregnancy characterised by poor maternal health. Her mother (a single parent) remembered her as a frail, sickly baby who was always a poor eater. During her first 18 months, Judith was twice admitted to the children's ward because of poor weight gain and dehydration. No organic disorder was found to account for her low weight. At home, Judith was disruptive during mealtimes. Her mother did not expect her to enjoy or take part in other family activities. Similarly at play group her behaviour was difficult to control, and it was noted that she did not relate appropriately to the other children.

As part of the assessment, the mother kept a detailed food diary and the family were offered family therapy focusing on mealtime behaviour. Over the course of treatment, Judith was expected to sit and eat at regular mealtimes. She gradually began to anticipate meals and the therapist encouraged the mother and Judith to share activities at other times. The amount of time spent in confrontation over eating reduced greatly and the mother was visibly more relaxed. The last two treatment sessions focused on some other aspects of Judith's behaviour and considered the mother's anxieties about Judith's admission to primary school. At follow-up Judith had successfully started school and was continuing to eat regular meals with the family.

Pica

This is defined as the persistent eating of non-nutritious substances such as soil, paint chippings, inedible plants, etc. It is common for toddlers and young children occasionally to mouth or chew inappropriate objects. Pica occurs more frequently in young deprived children, in older mentally handicapped children, and in children with pervasive developmental disorders. The dangers of eating such substances can include accidental poisoning (such as lead poisoning). Iron deficiency and pica have been shown to be associated. For some children the anaemia may be primary, but for all children with pica treatment of any associated anaemia may directly improve development and pica (Arbiter & Black, 1991).

Obesity

Children who consistently eat too much are at risk of becoming obese. Standardised weight and height charts must be used to make the diagnosis. Obesity can then be defined as being 20% heavier than the expected weight for a given height and sex (Tanner & Takaishi, 1966). However, both objective and subjective criteria are important when considering overweight children. Such children are more at risk of having poor social and peer relationships. This is discussed in more detail in Chapters 8 and 9.

Encopresis (faecal soiling) and enuresis

Since children with these problems are not usually brought to the attention of the child psychiatric service until aged five or six years, the modes of presentation, investigations and management are discussed in Chapter 8.

Constipation

Constipation is preventable by educating parents in non-punitive or coercive toilet training (Woodmansey, 1967).

Attention deficit disorder (hyperkinetic syndrome)

The hyperkinetic disorders (as defined in ICD-10) are a rare group of disorders occurring more frequently in boys than girls; they are often associated with delays in cognitive development and motor clumsiness (Taylor, 1986). The behaviour disturbance is characterised by overactivity, restlessness and lack of attentiveness, but is not usually diagnosed until early school age. However, characteristically these features are frequently seen in the first five years and, in the most severe cases, are pervasive in different situations (Sandberg *et al*, 1978).

Bearing in mind the wide normal variation of behaviour and activity levels among preschool children and the knowledge that individual differences for this age group are not stable over time, it is important to note that large numbers of parents, at some time during their child's preschool years, will complain that their young children are overactive. For these reasons it is not surprising that a clear hyperkinetic syndrome has not been validated in this young age group. However, the complaint of overactivity (e.g. in a child attending a day nursery) does need to be taken seriously and indeed such overactivity may predict later antisocial disorder (Richman *et al*, 1982).

From the age of three years the normal course of development involves a reduction of general levels of activity in some settings, but not all. The appropriate modulation of activity can therefore be impaired by developmental delay of whatever cause. Restlessness becomes more of a problem as a child enters schooling, when successively greater demands are made on his/her powers of attention and self-control. These continuities between the early years and later outcomes suggest that for the group of children who do not simply 'grow out of it', persisting difficulties may influence their personality development, sometimes to the point of pathology.

Assessment, treatment and outcome

This disorder is considered in more detail in Chapter 8, but for the preschool period, as with older children, assessment is based on a detailed history, including descriptions of behaviour in a number of settings, and examination of the child. Descriptions of behaviour need to be taken from both parents and other adults, such as play group leaders or teachers. Attention must also be paid to any associated learning, perceptual or behaviour difficulties and to family and social circumstances.

Factors interact to cause hyperactivity and its course is largely determined by complicating adversity. For these reasons, diagnosis is not the only consideration which influences treatment and management. There is a range of available treatments, including psychological, behavioural, dietary and drug treatments. Many of these require the cooperation and interest of the child, parents and teachers. Counselling, explanation, advice and support are therefore of particular importance if specific treatments are to follow – with or without drug treatments. Indeed, the key to long-term improvement is likely to be the child's own development of self-control, self-motivation and self-esteem.

Specific developmental disorders

The specific developmental disorders of speech and language, together with the specific developmental disorders of scholastic skills and motor function, and the mixed specific developmental disorders, are described in Chapter 2.

Pervasive developmental disorders

This group of disorders, as defined in ICD–10, is characterised by qualitative impairments in reciprocal social interactions, patterns of communication (including use of words, language and non-verbal communication) and by a restricted, stereotyped, repetitive repertoire of non-adaptive interests and activities. For all of the disorders included in this group, the diagnosis is primarily defined in terms of deviance. However, developmental delay is almost invariable. Despite the general acceptance of the diagnostic validity of these disorders, the aetiology in most cases is not known and there remains uncertainty about the diagnostic subdivisions and boundaries. Onset is usually in infancy or early childhood although, for some conditions such as childhood disintegrative disorder, there is a phase of normal development.

Young children suspected of suffering from a pervasive developmental disorder require a detailed systematic assessment including developmental history, obstetric and medical history, detailed family history, direct observation and detailed psychometric and neurodevelopmental examination. The need for further physical investigations should then be guided by the information obtained. The presence of specific features and the differentiation of static and progressive disorders will influence practice (see below).

Infantile autism

Infantile autism, an organic neurodevelopmental disorder involving cognitive and social deficit, was first described by Kanner (1943). It has a prevalence rate of approximately four per 10 000 population (Lotter, 1974), is three to four times more common in boys than girls (Smalley *et al*, 1988) and does not show any social class bias (Gillberg & Schaumann, 1982).

Modes of presentation

For most children, there is no clear period of normal early development. For the diagnosis to be made there needs to be evidence of delay or deviant development within the first three years of life.

Speech and language

Approximately 50% of autistic children do not develop any useful speech. For those children with speech, there is usually evidence of delay in both their expressive language and their understanding of speech. There is also usually a lack of appropriate social use of language and an inability to take part in conversation.

Speech is often stilted and may lack emotional expression. There may also be accompanying abnormalities such as the use of invented words (neologisms), unusual phrases (stereotyped phrases and metaphorical speech) or a persistent, rather mechanical repetition of sounds or words that the child has heard spoken by others in the past (delayed echolalia). Sadly, for most autistic children, whatever their level of acquired language, the principal difficulty seems to be an inability to use their own language to communicate flexibly and with meaning. Often there is an additional lack of the expected gestures which usually accompany speech and which add emphasis and meaning. As the child moves to middle childhood and adolescence, the language and communication abnormalities may well vary; this is considered in Chapter 8.

Social abnormalities

As babies they may be described as passive and generally unresponsive or quiet. They may be slow to develop a social smile and will usually not use anticipatory gestures such as putting up their arms to be lifted. They may resist cuddling and their parents' gestures of affection or lay passively in their mother's arms. As toddlers they are unlikely to show spontaneous affection and do not take part in family activities. They may avoid eye contact and prefer to be left on their own. They will not show normal separation anxiety or joy on reunion and are very unlikely to come spontaneously for comfort. They may be described by their parents as very brave or apparently less troubled by pain than other children. Once again, the social abnormalities will vary throughout childhood, the common thread being an inability to understand and respond to ordinary social and emotional cues. For even the most able of autistic children, it is their inability to use their own initiative in a social situation and their lack of reciprocity which hampers any attempt at gradual independence.

Behavioural abnormalities

In addition to these difficulties, the young autistic child will have a restricted repertoire of repetitive, non-adaptive behaviour and activities. Some of these include unusual preoccupations, a repetitive interest in parts of objects (such as spinning the wheels of a toy car rather than playing with the whole car), a tendency to impose rigidity or routine on a wide range of aspects of daily life, unusual attachments to odd or non-soft objects, and a tendency to manneristic behaviour, particularly involving the hands and upper limbs.

Case example
Stuart, aged four years, was born at term by normal delivery and was described as a very placid, easy baby, who did not cry and was a slow eater.

His parents became concerned when he was approximately two years old because he was not developing speech and showed no interest in play. At four years his non-verbal cognitive skills were within the average range but he showed marked delay in language development.

Motor development was within normal limits. As a baby he made no communicative sounds but enjoyed being cuddled and sitting on his parents' lap. By the age of three, although he made some attempt at pointing, his parents had to guess all his needs. He made two sounds, one happy and the other distressed. He would take an adult's hand when he wanted something but made no clear communicative gestures. He showed oversensitivity to regular household noises. It was always difficult to get his attention. He had no understanding of stories, preferring to flick the pages and pick out his favourite picture.

He showed no wariness of strangers and would simply wander off if something took his interest. He would approach his parents for some comfort but showed little interest in other people or their activities. His facial expressions were often inappropriate and his behaviour markedly disinhibited. He had no understanding of shared interests or enjoyment and no creative or imaginative play.

He had many unusual, repetitive preoccupations. These included a fascination with water (he would watch water flowing down the plughole or toilet and would lie down in puddles); he repetitively turned light switches on and off, and tore paper into strips and lined it up on the floor. He became very distressed if interrupted. He had a variety of attachments to unusual objects, such as a bottle of lentils. Finally, he had an unusual sensory interest in the feel of hair and plastic, and some manneristic behaviour including finger flapping at the edge of his peripheral vision and spinning in a complicated way. He was diagnosed as having infantile autism.

Aetiology

There is no single cause or aetiology to account for cases of autism. However, for some rare cases, there does seem to be an association with some physical factors such as infections (e.g. congenital rubella and cytomegalovirus), some perinatal factors, and some rare medical and genetic conditions. These include the fragile X chromosomal anomaly, single-gene disorders such as phenyl-ketonuria (an autosomal recessive disorder usually associated with mental retardation) and tuberose sclerosis (an autosomal dominant condition in which the children often show autistic-type behaviour). More recently, association has also been described with neurofibromatosis. However, with systematic psychiatric evaluation and more standardised assessment, it may be that the associations originally reported are in fact less strong or clear cut than was initially suggested (Rutter, 1990).

In the last 10 to 15 years a number of twin and family studies have indicated that genetic factors play a major role in autism, both in terms of the risks for autism *per se* and for a range of social and cognitive abnormalities (Bolton & Rutter, 1990).

Despite the recognition that autism is an organic neurodevelopmental disorder, there are few consistent or replicated findings on brain imaging and other neurophysiological studies. More precise information may become available in the near future.

The cognitive abnormalities are not secondary to social withdrawal – the pattern is different from that in most cases of general mental handicap. Language and language-related skills involving deficits in sequencing, abstraction and symbolic meaning are frequently present (Rutter, 1983). Recent neuropsychological research has demonstrated social cognitive deficits and impairments in the autistic individual's ability to appreciate that other people's beliefs may differ from their own, and to identify and understand socio-emotional cues (Baron-Cohen, 1989; Hobson, 1990).

Investigation and treatment

For any child with a possible pervasive developmental disorder, a full and detailed neurodevelopmental assessment is needed, including a systematic family history, and psychological testing. This type of standardised assessment facilitates the diagnosis of disorders such as Rett's syndrome (Olsson & Rett, 1987).

Careful consideration needs to be given to family factors relevant to the planning of treatment and support that will be offered to the family. Families require some continuing professional availability to alleviate distress and promote coping skills. Parents should be reassured that their behaviour has not caused the condition and that they can help their child despite the chronic and socially disabling nature of the condition.

There is no cure for autism and treatment approaches are most successful for the management of non-specific behavioural problems and have least impact on language skills and, to date, no effect on the overall intellectual functioning of the child.

Current treatment includes behavioural and educational methods in addition to family support. Such treatment programmes require an accurate appraisal of the child's skills and difficulties, conducted as far as possible in the child's natural environment. Autistic children have problems in generalising learning from one setting to another. Parents have a very important role acting as 'co-therapists'. Generally, a series of small steps change the child's behaviour with the minimum of distress – the so-called principle of 'graded change' (Le Couteur, 1990).

At present there is no specific drug or other treatment which has been shown to affect the underlying disorder, despite some strong therapeutic claims which have received considerable media coverage.

Rett's syndrome

This is a deteriorating condition (Ollson & Rett, 1987) currently only described in girls, and characterised by the progressive loss of acquired abilities (behavioural, social and psychomotor). It follows apparently normal development in the first one to two years of life, and is associated with gradual social withdrawal, signs of dementia, stereotyped hand-washing movements, and loss of purposeful hand use and broad-based stance ataxia. These young girls develop profound mental handicap and despite normal head circumference at birth, show a later deceleration of head growth. The prognosis is poor; sufferers develop at a very slow rate, and have severely reduced mobility with a risk of kyphoscoliosis and limb contractures. Further assessment, treatment and management of this rare condition will be considered in more detail in another book in the College Seminars series.

Childhood disintegrative disorder (Heller's syndrome; disintegrative psychosis)

This extremely rare disorder (Corbett *et al*, 1977; Evans-Jones & Rosenbloom, 1978; Hill & Rosenbloom, 1986), seen in both boys and girls, is characterised by an apparently normal development up to at least the age of two years, followed by a definite loss of previously acquired skills. This deterioration is frequently accompanied by a general loss of interest in the environment and qualitatively abnormal social functioning. Usually, there is a profound regression, with loss of language, regression of play, and loss of social skills and adaptive behaviour. Frequently, affected children lose control of bowel and bladder and sometimes motor control deteriorates. Typically these difficulties will be accompanied by the emergence of stereotyped, repetitive motor mannerisms and an autistic-like impairment in social interaction and communication. This impairment has similar deviant qualities to those seen in autism, rather than simply intellectual deterioration. However, despite this overlap of clinical features, the findings of Volkmar & Cohen (1989) indicate that at present disintegrative disorders should be considered as a separate subcategory of the pervasive developmental disorders.

Usually there is a lack of evidence of any identifiable organic disease, although in the literature there are clinical case reports of an associated encephalopathy such as metachromatic leucodystrophy and Addison–Schilder's disease. The condition is, however, presumed to be organic in origin and for some cases the deterioration is fatal. For others, however, the loss of skills may be followed by a degree of recovery and the development of a steady state of disability.

Asperger's syndrome (schizoid disorder of childhood)

This ICD-10 diagnostic category, described by Wing (1981), Gillberg & Gillberg (1989) and Green (1990), is also called 'schizoid disorder of childhood' (Wolff & Barlow, 1979). It is currently used for children suffering from the same type of qualitative impairment in reciprocal social interaction as is seen in autistic children. Sufferers also show a range of restrictive, repetitive and stereotyped interests and non-adaptive activities. Intelligence is usually within the normal range. In addition, despite an apparent absence of delay in early language development and appropriate use of grammar and vocabulary, there are frequent oddities in the ways language is used for communication. The prosody is often peculiar, such that everything might be said in a staccato or a monotonous, almost mechanical drone, and facial and gestural expressions of emotion can also be abnormal (Wing, 1981).

The reported prevalence is 2.6–3.0 per 1000 children, with a male preponderance (Wing & Gould, 1979; Gillberg & Gillberg, 1989). However, Gillberg & Gillberg included subjects with delayed language development or moderate impairment of language comprehension. There is uncertainty as to whether in fact these children should be considered as suffering from a mild variant of autism; certainly their difficulties should be considered along a continuum of disturbance, until further data are available to clarify these diagnostic uncertainties. In relation to presentation, assessment and management, there are clearly links and overlaps with the needs of autistic children.

Modes of presentation

Concerns may not be expressed by parents or professionals working with young children until about the age of three years when, despite a relatively normal early language development, the child may be noted to lack warmth and interest in social relationships. The speech abnormalities referred to above and the social difficulties may not appear disabling until the child gets older and enters more socially demanding environments such as school. For these reasons, Asperger's syndrome is also considered in Chapter 8.

Investigations and treatment

Assessment will involve, as it does for other pervasive developmental disorders, taking a full developmental history considering in detail social, emotional and behavioural problems, in conjunction with a physical examination and further investigations as appropriate. Some of these children are clumsy. The psychotherapeutic, behavioural and educational needs of this rare group of children are considered in Chapter 8.

Disorders of social functioning

As referred to above, the earliest social relationships for young children are with the parents. These are of crucial importance for the well-being and optimal development of infants and preschool children. The quality of these special social relationships or 'attachments' have been linked with personality development, feelings of self-esteem and self-worth, and later independence.

Bowlby (1969) originally described attachment to the mother as an adaptive biological process which ensures the infant's needs are met. From six to eight months of age, infants develop selective attachments to particular individuals to whom they will go to in preference to all others. So despite the acknowledgement of the central role of the mother, the feelings and behaviour attributed to the attachment process are usually experienced by all family members to varying degrees throughout the child's early life. As the child gets older, these feelings remain present but are experienced less intensely.

These emotional attachments have been extensively studied. Ainsworth *et al* (1978), assessing the effects of experimental brief separations and reunions of infants and their mothers (the 'strange situation procedure') described three different types of attachment – securely attached, anxiously attached, and anxious–avoidantly attached. There is controversy over whether this type of classification is the best way to describe the different types of attachment behaviour. However, there is general acceptance that the quality of the selective attachments is important for the well-being of the developing child. Child psychiatrists are often asked to comment on the strength and quality of these attachments with parents, particularly in connection with child placement and contact in the assessment of the risk of child abuse.

Reactive attachment disorder

A constellation of social, emotional and behavioural difficulties is recognised by professionals to be a probable consequence of severe parental neglect, abuse or mishandling. Some young infants and children who have experienced severe parental neglect show a characteristic pattern of social relationships and emotional disturbance, sometimes in association with growth failure. Despite criticism of the diagnostic validity of this syndrome (Rutter & Schaffer, 1980) this constellation of behaviours is accepted as a possible marker of disturbed emotional development and has been included as a separate diagnostic category in ICD-10. However, disagreements remain about the precise defining qualities of this diagnostic category.

Modes of presentation

A key feature is a persistently abnormal pattern of relationships with carers present since before the age of five years. These children may lack an age-appropriate interest in their primary carer(s) and may respond with a mixture of approach, avoidance and resistance to comforting. These contradictory or ambivalent social responses extend across different social situations but may be seen especially at times of parting or reunions. In contrast, with less familiar adults, they may show an apparent indiscriminate sociability with inappropriate requests for attention and displays of affection. This pattern of behaviour varies with changes in the child's emotional circumstances.

Emotional disturbance may include fearfulness and hypervigilance ('frozen watchfulness') that is unresponsive to comforting. Some children may appear miserable, lack emotional responsiveness and withdraw, or in contrast, show aggressive reactions to their own or others' distress.

In general, although such children show an interest in their peers, their social play and interaction is hindered by their negative emotional responses.

Case example

Claire, aged five, was the sister of a four-month-old baby who was admitted to a general paediatric ward for assessment and investigation for failure to thrive. Claire was not causing her parents any concern but aroused concern in the social worker. She had been born prematurely, had been difficult to feed and cried frequently during infancy. She was quiet and politely spoken but would occasionally become aggressive if she thought her mother was upset. She was also very good at occupying herself and 'not troubling' her parents.

She presented as a miserable, silent, watchful and fearful child. She did not offer any spontaneous comments and would look towards her parents, as if for permission, before making any response to social overtures from other adults. She did not show an age-appropriate interest in either of her parents and did not approach them for comfort.

This combination of unusual social relationships, hypervigilance and misery alerted the professionals to the need to assess the quality of parenting experienced by both daughters in this family.

Aetiological factors

Prematurity, congenital malformations and the specific temperamental characteristics of the young infant have been shown to influence parental attitudes and child rearing. For instance, infants with irregular feeding or sleeping patterns may be difficult to soothe. This in turn may reduce the opportunity for enjoyable parent–child interactions and may predispose to attachment problems.

Parental factors may include the physical or mental health of the primary carers. A major psychiatric disorder such as depression or psychosis may interfere with the parent's ability to respond to the infant. Similarly, serious personality disorders may affect the quality of care. Wolkind (1977) and others have also highlighted the importance of the early experiences of the primary carer; factors such as early emotional or physical abuse and poverty may affect the ability of parents to look after their own infants. Finally, parents attempting to rear a difficult or disabled infant may experience difficulties in relating to the infant while at the same time experiencing grief, guilt, disappointment and loss of their 'wished-for' child (Wolkind & Kruk, 1984) (see Chapter 11).

The differential diagnosis will include mental retardation and pervasive developmental disorders such as autism. Children with severe disturbances in their early attachments may lack reciprocity in their social interactions. However, unlike autistic children, these disturbances will not be as pervasive and would occur in the absence of other deviant aspects of communication development and without the repetitive, stereotyped, non-adaptive activities more usually seen in autism.

Investigation and treatment

The quality of developing infant–parent relationships is dependent on many factors. Therefore, a detailed developmental history and assessment is necessary, focusing on the developing infant and parenting and family factors.

The professionals need to work with parents to ensure that the young child is provided with a safe, caring and containing environment. All decisions should be made in the 'best interests of the child'. The aims of treatment, wherever possible, will be to build on the strengths and abilities of the biological parents or other caring adults and to facilitate the development of parenting skills. Under some circumstances, however, it may be necessary to search for alternative carers. The child, in a more facilitating environment, may need individual psychotherapy to restore normal development (Boston & Szur, 1990).

Social disinhibition syndrome, primary attachment disorder

Modes of presentation

These children seem to be unable to make specific attachments to their principal carer(s) and display persistent abnormal social functioning, often despite important changes in their circumstances. From the preschool years, they tend to show superficial, clinging attachments to any adult whom they may come in contact with, however briefly. Later, the indiscriminately 'friendly' behaviour may be accompanied by other attention-seeking behaviour, overactivity, emotional lability, poor toleration of frustration and aggressive behaviour.

Aetiological factors and assessment

This constellation of behaviours is recognised clinically as being associated with children with disrupted early experiences – such as transfer to a series of institutions or foster-home placements or grossly inadequate parental care. As with the previous syndrome, the diagnostic validity of this behavioural syndrome has not been established, but it has now been included, as a separate category, in ICD-10. These clinical features may occasionally also be seen in the offspring of well functioning families and some children with brain damage may present with an inability to develop specific attachments.

The assessment involves a detailed developmental history of the child, the family and their social circumstances, and direct observation of the child's behaviour. An assessment of the child's reaction to the child psychiatrist or other professional in a relatively contained clinical situation may provide important information, which will complement the details derived from the history taken and other available reports.

Treatment

The guiding principle of treatment will be the improvement or establishment of a settled, consistent environment for the child, with access to a limited number of adult carers. However, difficulties with developing relationships may well persist and, for older children, this increases the risk of further disruption and breakdown of foster or prospective adoptive placements. The long-term prognosis for children placed in permanent adoptive families after many years in institutionalised care tends to be good in terms of a reduction of behavioural disturbance but less clear cut with regard to personal and intimate relationships. Overall, the number of children experiencing prolonged periods of institutionalised care in very early childhood has decreased since the important policy-informing work of Tizard (1977), and others. However, for many young children who may have experienced severe early abuse there is still the risk of repeated breakdowns of foster placements (Crittenden, 1985).

Preschool behavioural adjustment disorders

This cluster of behavioural problems includes high levels of activity and aggression. These problems may vary from one social circumstance to another but are ones that parents and other caring adults may find difficult to control. These behaviours are more common in boys but do not show a consistent social-class bias.

Richman *et al* (1982) reported that 11% of children in this age group were described as being difficult to control, 5% had frequent temper tantrums, 13% were active and restless, and 9% attention seeking. Additional problems secondary to overactivity and restlessness may include failure to develop regular eating and sleeping patterns. This in turn may increase the risk of further temper tantrums.

Case example

Kevin, aged two years, was referred by his health visitor to the under-fives assessment team. He had been described as always a restless baby who, during the course of his first year of life, had lived with various relatives in his extended family. Currently his mother (a single parent) was finding his behaviour very difficult to control and complained that he was overactive, refused to obey her, and was often aggressive towards her, with biting, swearing and repeated temper tantrums when thwarted. His play and interests were limited and repetitive. At playgroup he was disruptive and aggressive towards staff and children. The adults found him difficult to manage. During the assessment, it became clear that Kevin's mother felt unsupported and criticised by her own parents. Gradually with therapeutic support from the psychiatric social worker and a twice weekly placement for Kevin and his mother at the local social services family centre, Kevin's behaviour became more manageable and his mother was able to talk more positively about some joint games and activities that they shared.

E

Assessment

The assessment needs to allow the parent(s) or primary carer(s) an opportunity to share the precise nature and severity of the problems they are experiencing. There may well be variation across the social settings but this should not detract from the serious socially handicapping and isolating nature of the behavioural disturbance.

As with other disorders in the preschool years, as well as focusing on the presenting behavioural disturbance, it is important to assess other factors. The emotional state of the child, particularly anxiety and insecurity, may well lead to excessively clinging behaviour or an unwillingness to tolerate any separation from the principal carer (see below). Such children may also have additional developmental difficulties, including enuresis and delays in speech and language. Finally, consideration of temperamental characteristics may allow a more detailed discussion of the young child's longer-term needs. This may be a new experience for parents who are otherwise overwhelmed by the present behavioural difficulties.

Assessment will also incorporate consideration of the parenting skills and the behaviour management strategies employed by each individual family.

The differential diagnosis needs to exclude hyperkinetic syndrome and infantile autism.

Management and treatment

Richman *et al* (1982) indicated that two-thirds of these children continue disturbed during their early school years. However, early clinical interventions focusing on specific behavioural difficulties and parent–child relationships may be successful. A variety of therapeutic approaches can be considered, including behaviour modification for discrete management problems, often in the context of family interviews or mother–child interviews. This therapeutic work may also provide an educative role by allowing parents to gain insights into the developmental needs of their children.

Other professionals may be required to provide additional resources and support for children and families living in, for example, overcrowded accommodation. Changes in housing, providing preschool nursery placements, and links with other families in similar situations may help alleviate some of the stress and burden for young and inexperienced families (Kolvin *et al*, 1988).

Emotional disorders

Many of the emotional disorders of early childhood are exaggerations of normal developmental trends but are considered as separate syndromes if the symptoms persist longer than expected and are so severe that social functioning and development are impaired. The headings below follow ICD-10 categories.

Separation anxiety disorder

It is appropriate for toddlers and preschool children to show some anxiety over real or threatened separations from those to whom they are attached. However, for some young children, this anxiety becomes a major source of fear or persists beyond the appropriate age. The intensity of this fear may then impair the child's normal social development and affect family functioning and so be considered as a separation anxiety disorder.

Extreme anxiety may be seen in a number of different ways. There may be a preoccupying worry that something might happen to the principal attachment figure (usually the mother) or that something might separate the child from him or her. The child might refuse to attend play group or school or to go to sleep at night, and may experience repeated nightmares or physical complaints such as nausea, stomach aches or headaches or vomiting. Finally, the child may show excessive distress with crying, misery, tantrums or social withdrawal.

Phobic disorder of childhood

Specific fears are common in the preschool period. In the first three years these are usually related to actual events. Richman *et al* (1982) reported between 2% and 3% of three-year-olds had worries and 9% had between three and six specific fears. These included fear of the dark, thunder, insects and animals.

Most fears persist for a matter of weeks or months and usually resolve spontaneously with limited interference in the child's life. With increasing age, fantasy and imagination begin to play a greater part in the focus of fears.

For some children, although their fears do initially seem appropriate for their preschool developmental phase, the degree of accompanying anxiety is clearly abnormal and adversely affects their general social and emotional development.

Social sensitivity disorder

This is a persistent and recurrent fear of or avoidance of strangers (adults or peers). Affected children usually have appropriate specific selective attachments to their parents or carers. However, this avoidance of social encounters is beyond the normal wariness seen from approximately six months and which continues throughout early childhood. For these children, the fear is of sufficient intensity to restrict their ability to take part in their expanding social environment.

Sibling rivalry disorder

Many young children experience some emotional disturbance following the birth of a younger sibling. This disturbance is considered a clinical disorder if there is evidence of persistent jealousy or rivalry and emotional disturbance is sufficient to impair psychosocial performance (Dunn & Kendrick, 1982). The problem usually emerges within the month after the birth of the sibling.

Aetiological factors and assessment

For all these emotional disorders, it is important to clarify both the duration of the anxiety and fear and the degree of social disability experienced by the child. It is also necessary to ascertain the coping mechanisms that the child has already learned to use. This information is then related to the developmental status of the child and his or her own constitutional and temperamental characteristics. The experiences of other family members are relevant. Genetic factors, parental behaviour and communication of their own anxieties must also be ascertained. Finally, a knowledge of family social adversity and other possible anxiety-provoking stresses is useful.

Treatment

For all these emotional disorders the common aims of treatment should be to reduce anxiety-provoking stress, to help the child and family understand the nature and function of the fears and anxieties they have experienced, and to enhance their own coping mechanisms.

The focus of therapeutic work is frequently to encourage parents to ensure that the child is not exposed to unnecessary stress and is helped to learn to cope more appropriately with ordinary, inevitable stresses. Brief focused counselling with families may facilitate an understanding of the way anxieties can be transmitted within a family and how these fears may contribute to a child's feelings of insecurity. Behavioural methods can be used for some specific fears. Role rehearsal of activities and watching others 'model' a feared activity can also be helpful.

For most children, both anxiety and phobic states have a good prognosis. Some intense reactions are short lived, while others may last two to three years. Children with anxiety reactions are sometimes prone to further episodes in adolescence and adult life. For all affected children, encouraging the development of their own coping skills has the potential for helping them deal with anxieties in the future. In older children, anxieties and fears may contribute to an irrational fear of school – the core symptom of school refusal (see Chapter 8).

Obsessive-compulsive conditions

Hersov (1985) reported that simple rituals are relatively common in preschool children, especially among those who are shy and conscientious. However, once again, they often fade away as long as they do not become the focus of parental attention. Disorders of this kind are much more clinically significant in older children and are reviewed in Chapters 8 and 9.

Depression

Clinical and research work has focused, in recent years, on the understanding of depression in childhood (Chapters 8 and 9). For preschool children uncertainties remain as to whether the normal grief reactions and protest–despair–detachment sequence noted by Bowlby (1969) and later workers, seen in children, for example, admitted alone to hospital, should be included within the depressive syndrome. The possibility of a discrete depressive syndrome in this young group remains an intriguing area for further research and clinical initiatives.

Although children of this age cannot express feelings of depression, their behaviour may suggest a depressive state. They may refuse food, not sleep properly, or appear tearful, unhappy and insecure. There may also be evidence of mild developmental retardation. The emotional state of all young children must be considered when taking a detailed developmental history (see above). This information needs to be considered in conjunction with an understanding of the cognitive and developmental status of the child, his or her family relationships, and the wider social context.

Management and assessment of depression are dealt with in Chapters 8 and 9.

Conduct disorder

Some young children do experience a combination of severe behaviour difficulties including overactivity, aggression and disturbed social relationships. These are usually considered (as described above) as separate clinical syndromes and not using the general catch-all category of 'conduct disorder', which is more usually used for school-aged children and adolescents.

Gender identity disorders

Most children have, by the age of three to four years, developed a definite gender identity. This then usually remains fixed. Normally, the physical appearance at birth immediately establishes the gender of the child. However, during early development, in addition to the designated sex at birth, the child's postnatal environment and experiences – including sex-typed behaviour and the attitudes of parents and others who might reinforce such behaviour – do play a central role in normal gender identity development. Sex chromosomes and postnatal hormones, in contrast, seem to have little direct effect on gender identity. Prenatal hormones may influence sex-related behaviour, for example so-called tomboyish behaviour in girls exposed to increased levels of prenatal androgens, but the effects are in degree and not on the gender identity *per se* (Ehrhardt & Baker, 1974).

Throughout the preschool years, genital interest and play and sexual exploratory play are common. Masturbatory activities are possibly more common in boys than girls. Gender identity disorders, as defined by DSM-III-R (American Psychiatric Association, 1987), are characterised by the persistent distress (in the prepubertal child) about his or her assigned sex and the desire to be of the other sex. This disorder is described as a profound disturbance of the normal sense of 'maleness or femaleness'. The disorder is more frequent in boys than girls.

Aetiology

The prevalence of this disorder is unknown, but it has been suggested that approximately 3–4% of children may experience gender identity difficulties. Biological factors may be relevant (Rutter, 1980*b*), but psychological factors appear to be of over-riding importance. Bradley (1990) summarises and postulates some of the current thinking regarding the relevant individual and family factors. The mechanism involves an interplay between a sensitive child and parents who might have their own unresolved gender identity conflicts and marital conflicts. This coming together of factors may endorse the child's anxieties about his or her own gender identity and lead to an encouragement of cross-sex behaviour and secrecy about their own gender uncertainties.

Investigation and treatment

Parents will usually present their children at the age of three to four years. Careful and thoughtful history taking may not only elicit a long history of concern about their child's gender identity but occasionally the behaviour may have become more noticeable following an early family traumatic event. Alternatively, the child's behaviour may lead to identification of disorder at school entry.

For preschool children treatment is usually with the parents to consider the child's uncertainty and lack of security regarding their biologically determined gender identity. In addition, some authors recommend that parents are positively encouraged to limit the child's cross-sex behaviour.

For older children, individual psychotherapy may provide them with an opportunity to understand the feelings that may have led to the cross-sex behaviour. Green *et al* (1985, 1987), following up a group of prepubertal so-called 'feminine boys', found that most evolved a bisexual or homosexual orientation when reassessed in adolescence and early adult life. The cross-gender behaviour in boyhood identified by this study included doll play, feminine role playing, avoiding rough and tumble play and sports, a desire to be a girl, and preferring girls as friends. The long-term prognosis of these boys, presenting early, was overall thought to be poor.

Summary and conclusions

The preschool years are a time (for children, families and the professionals involved in their care) of rapid developmental change, from virtual total dependence upon adult carers to increasing autonomy and partial independence. The clinical syndromes of early childhood need to be considered within this context and any proposed interventions planned as adjuncts to promote and facilitate development.

A review by McGuire & Earles (1991) endorses the need to assess a child's skills and difficulties within a framework that also considers his or her developmentally appropriate abilities and specific social context.

References

Ainsworth, M. D. S., Blehar, M. C., Waters, E., *et al* (1978) *Patterns of Attachment: A Psychological Study of the Strange Situation*. Hillside: Lawrence Erlbaum.

American Psychiatric Association (1987) *Diagnostic and Statistical Manual of Mental Disorders* (3rd edn, revised) (DSM–III–R). Washington, DC: APA.

Arbiter, E. A. & Black, D. (1991) Pica and iron deficiency anaemia. *Child Care, Health and Development*, **17**, 231–234.

Baron-Cohen, S. (1989) The autistic child's theory of mind: a case of specific developmental delay. *Journal of Child Psychology and Psychiatry*, **30**, 285–297.

Bolton, P. & Rutter, M. (1990) Genetic influences in autism. *International Review of Psychiatry*, **2**, 67–80.

Boston, M. & Szur, R. (1990) *Psychotherapy with Severely Deprived Children*. London: Karnac Books/Maresfield Library.

Bowlby, J. (1969) *Attachment*. London: Hogarth Press.

Bradley, S. J. (1990) Gender dysphorias of childhood and adolescence. In *Psychiatric Disorders in Children and Adolescents* (eds B. D. Garfinkle, G. A. Carlson & E. B. Weller). London: W. B. Saunders.

Corbett, J., Harris, R., Taylor, E., *et al* (1977) Progressive disintegrative psychosis of childhood. *Journal of Child Psychology and Psychiatry*, **18**, 211–219.

Cox, A. D., Pound, A., Mills, M., *et al* (1991) Evaluation of a home visiting and befriending scheme for young mothers. *Journal of the Royal Society of Medicine*, **84**, 217–220.

Crittenden, P. M. (1985) Maltreated infants: vulnerability and resilience. *Journal of Child Psychology and Psychiatry*, **26**, 85–96.

Dowdney, L., Skuse, D., Heptinstall, E., *et al* (1987) Growth retardation and developmental delay amongst inner-city children. *Journal of Child Psychology and Psychiatry*, **28**, 529–541.

Dunn, J. & Kendrick, C. (1982) *Siblings: Love, Envy and Understanding*. Cambridge: Harvard University Press.

Ehrhardt, A. A. & Baker, S. W. (1974) Fetal androgens, human central nervous system differentiation and behaviour sex differences. In *Sex Differences in Behaviour* (eds R. C. Friedman, R. M. Richart & R. L. Van de Wiele). New York: Wiley.

Evan-Jones, L. B. & Rosenbloom, L. (1978) Disintegrative psychosis in childhood. *Developmental Medicine and Child Neurology*, **20**, 462–470.

Fraiberg, S. (ed.) (1980) *Clinical Studies in Infant Mental Health. The First Year of Life*. New York: Basic Books.

Gillberg, C. & Schaumann, H. (1982) Social class and infantile autism. *Journal of Autism and Developmental Disorders*, **12**, 223–228.

────── & Gillberg, C. (1989) Asperger's syndrome - some epidemiological considerations: a research note. *Journal of Child Psychology and Psychiatry*, **30**, 631-638.

Graham, P. (1986) *Child Psychiatry: A Developmental Approach*. Oxford: Oxford University Press.

Green, J. (1990) Is Asperger's a syndrome? *Developmental Medicine and Child Neurology*, **32**, 743-747.

Green, R. (1985) Gender identity in childhood and later sexual orientation: follow-up of 78 males. *American Journal of Psychiatry*, **142**, 339-341.

────── , Roberts, C. W., Welhams, K., *et al* (1987) Specific cross-gender behaviour in boyhood and later homosexual orientation. *British Journal of Psychiatry*, **151**, 84-88.

Hersov, L. (1985) Emotional disorders. In *Child and Adolescent Psychiatry: Modern Approaches* (2nd edn) (eds M. Rutter & L. Hersov). Oxford: Blackwell Scientific.

Hill, A. E. & Rosenbloom, L. (1986) Disintegrative psychosis of childhood; teenage follow-up. *Developmental Medicine and Child Neurology*, **28**, 34-40.

Hinde, R. A. (1982) Attachment: some conceptual and biological issues. In *The Place of Attachment in Human Behaviour* (eds C. M. Parkes & J. Stevenson-Hinde), pp. 60-76. New York: Basic Books.

Hobson, P. (1990) On acquiring knowledge about people and the capacity to pretend: response to Leslie (1987). *Psychology Review*, **97**, 114-121.

Kagan, J. (1979) The form of early development. Continuity and discontinuity in emergent competencies. *Archives of General Psychiatry*, **36**, 1047-1054.

Kales, A., Soldatos, C. R., Bixler, E. O., *et al* (1980) Hereditary factors in sleep walking and night terrors. *British Journal of Psychiatry*, **137**, 111-118.

Kanner, L. (1943) Autistic disturbance of affective contact. *Nervous Child*, **2**, 217-250.

Kolvin, I., Miller, F., Fleeting, M., *et al* (1988) Social and parenting factors affecting criminal-offence rates. Findings from the Newcastle Thousand Family Study (1947-1980). *British Journal of Psychiatry*, **152**, 80-90.

Lask, B. (1988) Novel and non-toxic treatment for night terrors. *British Medical Journal*, **297**, 592.

Le Couteur, A. (1990) Autism: current understanding and management. *British Journal of Hospital Medicine*, **43**, 448-452.

Lotter, V. (1974) Factors related to outcome in autistic children. *Journal of Autism and Developmental Disorders*, **4**, 263-277.

Matthews, B. & Oakley, M. (1986) Triumph over terror. *British Medical Journal*, **292**, 203.

McGuire, J. & Earles, F. (1991) Prevention of psychiatry disorders in early childhood. *Journal of Child Psychology and Psychiatry*, **32**, 129-154.

Minde, K. & Minde, R. (1981) Psychiatric intervention in infancy; a review. *Journal of the American Academy of Child Psychiatry*, **20**, 217-238.

────── & ────── (1986) *Infant Psychiatry. An Introductory Textbook*. Developmental Clinical Psychology and Psychiatry Series, vol. 4. Beverly Hills: Sage.

Ollson, B. & Rett, A. (1987) Autism and Rett syndrome: behavioural investigations and differential diagnosis. *Developmental Medicine and Child Neurology*, **29**, 429-441.

Richman, N. (1981) A community survey of one to two year olds with sleep disturbance. *Journal of the American Academy of Child Psychiatry*, **20**, 281-291.

────── (1985) A double-blind drug-trial of treatment in young children with waking problems. *Journal of Child Psychology and Psychiatry*, **26**, 591-598.

────── , Stevenson, J. & Graham, P. (1982) *Pre-school to School: A Behavioural Study*. London: Academic Press.

Rutter, M. (1980*a*) The long-term effects of early experience. *Developmental Medicine and Child Neurology*, **22**, 800-815.

—— (1980*b*) Psychosexual development. In *Scientific Foundations of Developmental Psychiatry* (ed. M. Rutter). London: Heinemann Medical.

—— (1983) Cognitive deficits in the pathogenesis of autism. *Journal of Child Psychology and Psychiatry*, **24**, 513–531.

—— (1990) Autism as a gender disorder. In *The New Genetics of Mental Illness* (ed. P. McGuffin). London: Heinemann Medical.

—— & Schaffer, D. (1980) DSM-III: a step forward or back in terms of the classification of child psychiatric disorders? *Journal of the American Academy of Child Psychiatry*, **19**, 371–394.

Sandberg, S., Rutter, M. & Taylor, E. (1978) Hyperactive disorder in clinical attenders. *Developmental Medicine and Child Neurology*, **20**, 279–299.

Skuse, D. (1984) Extreme deprivation in early childhood. II. Theoretical issues and a comparative review. *Journal of Child Psychology and Psychiatry*, **25**, 543–572.

—— (1985) Non-organic failure to thrive: a reappraisal. *Archives of Disease in Childhood*, **60**, 173–178.

Smalley, S., Asarow, R. & Spence, M. (1988) Autism and genetics: a decade of research. *Archives of General Psychiatry*, **45**, 953–961.

Tanner, J. M. & Takaishi, M. (1966) Standards from birth to maturity for height, weight, height velocity and weight velocity: British children in 1965. *Archives of Disease in Childhood*, **41**, 454–471.

Taylor, E. (ed.) (1986) *The Overactive Child*. Clinics in Developmental Medicine, no. 97. Oxford: Blackwell Scientific.

Tizard, B. (1977) *Adoption: A Second Chance*. London: Open Books.

Volkmar, F. & Cohen, D. J. (1989) Disintegrative disorder or "late-onset" autism. *Journal of Child Psychology and Psychiatry*, **30**, 717–724.

Wing, L. (1981) Asperger's syndrome: a clinical account. *Psychological Medicine*, **11**, 115–129.

—— & Gould, G. (1979) Severe impairments of social interaction and associated abnormalities in children: epidemiology and classifications. *Journal of Autism and Developmental Disorders*, **9**, 11–30.

Wolff, S. & Barlow, A. (1979) Schizoid personality in childhood: a comparative study of schizoid, autistic and normal children. *Journal of Child Psychology and Psychiatry*, **20**, 19–46.

Wolkind, S. N. (1977) Women who have been "in care" – psychological and social status during pregnancy. *Journal of Child Psychology and Psychiatry*, **18**, 179–182.

—— & Kruk, S. (1984) From child to parent: early separation and the adaptation to motherhood. In *Longitudinal Studies in Child Psychology and Psychiatry: Practical Lessons from Research Experience* (ed. A. Nicol). Chichester: Wiley.

Woodmansey, A. C. (1967) Emotion and the motions: an enquiry into the causes and prevention of functional disorders of defaecation. *British Journal of Medical Psychology*, **40**, 207–223.

World Health Organization (1992) *ICD-10 Classification of Mental and Behavioural Disorders. Clinical Descriptions and Diagnostic Guidelines*. Geneva: WHO.

8 Clinical syndromes in middle childhood
Mark Berelowitz & Julia Nelki

---

*Emotional problems ● Post-traumatic stress disorder ● Conduct disorder ●
Hyperactivity, hyperkinesis and attention deficit disorder ● Developmental
problems ● Eating disorders ● Psychoses ● Sexual problems ● Conclusion*

Middle childhood refers to the period between starting primary school and
reaching puberty or adolescence. It is a time of considerable social challenges
for the child, who at this stage enters much more fully into a social world
outside the family. This period lacks the considerable and rapid biological
developments of early childhood and early adolescence, and is characterised
by a low mortality rate. Certain child psychiatric disorders will have their onset
at this time. But perhaps more importantly, it is a time when disorders are
likely to become more apparent, especially in the classroom, where educational
and social difficulties will manifest themselves.

The most important challenge of this period is starting school. The child
will learn to work with and accept instruction and discipline from unfamiliar
adults, and will share with and compete with peers. Opportunities for learning
expand, and these go hand in hand with the formal assessment of abilities,
with the consequent possible readjustment of expectations.

The commonest disorders of middle childhood are disturbances of emotion
and conduct (or behaviour), affecting 7% of children in inner cities, and
accounting for well over 80% of all child psychiatric problems (Rutter *et al*,
1975). Some of the disorders discussed within this chapter are given in Box 8.1.

With all disturbances of childhood one has to remember that the 'form' of
the disorder, that is, the way in which it presents, will depend very much
on the child's age and stage of development. This is particularly important
in middle childhood, when children's verbal fluency might mistakenly lead
one to expect that they will describe their feelings and worries in adult terms.
Also, as with most child psychiatric problems, it is common to find that there
are circumstances in which the child is free of symptoms.

Emotional problems

Anxiety disorders

Modes of presentation

Anxiety in this age group is unlikely to take its adult form of sweating,
palpitations, dry mouth, and depersonalisation and derealisation.

Box 8.1   Some disorders of middle childhood

Emotional disorders
  Anxiety disorders
  Fears and phobias
  Depression
  School refusal
  Obsessive-compulsive disorder
  Elective mutism
  Hysteria
  Recurrent abdominal pain
Conduct disorder
  Fire setting
  Stealing
Attention deficit/hyperactivity
Developmental disorder
  Enuresis
  Soiling
  Tic disorders
  Childhood dementia
Psychoses
  Schizophrenia
  Manic-depressive illness
  Organic psychoses

The child may be frightened to go out to school or to be left alone. He or she may have difficulties sleeping, and startle easily. There may be physical complaints with no apparent organic cause, such as stomach ache, headache and sickness. The child may slip back to behaviour more appropriate to a previous developmental stage, such as enuresis, soiling and clinginess, or might ruminate excessively, develop some new obsessions, or try to avoid anxiety-provoking situations. In some cases the anxiety may be severe enough to affect concentration and interfere with learning. It is important, however, for parents and professionals to recognise that some anxiety is entirely appropriate at this stage, and that learning to cope with the anxiety engendered by separation or competition is part of normal development. One would expect a child to have some anxiety on entering a new social situation. And, as with adults, a tolerable degree of anxiety may enhance performance.

Aetiology

The precise aetiology will vary from case to case. Genetic factors (Graham & Stephenson, 1985) may be important. Parental overprotectiveness, possibly as a result of the parents' own experiences or following the illness or death of another child, may sometimes increase the child's anxiety, as may specific events, such as the death of a sibling, family break-up, or witnessing or experiencing some acutely traumatic episode. Chronic family stressors, such as overcrowding, poverty, and marital discord are also risk factors.

Assessment

The history should take into account the duration of the problem, its effect on the child and on other family members, acute and chronic family stresses (marital discord, death of a grandparent), and areas of coping or good functioning. Is the disorder discrete, or is it occurring in conjunction with another problem? What (successful and unsuccessful) measures have been taken to deal with it?

Management

In general, treatment should be aimed at reducing avoidable stresses, improving coping, and helping the family develop a sympathetic but firm attitude to the child's problems. In practice this may be provided through anxiety management training, family therapy or short-term focal therapy for the child. Individual psychotherapy may also be helpful in selected cases.

Case example

Julian was referred by his parents at the age of nine. From the age of seven he had become increasingly anxious at school, to a degree which affected his learning. He had also begun to wet the bed. At home his normal politeness was now punctuated with rudeness and distress. His father felt very let down by Julian, and felt he was avoiding challenging boyish activities which the two of them might have enjoyed together.

It emerged that the paternal grandfather had died when the father was seven, from untreated hypertensive heart disease, at which time the material circumstances of father's family had deteriorated markedly. Furthermore, when Julian was six, his father had undergone a routine medical examination, and was found to be moderately hypertensive himself. This had caused both parents considerable anxiety, which they believed had been kept from the children. Julian and his younger brother and sister refuted this – they knew all about dad's medical history.

An additional feature was that both parents, but especially the mother, treated Julian as a young adult, and entered into very protracted discussions with him about the pros and cons of their child-rearing practices. This was intended to reduce his anxiety, but instead had the reverse effect.

Family therapy sessions were offered. Firstly, the family's anxieties about the father's illness were explored. The hypertension was in fact well controlled, but the father had unwittingly behaved as though he might die soon, and had withdrawn somewhat from close contact with Julian. The family was helped to realise that the father was not in imminent danger of dying, and that he had a great deal to offer Julian emotionally.

Secondly, the father was given the main role in dealing with Julian's enuresis and a simple behavioural programme initiated (see below and Chapter 10).

Thirdly, the parents were helped to be less nervous about dealing with Julian firmly. For example, they made it plain to him that they were satisfied with his school, and that they intended to help him settle down there rather than transfer him to an inferior school (something which he had requested). Julian responded well to this (somewhat to his parents' surprise), and he became considerably less anxious, and enjoyed school more. He and his father also enjoyed their times together much more.

Fears and phobias

Phobias are conditions in which there is an unrealistic and inappropriate fear of certain objects or situations. Middle childhood is a time when specific fears (e.g. of the dark or of animals) lessen, although specific fears of school and other social situations are the commonest at this age and affect boys and girls equally. Animal phobias, which are far less common, are more likely to be found in girls and usually originate from preschool times. About 2% of children are affected, although phobias are rarely the prime reason for referral.

Aetiology

Little is known about the precise origins of phobias. They may be shared by other family members, so that the child learns from an early age to fear a specific phenomenon or object. Sometimes the phobia appears to be a more socially acceptable expression of another anxiety, which might be to do with the child's view of his or her place in the family. Freud's celebrated case of Little Hans is one such example (Freud, 1909). Children who have suffered an acute or chronic trauma may develop specific fears (e.g. of going into the park where the traumatic incident took place).

Assessment

One should take a detailed history of the fears and their nature, and look for any precipitant or obvious cause. The family's response to the child's feelings is important, and may give some pointers as to why the symptom has persisted.

Management

If the phobia is the only symptom then behavioural methods are usually used, in the form of desensitisation to the feared situation, with the child alone or with the whole family. Modelling, using other children or parents to demonstrate normal behaviour, and relaxation techniques may also be helpful. If the symptom is part of a more widespread emotional disorder, family or individual therapy may be indicated.

Outcome

Most tend to improve even if untreated.

Depression

Childhood depression has been the subject of intensive study in the last decade, and it is now well established that prepubertal children can experience depression (Angold, 1988*a,b*). The prevalence rises with increasing age and is much more common in adolescence than in middle childhood.

Modes of presentation

This varies considerably with age. In middle childhood one is unlikely to find evidence of a persistent depressed or dysphoric mood, and the 'vegetative' symptoms of adulthood are most uncommon. Younger children are likely to have feelings of sadness or helplessness, and older children may complain of being unfairly treated or unloved. Anhedonia and boredom may be prominent. Other features include social withdrawal, anger and irritability, somatic complaints, deterioration in school work, and sleep difficulties.

At this age it is slightly more common in boys, although as adolescence approaches it becomes more common in girls. Attempted and completed suicides are rare, but do occur.

Depressive feelings are common both in normal children and in children with other evidence of psychiatric disorder (Rutter *et al*, 1970). In certain cases it may be an entirely normal and indeed adaptive response to external circumstances such as bereavement. Careful clinical assessment may be needed to distinguish between such a state and a frank depressive syndrome.

Aetiology

Children of parents with depressive illnesses are at risk for a wide spectrum of child psychiatric disorders, including depression (Angold, 1988*a*). There is evidence that disturbing events such as divorce, especially in the context of continuing parental conflict, lead to depressed mood and anxiety in children but not specifically depressive disorder. The precise link between loss and depression in children is not clear, although life events are a non-specific precipitant of emotional and conduct disorders, including depression (Goodyer, 1990).

Assessment

The diagnosis of depressive disorder requires the identification of the symptoms described above. The child will be unlikely to say outright that he or she is depressed. A sensitive clinical history is essential. Physical illness, normal bereavement reactions and ordinary sadness should be excluded. Precipitating factors, especially losses, should be identified. Attention should be paid to the child's physical well-being, and the small but real risk of attempted suicide or self-destructive behaviour should not be forgotten. Possible hidden factors, such as sexual abuse, are unlikely to become evident unless the possibility is borne in mind and the child is seen on his or her own.

Management

There are a number of treatment options, but the efficacy of specific treatments remains unproven. In the majority of cases one will not need to take special measures to ensure the child's safety (because suicide is so uncommon in this age group and because supervision of the patient by the family is easier than in older age groups). It is helpful to explain to the child and the parents that children do become depressed, and that the condition is treatable. Family therapy may help the family to become less hostile and more sympathetic towards the child. Cognitive therapy is of proven efficacy with adults, and may well be helpful to children too. Individual psychotherapy is useful where conflicts are primarily internal and family support is lacking. Pharmacotherapy is not widely used except for the more severe cases.

Outcome

It seems that most depressed children will be amenable to treatment or will improve spontaneously. A small proportion of children become recurrently and chronically depressed. However, the fact that the validity of the diagnosis in this age group has only recently been established means that we should learn much more about the natural history of the disorder over the next decade.

School refusal

Non-attendance at school is divided into two broad categories, truancy, which is a conduct disorder (discussed later), and school refusal, which is viewed as an emotional disorder (Hersov, 1960*a,b*). Although many children do not like going to school and about one in ten of all pupils do not attend school at any one time, the prevalence of school refusal is low (less than 3% of all children with psychiatric disorders on the Isle of Wight; Rutter *et al*, 1970). Boys and girls are affected equally.

Mode of presentation

The child (usually gradually) becomes unable to go to school, or to stay in school once there. He or she may express a willingness to attend in principle, but this is not carried through in practice. Commonly the child complains about school being upsetting, or about the journey being difficult. Some children begin to move increasingly slowly in the morning, delaying getting ready for school. If pressed, they may panic. Other children develop somatic complaints which justify non-attendance.

The disorder is most common at the start of primary school, at five, at the time of secondary transfer, at 11, and at about 15 years. It is sometimes of acute onset, and may follow illness in the child, bereavement, or any disruption in the school setting.

The child does not wander the streets, or spend time with friends. He or she is more likely to stay at home, helping mother about the house or watching videos. The parents will often support in principle the idea of school attendance, but may at the same time justify the child's non-attendance on various grounds (e.g. journey too far, school too big).

Aetiology

Separation anxiety, in which the child is greatly distressed by the mother's absence, usually underlies school refusal (Hersov, 1960*a*,*b*). This may be the result of overt stresses such as maternal illness or a history of marital violence, or it may be an enduring characteristic of the mother–child relationship. Gittelman-Klein & Klein (1980) found separation anxiety to be a marked feature in over 90% of the 45 children they studied. Depressed mood and other emotional symptoms occur in about half of school refusers (Kolvin *et al*, 1984; Bools *et al*, 1990).

The evidence for 'school phobia' is less strong (Waldron *et al*, 1975), but the possibility of deficiencies in the school environment should not be ignored (bullying, lack of supervision, lack of adequate toilet facilities). Hersov (1960*a*,*b*) found that families of school refusers, as compared with those of truanting children, were smaller, with more parental neurosis, less experience of maternal separation in childhood and more overprotection. Twenty per cent of mothers had a psychiatric disorder, usually a depressive illness. Bools *et al* (1990) found two-thirds of the parents of school refusers had been treated for psychiatric disorder at some time, including one-third at the time of the study. Truanting children were from a lower socio-economic group, with inconsistent parental discipline, frequent paternal absence and other antisocial behaviour.

Assessment

It is particularly helpful to see the whole family together. Attitudes to separation, and the ability to cope with anxieties associated with separation, should be carefully examined. Are the siblings more successful at going to school and, if so, why? One needs to enquire about parental illness, about current or previous marital violence, and about precipitating factors in the child or the school (illness, change of teacher, loss of a friend). A report from the school about the child's academic ability is essential, as academic failure may be a contributing factor. If there are physical symptoms, a single thorough physical examination should be carried out and the minimum of necessary special investigations completed as soon as possible.

Management

The main principle of treatment is to get the child back to school as soon as possible. Many cases of school refusal are dealt with by general practitioners or by education social workers. By the time a referral is made to child psychiatry the child may have been out of school for weeks or months. A simple approach of helping the parents apply consistency and firmness in getting the child back to school will often suffice. The parents will need to cooperate in ensuring that the child gets a good night's sleep, is dressed and eats breakfast on time, and is escorted right into school. If the child leaves school prematurely, he or she should be taken back in the same way. The programme must be coordinated with the education social worker and the class teacher. It can be disastrous to get children into school, and then find that the staff were not expecting them.

Where there are family difficulties these should be dealt with as part of the programme. For example, if the child is worried about the mother's health, the father may need to indicate by words and actions that he will take more care of her and that the child need not worry unduly.

Berney *et al* (1981) found more than 40% of school refusers to be significantly depressed. They studied the effect of adding clomipramine to the standard psychotherapeutic treatments for school refusal, and found that the medication produced no discernible benefits and had no effect on mood or on separation anxiety.

In more refractory cases return may be made easier by attendance at special small units as an interim measure. Home tuition is a last resort. If the parents are unable or unwilling to take part in a structured programme, residential schooling may be indicated.

Individual psychotherapy to explore persistent anxieties may be offered once the child is back at school. The admission of school refusers to in-patient units is now most uncommon. The prognosis is better in those who are younger, and where the problem is picked up quickly.

Case example
Jackie, aged six, was referred because of non-attendance in the second year of school. She lived alone with her mother, and had little contact with her father, who now had a new family. There had been no problems in the first year of school. At the beginning of the second year Jackie began to complain bitterly to her mother about the school – she said that she did not like her new teacher, and that she was being bullied. She asked to go to another school. In the meantime she preferred to stay at home with her mother, or go shopping with her rather than go to school. Her mother was socially isolated, and Jackie appeared to be her closest friend. A meeting was held at school, where it was established that Jackie

was not being bullied. However, she very much missed her teacher from the first year, who was now away on maternity leave.

The treatment plan combined a number of different elements. The education social worker assisted the mother in preparing Jackie for school in the morning and in getting her to school and into the classroom. Her mother particularly needed help in being firm, and in not giving in too quickly. The class teacher gave Jackie extra attention for the first few weeks. If Jackie became very upset at school, she could telephone her mother once only, but her mother would not take her home. The mother was encouraged to expand her social network. She was put in touch with a women's group, and also became more friendly with a female cousin who had a child of the same age. When the former teacher's baby was born, Jackie sent her a card, and was very pleased to receive a personal reply. Her attendance at school improved substantially, but she continued to be described by teachers as not really enjoying her time at school very much.

Obsessive-compulsive disorders

Obsessions are persistent, intrusive and repetitive thoughts. Compulsions are ritualised stereotyped behaviours. These are rare conditions, affecting approximately 1% of clinic populations and 0.3% of the general population, although obsessive features may frequently accompany other psychiatric disorders such as depression, anorexia nervosa, autism, Asperger's syndrome and tics. Middle childhood is often the time of onset.

Mode of presentation

Mild obsessions, magical thoughts and rituals are a normal part of development, especially at this age. In some children they may increase in frequency and intensity and become handicapping. The onset is usually insidious. The child is not able to stop the behaviour, and other people, especially parents, may be drawn into colluding with the rituals.

Aetiology

The condition runs in families, with 5% of parents having the disorder themselves, and about two-thirds having obsessional traits. The link may be genetic or environmental.

Assessment

A detailed account of the symptoms is needed, with a diary of their timing and pattern. Normal ritualised behaviour can be differentiated from an obsessive-compulsive disorder by not being experienced as unpleasant or overwhelmingly compulsive. A systemic assessment will take into account the effect of the symptoms on the family. Other stresses, symptoms of anxiety or psychiatric disorder need to be looked for in all family members.

Management

Behaviour therapy, using response prevention, modelling and real-life exposure, is the most successful method to date, although psychotherapy for the child, with counselling for the parents, is still used at times in spite of its limited success. Family therapy may help if there are family stresses. Antidepressants have been tried with limited success although improvements have been reported with clomipramine (Flament *et al*, 1985).

Outcome

The prognosis is better when the obsessional symptoms are part of an affective illness than when of a pure obsessive–compulsive disorder. Those with a shorter history before referral do better than those with long-standing symptoms. Many patients will continue to have symptoms that require further episodes of treatment.

Elective mutism

This is a condition in which the child speaks in some situations and not in others (Kolvin & Fundudis, 1981). The child has the ability to speak, but does not do so in certain circumstances or with certain people. The child usually has little control over this, and so the term 'selective mutism' might be more accurate. It is very rare (0.8/1000 children), and is more common in girls.

Mode of presentation

Mutism characteristically develops after the onset of relatively normal speech, although about 50% of children have a history of minor speech problems. Shyness and various emotional and conduct symptoms are common. Children are often shy and stubborn. Mutism often starts with the onset of school.

Aetiology

Minor abnormalities on electroencephalography are common, as is a history of minor or major psychiatric problems in the parents. It is commoner in families where the parents' first language is different from that of the child. In a substantial number of cases there is a history of a traumatic incident, although it is not clear whether these cases should be given a separate diagnosis of a 'traumatic mutism'.

Assessment

Transient mutism, which is linked to separation anxiety and which may be a short-term response to a new situation, should be excluded. It is essential that one establishes that hearing, as well as language comprehension and production, are normal.

Management

The patients are probably quite heterogeneous, and treatment should be individually tailored. Family work is helpful to look at communication patterns and separation difficulties. Behavioural methods can be used to reinforce the child for speaking in new situations.

Outcome

Less than half had improved after five or ten years, even with intensive treatment (Kolvin & Fundudis, 1981). The prognosis is poor if mutism is still present at the age of ten and if there are family psychiatric difficulties.

Case example

Samira was referred by an educational psychologist at the age of nine. Since starting primary school she had never spoken to members of staff, although she did speak to friends, and to her family at home. She was of normal intelligence, and her academic work was good.

She was the youngest child of a devout Muslim family, who immigrated to Britain when Samira was two. Her mother never learned to speak English properly, although her father was fluent, having served in the British Army abroad. An older sister had minor speech problems and was very shy. During the assessment interview Samira spoke only to her mother.

There was a history of marital discord and intrafamilial violence. An older sibling had left home after a beating from the father. Her father did not believe that Samira was learning anything at school, and so he would get her up at 5 a.m. every day to teach her mathematics, and would study with her again in the evening until 11 p.m.

A more serious history of violence to the children emerged, and the mother reported this to social services. Care proceedings were initiated, and the father moved out of the home. However, care proceedings were dropped when the mother withdrew her allegations and allowed the father back into the home. The parents refused to bring Samira to the psychiatric clinic, but agreed to her having play therapy with a community psychiatric nurse at school. These sessions initially progressed well, with Samira using drawing and play to express herself. The therapist began to get a picture of a girl who was exposed to much parental discord, some physical abuse, as well as substantial conflict between the practices of her family and of the wider society. However, despite her obvious interest in the treatment, Samira then stopped attending school altogether. As the parents refused to bring her to the clinic, the matter was referred back to social services for further investigation.

Hysteria (conversion disorder)

In hysterical conversion disorders there is a loss of physical functioning which has a psychological rather than an organic cause. It is very rare in this age group, where it is equally common (or uncommon) in boys and girls.

Mode of presentation

Children most commonly present with disorders of gait or loss of limb function. Pseudoseizures have been reported in association with incest (Goodwin *et al*, 1979).

Aetiology

Most of the different theories about the aetiology have in common the notion that some advantage accrues to the child through the development of the symptom, either by reduction in anxiety, or by the increased care and decreased responsibility that go with the sick role. This should not be taken to mean that the symptoms are under the child's conscious control.

Assessment

A careful history, physical examination and observation will establish the diagnosis in many cases. However, some cases are enormously complex, and may require admission to an in-patient unit for diagnosis. The possibility of sexual abuse should not be forgotten.

Management

Most forms of treatment involve taking the child's predicament seriously, dealing with it sympathetically, and helping the child and family reduce the secondary advantages of the sick role and increase the advantages of 'wellness behaviour'. This can be done by a combination of individual, family and behavioural methods. In many cases it is helpful to combine physical and psychological treatments.

Outcome

A follow-up study at the Maudsley Hospital of 28 children previously diagnosed with hysteria (Caplan, 1970) showed that 46% were found to have an organic illness related to the symptom that was not recognised on admission. Amblyopia was the commonest complaint that turned out to have a physical cause.

Case example

Sarah, aged nine, was brought one morning to casualty by her father, with acute weakness in her right arm. This had developed after she had bumped her arm lightly against the basin while brushing her teeth in preparation for going to school. Neurological examination revealed that there was loss of power in the arm, but the pattern of the weakness was unusual, and there were no other symptoms. She was right-handed. The casualty officer interviewed Sarah and discovered that she was supposed to be taking a history examination that morning, for which she believed she had not prepared adequately. She was afraid that her father would be very angry if she did badly in the examination. When the casualty officer offered to help her explain this to her father, the weakness reduced considerably, and she was totally free of symptoms at a follow-up appointment one week later. Sarah and her family declined any further child psychiatric or neurological follow-up.

Recurrent abdominal pain

Recurrent abdominal pain with no organic cause occurs in about 25% of 5–6-year-old children (Faull & Nicol, 1986). It affects boys and girls equally and frequently accompanies emotional disorders, particularly school refusal. However, it is also common in children without obvious psychological difficulties.

Mode of presentation

The child complains of severe diffuse recurrent abdominal pain, lasting a few hours. The cyclical nature of the pain in some cases, and the fact that it may be accompanied by vomiting and headache, has led to it being called by some the 'periodic syndrome' or 'abdominal migraine'. It is usually poorly localised, and without other features of an acute abdominal disorder. Attacks may be triggered by stress and often subside after rest.

Aetiology

The aetiology and mechanisms whereby pain is produced are unknown. Garber *et al* (1990) found that children with recurrent abdominal pain of any cause and their families have more psychiatric problems than normal controls; their mothers were significantly more anxious than mothers of healthy children and children with organic pain.

Faull & Nicol (1986) and Davison *et al* (1986) found recurrent abdominal pain to be associated with temperamental difficulties, and possibly with lack of communication between the parents.

Assessment and management

Careful coordination between the paediatrician, the general practitioner and the child psychiatrist is essential. A single thorough physical examination and a careful individual and family psychiatric history will be necessary. Medical investigations should be done only if the doctors believe them to be truly necessary.

Establishing the cause, and being frank about areas of uncertainty, is part of the treatment. Many cases will have no apparent cause or precipitant. Individual and family anxieties should be dealt with by the appropriate form of psychotherapy – the reaction of other family members to the pain, and to the uncertainty about its origins, may have a considerable influence on outcome. The short-term prognosis is good, but in many cases the problem recurs in adult life.

> **Case example**
> Brian, aged nine, suffered diffuse acute abdominal pain when his father was dying of stomach cancer. This led to him taking more time off school and staying at home, where his mother was nursing his father and younger sister. He could not talk about his father's illness with anyone. His pain started after the cancer had been diagnosed and no organic cause was found. He had suffered asthma as a younger child. He had always had a difficult relationship with his father, who had spent some years away from his mother and the children. The family were seen together, and Brian was also seen on his own. Brian initially talked only about his physical pain, but as he and his family became better able to face his father's imminent death, his physical pain decreased and his sadness increased.

Post-traumatic stress disorder

It is increasingly being recognised that children suffer from post-traumatic stress disorder, and that the condition is amenable to treatment. The form of the disorder will depend on the nature of the trauma, and the child's age and stage of development. The term is most commonly used to apply to acutely traumatic events, but may also have some relevance for chronic stresses such as child sexual abuse (Terr, 1991).

Mode of presentation

The characteristic features are anxiety, fearfulness, and recurrent intrusive memories and dreams of the traumatic event. Sleep disturbance and avoidance of reminders of the incident are common.

Assessment and management

The diagnosis depends on identifying the trauma and the consequent symptoms described above. The child and family should be allowed in the first instance to recall and re-tell the details of the trauma. Subsequent treatment can follow a behavioural or a focal psychodynamic approach. A developmental perspective is essential, as symptoms may recur at the time of developmental milestones.

Conduct disorder

Conduct disorder refers to severe and persistent antisocial behaviour. It is much more common in boys. Social norms will influence the diagnosis. (Delinquency is a legal term referring to those forms of antisocial behaviour that break the law.)

Mode of presentation

Features include excessive fighting, disobedience, tantrums, stealing, destruction of property, cruelty (especially to animals), fire setting or truanting. Antisocial behaviour may be specific to a situation or pervasive, and the acts may be carried out alone (unsocialised conduct disorder) or with a peer group (socialised conduct disorder). Emotional problems are often present as well.

Aetiology

Children with conduct disorders tend to come from disadvantaged backgrounds with a history of violence, mental illness, death or abandonment. Aggression may be a family characteristic, and the families are often chaotic, with inconsistent parenting and lack of supervision. Discipline tends to be coercive rather than consistent, firm and facilitating. Antisocial behaviour and alcoholism are common in the parents.

Overactivity at three years is associated with antisocial behaviour in middle childhood (Richman *et al*, 1982). There are close associations with hyperactivity (Taylor, 1983) and with specific reading retardation (Rutter *et al*, 1970).

Mode of presentation

There is typically a history of persistent annoying or antisocial behaviour which has driven the school or parents to despair. All methods of discipline are thought to have failed, and the parents often make use of escalating degrees of severe physical chastisement (which also produces no improvement).

Assessment and management

A careful history of the problem behaviour and the parents' response to it is essential, as is a full family history of antisocial problems. Educational ability should also be assessed. One should enquire about associated problems, especially depression, and about precipitating factors. Areas of good functioning and personal achievement should not be forgotten.

Treatment is difficult, and the prognosis is poor. In a study of clinic attenders, about one-third of boys with conduct disorder become delinquent adults (Robins, 1966). Of women with three or more conduct problems in childhood, 85% had psychiatric problems as adults (Robins, 1986).

Few delinquent adults do not have a history of childhood conduct disorder. Children with good peer relationships do better; those with pervasive conduct problems, especially aggression, and with poor peer relationships, do worse.

Parent training is a popular form of treatment in the United States (Patterson, 1982). Behaviour therapy and family and individual psychotherapy may be useful for discrete problems. Consultation with the school and attempts to reduce scapegoating or labelling may also be helpful.

Case example

Alan, aged nine, was referred by his father and stepmother, with whom he was living. He was argumentative, ran away often, and was destructive of his and his father's property. His father was very critical of Alan's biological mother, with whom the boy spent his weekends, and in whose house he had contracted head lice. Alan tended to run away when his mother's boyfriend dropped him off at his father's house after access visits.

Parental discipline was remarkably inconsistent. When Alan repeatedly spat into his hand and threw the saliva onto the ceiling of his bedroom (covering the entire ceiling), the father cleaned it all himself, and made no comment to Alan. When Alan spent 50p of his own pocket money on sweets that the father disliked, the father kept him in for a month. Treatment, which combined parent training and family therapy, took three years. It was aimed at increasing parental consistency, and developing an appropriate tariff of punishments for misdemeanours. Considerable effort was also directed at improving communication between the estranged parents, so that the father would always know when to expect Alan home, and would ensure that he came indoors and settled down after returning from his mother.

The improvements were maintained by brief two-monthly follow-up appointments. Without these, relapses occurred.

Special forms of conduct disorder

Fire setting

Fire setting is an uncommon but dangerous and anxiety-provoking condition. It is best seen as a severe form of conduct disorder, with a younger peak age, very high male predominance and greater psychosocial disturbance (Jacobson, 1985).

Fire setters can be divided into a younger group who tend to set fires on their own and in the home, and an older group who operate in gangs and often show other antisocial behaviour. In only about 25% is fire setting the primary reason for referral.

There is usually a history of family disruption and breakdown, antisocial problems and alcoholism, and low intelligence in the parents.

Assessment and treatment are as for conduct disorder, although obviously careful attention must be paid to the safety of the child and the community. Vigilance may be required with regard to access to incendiary devices. Not surprisingly, children's wards and children's homes are reluctant to admit children with a history of serious fire setting.

In some younger children the behaviour may be less ominous, and will respond to guidance about fire safety.

Stealing

About 5% of primary-school children steal at least once (Wolff, 1967). They fall into two categories, with considerable overlap.

So-called 'comfort stealing' is the commonest presentation in this age group. Here the symptom comes into the category of conduct problems, but the underlying cause is emotional. Comfort stealing occurs in well socialised boys and girls who are in some respect feeling unloved. The stealing may be followed by lying. This may produce a hostile critical response from the parents, adding further to the child's sense of being unwanted. Typically the child will steal from a stepmother's purse, just as it becomes clear that she is now an established member of the family. Or the child may steal on being moved from the mother's home to the father's home, in cases where the parents are separated.

Treatment involves understanding the child's predicament, trying to get the parents to respond in a more sympathetic way, and to help the child find less provocative ways of attracting attention.

The second type of stealing, which is usually associated with other antisocial behaviour, occurs more commonly in adolescence, but is also to be found in this age group. The seminal work by Bowlby (1946) identified a history of emotional neglect and separation. This was confirmed by Rich (1956), who concluded that young children who steal are usually unhappy and isolated.

Hyperactivity, hyperkinesis and attention deficit disorder

In terms of classification this is a complex area, with a number of possibilities for confusion. As more is learned about the condition, changes in definition have taken place. A distinction is drawn in this chapter (where possible) between hyperactivity in general and the hyperkinetic syndrome in particular. Also, some attention is paid to the American notion of attention deficit disorder. Taylor *et al* (1991) and Schachar (1991) provide comprehensive and up-to-date analyses from the British and American perspectives, respectively.

Definition and presentation

The hyperactive child is restless, inattentive, overactive, impulsive, disruptive and distractible. The condition may best be seen as a dimension of behaviour. DSM-III (American Psychiatric Association, 1980) included the condition attention deficit disorder with hyperactivity (ADDH), a diagnosis which has been superseded by the DSM-III-R diagnosis of attention deficit hyperactivity disorder (ADHD) (American Psychiatric Association, 1987) – this requires the presence of overactivity and inattentiveness, with or without impulsiveness. The hyperactivity in question may be situational or pervasive. In the UK many of these children would be diagnosed as having a conduct disorder.

On the other hand, Taylor's group in the UK identifies a much more narrowly defined hyperkinetic syndrome in terms of severe, pervasive overactivity and inattentiveness at home and at school (Taylor *et al*, 1991).

Epidemiology

Attention deficit disorder with hyperactivity is found in at least 6% of the population, is more common in boys, increases with social adversity, and declines with age.

The point prevalence for the much more restrictive hyperkinetic syndrome is about 1.7%. Although Taylor *et al* (1991) studied only boys, and therefore drew no conclusions about gender, earlier studies suggest that the hyperkinetic syndrome is more common (about four times) in boys.

The prevalence of ADHD has not yet been studied, but is thought likely to be substantially above 1.7%.

Associated features

Taylor *et al* (1991) argue that hyperkinetic syndrome is an identifiable clinical entity, with specific associated developmental and cognitive features. The children tend to have low IQs, language delay, and clumsiness. The precise nature of the attention problem requires further study – it may not be an attention deficit *per se*, but rather a problem in exploring and integrating new knowledge effectively. Psychosocial adversity in general is not associated with hyperkinesis. However, poor parental coping and expressed criticism of the child are associated with persistence of the disorder.

With regard to ADDH and ADHD, cognitive impairment is more strongly associated with pervasive than with situational hyperactivity. In fact some children with situational hyperactivity have no impairment in respect of their cognitive functioning. Psychosocial and economic adversity is associated with increased prevalence.

Aetiology

Hyperactivity in general is more common in children with brain damage or mental handicap than in the general population. No specific causal links have been found. Perinatal risk factors may be important in the hyperkinetic syndrome.

There is modest support for a genetic influence. The role of food additives remains controversial, as does the possibility of immunological factors (Egger *et al*, 1985).

As noted above, continuing maternal criticism and hostility may be associated with persistence of the disorder.

Assessment

A careful account should be taken of all the symptoms. The diagnosis should not be based on one or two strong features alone, or on parent or teacher reports only. One should also try to distinguish co-morbid conditions such as conduct disorder and depression.

A full developmental history should be taken and attention should be assessed formally using the appropriate psychometric tests. Details of family relationships and interactions will be informative.

Management

Cognitive, behavioural, drug, family and supportive therapies all have a part to play. The family and school should be helped to understand the disorder and given appropriate information and support. The first line of treatment in the UK will usually be a combination of advice and behavioural intervention. The symptoms will often attenuate with age. Dietary modifications may sometimes produce improvements.

Stimulant drugs, such as methylphenidate (Ritalin), have an important part to play in treatment of the hyperkinetic syndrome, and will have an immediate effect on performance and concentration in a substantial number of children, as will certain antidepressants. Addiction is unlikely, but insomnia and diminished appetite and growth rate need watching.

The prescription of psychotropic drugs to children is uncommon in the UK, and those unfamiliar with the drugs and the disorder should seek appropriate advice about dosages and about the measurement of effectiveness.

Outcome

The prognosis is better if the disorder occurs on its own, responds to medication, and where the child has the benefits of normal intelligence and a supportive family. Antisocial problems worsen the prognosis, as do maternal criticism and depression.

Developmental problems

Enuresis

Enuresis is defined as the repeated involuntary passing of urine after the age of five with no organic cause. It may be diurnal or, as is more usual, nocturnal, primary (never been dry) or secondary (follows a period of dryness). Approximately 10% of children are still wet by night at five, and 5% at ten years. Enuresis is twice as common in boys. Bladder (and bowel) control can only occur when the relevant physiological maturation has taken place.

Mode of presentation

Many cases will be dealt with by the primary-care team. Brief episodes of enuresis in new or difficult situations are not uncommon and usually do not require treatment. Cases referred to child psychiatrists are probably more refractory or have associated emotional problems.

Referral may be via the school, parents, primary-care workers or paediatricians. Enuresis may be the primary complaint or may be associated with other problems. Social withdrawal or teasing can result. The strain on an impoverished mother of having to wash pyjamas and sheets every day should not be underestimated.

Aetiology

Seventy per cent of primary enuretics have a first-degree relative who was also enuretic. Both genetic and environmental family factors appear to have an effect. The environmental factors may include long-standing features, such as sustained conflict over toilet-training, family discord and social disadvantage; acute stresses are also important, including illness, hospital admission and the birth of a sibling (Douglas, 1973).

Enuresis is commoner in large working-class families and children living in institutions.

Most enuretic children are psychiatrically otherwise normal, but non-specific psychiatric problems are found in 20% of cases, particularly in girls and those with daytime enuresis. A history of urinary-tract infections is also associated (this may be a cause or a consequence). A low IQ may make it hard for a child to learn to use the toilet properly.

Assessment and management

This subject is well covered by Shaffer (1985). The onset and frequency of the problem, and of other developmental factors, should be noted. One should enquire about sleeping arrangements (can the child climb out of bed, find the light switch, and locate the toilet with sufficient ease?), and about the chronology of the acquisition of continence in other family members. A physical examination, mid-stream urine sample, and other examinations as necessary should be carried out by the relevant practitioner. Many cases will resolve without formal treatment.

The first stage of treatment is to establish a baseline, together with sensible advice, consistency, praise for dry nights, and attention to sleeping arrangements. This may be curative on its own. Increasing fluids by day, coupled with praise for good use of the toilet, is recommended by Foxx & Azrin (1973). The next stage is a 'star chart' - effectively a calendar on which the child places a sticker or star for every dry night. This requires some parental enthusiasm, and the goal should be steady improvement rather than instant cure. None of the above measures require any special equipment.

The 'bell and pad' (a form of enuresis alarm) has been shown to be effective with children from reasonably stable families (Dische *et al*, 1983). This works on the principle that water is a good conductor of electricity. When the child urinates, the urine completes an electric circuit between two strategically placed electrodes. This sets off a battery-operated alarm. This should wake both child and parent. The latter encourages the former to empty the bladder, and then they all return to sleep. This again requires motivation of both parent and child.

Tricyclic drugs and desmopressin have also been used, to limited effect. The mechanisms by which they work are unclear.

Family and individual psychotherapy are indicated where the primary problem is not toiletting. Focusing on the toiletting can however be helpful in resolving other problems which might not otherwise have been discussed.

The vast majority of enuretic children will become dry by early adolescence.

Soiling

'Faecal soiling' is the term used to describe all disorders of bowel function and control over the age of four in the absence of physical abnormality or disease. It includes: failure of bowel control; depositing the faeces in abnormal places by a child who has achieved control; excessively fluid faeces (e.g. constipation with overflow incontinence). The term 'encopresis' is often used to describe all these conditions. It is much more common in boys.

Aetiology

A combination of factors is likely. These may include coercive or premature attempts to toilet train the child, developmental delay, or family conflict and discord (Woodmansey, 1967). As with any other parent–child interaction where the child has some control over the outcome, this is a fertile area for the expression of feeling and for attracting both negative and positive attention.

The condition may be part of a more generalised emotional disturbance or parental neglect. Sexual abuse should always be considered. Rarely, the development of faecal incontinence may signify a developing psychosis or organic brain disorder.

Assessment and management

A joint approach involving paediatrician, psychiatrist and primary-care team is needed. It is essential to assess the degree of constipation, and to look for impaction and other anal or gastrointestinal pathology. A detailed history will establish whether the soiling is primary or secondary, whether it is due to lack of control (faeces usually solid), overflow (liquid), or depositing faeces in odd places, and what has been tried by the family.

The management will depend on the cause and nature of the problem. Physical obstructions and organic problems should be treated. Mild cases will respond to simple behavioural techniques (rewarding success and taking a low-key approach to failure). Contingency planning (for 'accidents' at awkward times) is essential. More refractory cases may require hospital admission for intensive retraining, possibly following the evacuation of immovable bowel contents. Substantial underlying problems (sexual abuse, psychosis, intellectual retardation) should be dealt with in the usual way.

This is an embarrassing and disruptive problem for children and families, and requires sympathetic handling. Whatever treatment is given, it is essential to remember that there is more to the child than just an anus and rectum, and efforts should be made to ensure that family life does not revolve only around this problem.

Case example

Natalie, aged five, was referred by a paediatrician after a year's history of chronic constipation with overflow. This had started after her parents' sudden separation. The soiling took place only when Natalie returned home from visiting her father.

Natalie was found to be severely constipated and needed admission for removal of a faecal impaction. A family interview established that the parents did not trust one another at all, were battling over custody, and were at cross-purposes in their handling of Natalie, who was herself preoccupied with cleanliness. She seemed to feel herself responsible for the marital breakdown.

The child psychiatric treatment included family sessions to resolve parental differences over the handling of the child, and to deal with the distress of the divorce. A behavioural programme was drawn up: Natalie would go to the toilet before leaving her father's house. On arrival at her mother's Natalie would be asked about her weekend in a sympathetic way which avoided criticism of her father. She would be encouraged to go to the toilet as part of this discussion. Lack of soiling was rewarded using a star chart. A copy of the chart was kept in both homes, and progress therewith discussed by both parents in Natalie's presence. The soiling soon resolved fully, although there was a brief self-limiting relapse when her father went on a long holiday with his girlfriend.

Tic disorders

Tics are rapid, involuntary, purposeless, repetitive movements.

Mode of presentation

The condition tends to involve the upper part of the body, particularly the face, neck and arms. Tics affect about 20% of children at some time in their lives (Shapiro & Shapiro, 1981). Most cases are transient, but the condition persists in about 1% of children. Tourette's syndrome is a rare condition in which vocal tics, often including obscenities, are present (Shapiro *et al*, 1973). All forms of tics are commoner in boys. The problem often begins at a time of stress, and may be associated with developmental delays.

Aetiology

This is unclear. There are postulated neurological (basal ganglia) and neurochemical (dopamine metabolism) abnormalities. The condition is invariably exacerbated by stress. There is still no convincing explanation for the obscene utterances associated with Tourette's syndrome.

Tic disorders and psychiatric illness are common in other family members. Two-thirds of the children have non-specific abnormalities on electroencephalography. Half have other psychiatric problems as well.

Assessment

The frequency, timing and patterns of the tics can be established with a diary. Neurological examination is usually indicated. The effect of the tics on family functioning, and vice versa, should be identified.

Management

Mild tics will usually resolve spontaneously, are best ignored, and should never be punished.

Where the tics are more complex, disabling, disruptive or persistent, a combination of behaviour modification, pharmacotherapy and psychotherapy should be offered. Massed practice, when the child is asked to practise the tic several times a day, enables the child to take some control, and is often effective. Haloperidol and pimozide are both effective in low doses. The latter has fewer side-effects, but may also be less effective. Psychotherapy may be helpful for dealing with precipitants and consequences of the disorder.

Autism and Asperger's syndrome

Autism

The nature of this condition is such that most cases ought to be detected in the preschool years. However, some cases go undetected for many years, and the possibility of autism should be borne in mind with any school-age child who is described as aloof, uncommunicative or unable to play. A comprehensive psychiatric, psychological and intellectual assessment is essential.

More commonly in this age group the issues will relate to school placement and family support. The vast majority of children with autism will need specialised schooling. The condition can place great strain on a family, and it is important to see that the marital relationship and the healthy siblings are not neglected. Some parents will seek genetic counselling – this is a matter for experienced professionals.

Asperger's syndrome

This intriguing disorder (Wing, 1981; Wolff, 1991) is best seen as part of an autism spectrum, with Asperger's syndrome being equivalent to high-level autism. The condition is rare (Wolff, 1991).

Children with Asperger's syndrome have many of the features of autism, but their relatively good verbal fluency and intelligence mean that the disorder will often go undetected. The salient features include impairment in reciprocal interaction; circumscribed interests; imposition of routine; non-verbal communication problems; and motor clumsiness. It should be considered in the differential diagnosis of aloof, uncommunicative children, and children with disabling obsessional symptoms and rituals.

Childhood dementias

These rare conditions all involve progressive loss of intellectual functioning, usually accompanied by personality changes. The school-age child may present with loss of literacy skills, for example. Other features may include autistic-like or schizophrenia-like symptoms. Fits may occur. The hallmark is progressive deterioration, and the prognosis may be very poor.

Investigation and initial management are best done by specialists. If the diagnosis is confirmed, the local services will have an important part to play in providing palliative treatment and hospice care, as well as family support.

Eating disorders

Anorexia nervosa

This is characterised by excessive dieting and weight loss, an intense fear of gaining weight, and a disturbed perception of body shape. It is accompanied by primary or secondary amenorrhoea or delayed onset of puberty.

Bulimia nervosa is not widely recognised in this age group.

Mode of presentation

Prepubertal anorexia nervosa is very uncommon. It is accompanied by primary amenorrhoea, growth retardation and delayed puberty. It is even less common in boys, who present with weight loss, fear of weight gain and delayed growth and puberty.

It is not easy to diagnose anorexia in this age group. There may be an insidious failure to gain weight, rather than an obvious weight loss. Secondary amenorrhoea, a key feature in older females, is obviously not relevant here. Puberty may be greatly delayed.

Aetiology

Jacobs & Isaacs (1986) compared post- and prepubertal anorectics and found more feeding and behavioural difficulties in the prepubertal group. There were also more family difficulties and major life events preceding the onset. Levels of overt sexual anxiety were similar.

Fosson *et al* (1987) found prepubertal anorexia to be a serious disorder. Depression was commonly present. There was often a delay in making the diagnosis. There was a surprisingly high number of boys (27%) in their sample.

Assessment and management

This is basically the same as for older children. Vigorous measures may be needed to ensure that enough weight is gained to make it possible for the child to enter puberty.

Outcome

In postpubertal anorectics, young age is usually a good prognostic feature. However this gradient does not appear to apply below puberty, and the prognosis in the prepubertal group is relatively poor.

Obesity

Obesity is defined as being 20% over the expected weight for height and sex. It is the commonest nutritional disorder in the Western world and is more common in girls than boys.

Mode of presentation

Many children are very sensitive about their weight and appearance at this age. Teasing may be sufficiently severe to lead to social isolation (Tobias & Gordon, 1980), and this may precipitate referral. Other cases will be picked up during routine examinations.

Aetiology

There are many factors leading to the development of obesity. Genetic factors probably play a part, although the evidence is conflicting (Brook *et al*, 1975;

Hawk & Brook, 1979). Organic causes are rare. An imbalance between caloric intake and energy output is the predominant cause, often compounded by bad eating habits.

Bottle-fed babies are more likely to be overweight in infancy and middle childhood than breast-fed babies.

Social and cultural factors have a considerable influence on family eating patterns and energy output, and on attitudes to obesity.

Assessment

The level of overweight and its duration need to be established. Family eating patterns and exercise levels need to be ascertained. The child's emotional state should be carefully assessed. If all the family members are overweight and do not wish to change their eating habits, the prognosis is poor.

Management

Lack of motivation to change ingrained habits may be a major problem. Dietary advice can be given and the child encouraged to exercise but this is often not sufficient. Belief systems about food, fatness and dieting may need to be explored with the child and the whole family. The attitude of the family to food and family eating habits may need to change before the child can lose weight. Modification of eating patterns by behavioural measures have been shown to be helpful with adults and adolescents.

In-patient treatment may be indicated where the child's physical health is suffering, or where the home environment is very resistant to change.

Outcome

About 40% of obese children will become obese adults (Stark *et al*, 1981), and the benefits of treatment are often not enduring.

Psychoses

The important conditions in this age group are schizophrenia, manic–depressive illness, and organic psychoses. All are rare, and require expert diagnosis and management.

Schizophrenia

Typical symptoms as found in adults may not be evident, and one may have to rely on indirect evidence of delusions and hallucinations (Garralda, 1984). The onset may be very insidious. A history of developmental delay is common (Zeitlin, 1986).

In-patient treatment, pharmacotherapy, special schooling and intensive parent counselling will be necessary.

Manic-depressive illness

This is much less common before puberty than after. The assessment and treatment of depression has been discussed above. Haloperidol is the treatment of choice for mania.

Organic psychoses

Delirium is common in children with febrile illnesses, but is of little psychiatric significance.

Cerebral infections and epilepsy can cause organic brain syndromes without progressive brain damage.

Poisoning (accidental or deliberate) should always be considered as part of the differential diagnosis (see also Chapter 11 – Munchausen by proxy).

Sexual problems

Children in this age group may be referred for excessive masturbation, precocious sexual behaviour and gender identity problems (feminine behaviour in boys seems to arouse more concern than tomboyish behaviour in girls).

Gender identity is probably firmly established by the age of four, if not sooner, and is unlikely to be amenable to efforts to alter it. Sex role identity (or sexual orientation) becomes established much later (Green, 1985).

Saghir & Robins (1973) found links between both 'tomboyism' in childhood and adult lesbianism, and between effeminate behaviour in childhood and adult male homosexuality. Effeminate behaviour in boys can be altered, by means of a behavioural approach or by individual and family psychotherapy. This is unlikely to affect ultimate sexual orientation.

When the presenting symptom is of precocious interest in sexual matters, or excessive masturbation, the possibility of sexual abuse (see above and Chapter 11) must always be considered. Hormonal disorders leading to precocious puberty should also be considered.

Conclusion

Middle childhood is marked by entry into the schooling system, and by participation in a wider world outside the family home. It is a time when individual, including intellectual, functioning will become more obvious. The serious and the common child psychiatric disorders will be apparent to the discerning eye. It is therefore a good time to attempt to detect and treat such disorders, before maladaptive patterns and family attitudes have become entrenched, and while there is still time for the child to make good use of his or her educational and social opportunities.

References

American Psychiatric Association (1980) *Diagnostic and Statistical Manual of Mental Disorders* (3rd edn) (DSM–III). Washington, DC: APA.
——— (1987) *Diagnostic and Statistical Manual of Mental Disorders* (3rd edn, revised) (DSM–III–R). Washington, DC: APA.
Angold, A. (1988*a*) Childhood and adolescent depression. I: Epidemiological and aetiological aspects. *British Journal of Psychiatry*, **152**, 601–617.
——— (1988*b*) Childhood and adolescent depression. II: Research in clinical populations. *British Journal of Psychiatry*, **153**, 476–492.
Berney, T., Kolvin, I., Bhate, S., *et al* (1981) School phobia: a therapeutic trial with clomipramine and short term outcome. *British Journal of Psychiatry*, **138**, 110–118.
Bools, C., Foster, J., Brown, I., *et al* (1990) The identification of psychiatric disorders in children who fail to attend school: a cluster analysis of a non-clinical population. *Psychological Medicine*, **20**, 171–181.
Bowlby, J. (1946) *Forty Four Juvenile Thieves*. London: Baillière, Tindall and Cox.
Brook, C. G. D., Huntley, R. M. C. & Slack, J. (1975) Influence of heredity and environment in the determination of skinfold thickness in children. *British Medical Journal*, ii, 719–721.
Caplan, H. L. (1970) *Hysterical 'Conversion' Symptoms in Childhood*. MPhil Dissertation, University of London.
Davison, I. S., Faull, C. & Nicol, A. R. (1986) Temperament and behaviour in six-year olds with recurrent abdominal pain: a follow up. *Journal of Child Psychology and Psychiatry*, **27**, 539–544.
Dische, S., Yule, W., Corbett, J., *et al* (1983) Childhood nocturnal enuresis: factors associated with outcome of treatment with an enuresis alarm. *Developmental Medicine and Child Neurology*, **25**, 67–80.
Douglas, J. W. B. (1973) Early disturbing events and later enuresis. In *Bladder Control & Enuresis: Clinics in Developmental Medicine 48/491* (eds I. Kolvin, R. C. Mackeith & S. R. Meadow). London: Heinemann, Spastics International Medical Publications.
Egger, J., Carter, C. M., Graham, P. J., *et al* (1985) Controlled trial of oligoantigenic treatment in the hyperkinetic syndrome. *Lancet*, i, 540–545.
Faull, C. & Nicol, A. R. (1986) Abdominal pain in six-year olds: an epidemiological study in a new town. *Journal of Child Psychology and Psychiatry*, **27**, 251–260.
Flament, M., Rappaport, J., Berg, C., *et al* (1985) Clomipramine treatment of childhood obsessive compulsive disorder. *Archives of General Psychiatry*, **82**, 977–983.
Fosson, A., Knibbs, J., Bryant-Waugh, R., *et al* (1987) Early onset anorexia nervosa. *Archives of Diseases in Childhood*, **62**, 114–118.
Foxx, R. M. & Azrin, N. H. (1973) Dry pants: a rapid method of toilet training children. *Behaviour Research and Therapy*, **11**, 435–442.
Freud, S. (1909) Analysis of a phobia in a five-year old boy. *Standard Edition of the Complete Psychological Works of Sigmund Freud*, vol. 10. London: Hogarth Press.

Garber, J., Zeman, J. & Walker, L. (1990) Recurrent abdominal pain in children: psychiatric diagnoses and parental psychopathology. *Journal of the American Academy of Child and Adolescent Psychiatry*, **29**, 648-656.

Garralda, M. E. (1984) Psychotic children with hallucinations. *British Journal of Psychiatry*, **145**, 74-77.

Gittelman-Klein, R. & Klein, D. F. (1980) Separation anxiety in school refusal and its treatment with drugs. In *Out of School - Modern Perspectives in School Refusal and Truancy* (eds L. Hersov & I. Berg). Chichester: Wiley.

Goodwin, J., Simms, M. & Bergman, R. (1979) Hysterical seizures: a sequel to incest. *American Journal of Orthopsychiatry*, **49**, 697-703.

Goodyer, I. (1990) Family relationships, life events and childhood psychopathology. *Journal of Child Psychology and Psychiatry*, **31**, 161-192.

Graham, P. & Stephenson, J. (1985) A twin study of genetic influences of behavioural deviance. *Journal of the American Academy of Child Psychiatry*, **24**, 33-41.

Green, R. (1985) Atypical sexual development. In *Child and Adolescent Psychiatry - Modern Approaches* (eds M. Rutter & L. Hersov). London: Blackwell.

Hawk, L. J. & Brook, C. G. D. (1979) Family resemblances of height, weight, and body fatness. *Archives of Diseases in Childhood*, **54**, 877-879.

Hersov, L. (1960*a*) Persistent non-attendance at school. *Journal of Child Psychology and Psychiatry*, **1**, 130-136.

—— (1960*b*) Refusal to go to school. *Journal of Child Psychology and Psychiatry*, **1**, 137-145.

Jacobs, B. W. & Isaacs, S. (1986) Pre-pubertal anorexia nervosa: a retrospective controlled study. *Journal of Child Psychology and Psychiatry*, **27**, 237-250.

Jacobson, R. R. (1985) Child firesetters: a clinical investigation. *Journal of Child Psychology and Psychiatry*, **26**, 759-768.

Kolvin, I. & Fundudis, T. (1981) Elective mute children: psychological development and background factors. *Journal of Child Psychology and Psychiatry*, **22**, 219-232.

——, Berney, T. & Bhate, S. (1984) Classification and diagnosis of depression in school phobia. *British Journal of Psychiatry*, **145**, 347-357.

Patterson, G. R. (1982) *Coercive Family Process*. Eugene: Castalia.

Rich, J. (1956) Types of stealing. *Lancet*, *i*, 496-498.

Richman, N., Stevenson, J. & Graham, P. (1982) *Preschool to School: A Behavioral Study*. London: Academic Press.

Robins, L. (1966) *Deviant Children Grown Up*. Baltimore: Williams and Wilkins.

—— (1986) The consequences of conduct disorder in girls. In *Development of Antisocial and Prosocial Behaviour: Research, Theories and Issues* (eds D. Olweus, J. Block & M. Radke-Yarrow). New York: Academic Press.

Rutter, M., Tizard, J. & Whitmore, K. (1970) *Education, Health & Behaviour*. London: Longman.

——, Cox, A., Tupling, C., *et al* (1975) Attainment and adjustment in two geographical areas. I. The prevalence of child psychiatric disorder. *British Journal of Psychiatry*, **175**, 493-509.

Saghir, M. & Robins, E. (1973) *Male and Female Homosexuality*. Baltimore: Williams and Wilkins.

Schachar, R. (1991) Hyperactivity. *Journal of Child Psychology and Psychiatry*, **32**, 155-191.

——, Rutter, M. & Smith, A. (1981) The characteristics of situational and pervasively hyperactive children: implications for syndrome definition. *Journal of Child Psychology and Psychiatry*, **22**, 375-392.

Shaffer, D. (1985) Enuresis. In *Child and Adolescent Psychiatry - Modern Approaches* (eds M. Rutter & L. Hersov). London: Blackwell.

Shapiro, A. K., Shapiro, E. & Wayne, H. L. (1973) The symptomatology and diagnosis of Gilles de la Tourette's syndrome. *Journal of the American Academy of Child Psychiatry*, **12**, 703-723.

—— & —— (1981) The treatment and aetiology of tics and Tourettes's syndrome. *Comprehensive Psychiatry*, **22**, 193-205.

Stark, O., Atkins, E., Wolff, O. H., *et al* (1981) Longitudinal study of obesity in the National Survey of Health and Development. *British Medical Journal*, **283**, 13-17.

Taylor, E. A. (1983) Drug response and diagnostic validation. In *Developmental Neuropsychiatry* (ed. M. Rutter), pp. 348-368. New York: Guilford.

—— (1985) Syndromes of overactivity and attention deficit. In *Child and Adolescent Psychiatry - Modern Approaches* (eds M. Rutter & L. Hersov). London: Blackwell.

——, Sandberg, S., Thorley, G., *et al* (1991) *The Epidemiology of Childhood Hyperactivity*. Maudsley Monograph no. 33. Oxford: Oxford University Press.

Terr, L. C. (1991) Childhood traumas: an outline and overview. *American Journal of Psychiatry*, **148**, 10-20.

Tobias, A. L. & Gordon, J. B. (1980) Social consequences of obesity. *Journal of the American Dietetic Association*, **76**, 338-342.

Waldron, S., Shrier, D., Stone, B., *et al* (1975) School phobia and other childhood neuroses: a systematic study of the children and their families. *American Journal of Psychiatry*, **132**, 802-808.

Wing, L. (1981) Asperger's syndrome: a clinical account. *Psychological Medicine*, **10**, 85-100.

Wolff, S. (1967) Behavioural characteristics of primary school children referred to a psychiatric department. *British Journal of Psychiatry*, **113**, 885-893.

—— (1991) "Schizoid" personality in childhood and adult life. I: The vagaries of diagnostic labelling. *British Journal of Psychiatry*, **159**, 615-620.

Woodmansey, A. C. (1967) Emotion and the motions: an enquiry into the causes and prevention of functional disorders of defaecation. *British Journal of Medical Psychology*, **40**, 207-223.

Zeitlin, H. (1986) *The Natural History of Psychiatric Disorder in Childhood*. Maudsley Monographs. London: Oxford University Press.

9 Clinical syndromes in adolescence
Les Scarth

Conduct disorders ● *Sexual problems* ● *Substance abuse* ● *Emotional disorders* ● *Tourette's syndrome* ● *Psychotic disorders* ● *Eating disorders* ● *Adolescent manifestations of childhood-onset disorders* ● *Conclusion*

Adolescence represents a way-station, or rather a series of way-stations, on the developmental journey between childhood and adulthood. Biological change, preset by the hormonal changes of adrenarche around seven or eight years of age, now surges forward, propelled by hypothalamic, pituitary and adrenal and gonadal hormone release, the most obvious effects being on growth, body shape and the development of secondary sexual characteristics. Boys become men, girls change to women, both physically and psychologically, over about five years. Mood is less stable; thinking becomes increasingly, but uncertainly, more complex. Social expectations and family roles change, with greater autonomy and respect being demanded and given.

In spite of its historical reputation for turmoil, both internal and social, for most adolescents this developmental epoch brings discomfort rather than disorder. Most adolescents 'find' themselves and like what they find. Most parents of adolescents are irritated by, rather than rejecting of, their offspring. A minority of adolescents suffer psychiatric disorders, but those who do cause

---

Box 9.1 Some disorders of adolescence

Conduct disorders
  Delinquency
  Stealing
  Truancy
  Fire setting
Substance abuse
  Tobacco
  Alcohol
  Solvents
  Cannabis
Emotional disorders
  Depression
  Self-harm
  Suicide
  Anxiety
  Obsessional disorders
Tourette's syndrome
Eating disorders

---

great (and justified) concern to their families and communities, being often difficult to contain and untrusting of authority. Early recognition of disorder with prompt treatment can be rewarding, as many of the disorders otherwise distort normal developmental processes. With assistance, most disturbed adolescents can be returned to a normal developmental path and become happy, responsible adults.

Some of the disorders discussed in this chapter are listed in Box 9.1.

Conduct disorders

These are the commonest disorders in adolescence, affecting 4–10% of adolescents (Kazdin, 1987). Many of the disorders will have begun in middle childhood, particularly those in boys, those associated with parental psychopathology, and even more so, those linked to specific reading difficulties. Conduct disorders beginning in adolescence may have less strong links with the first two of these factors (White, 1989).

The presenting features will be socially disapproved behaviour, outside the normal range in terms of frequency and severity. Such behaviour will be relatively impervious to modification by the normal range of sanctions available within families, schools, or the community.

Boys are more commonly affected than girls. A half to a third of these disorders are present from childhood, and are likely to be associated with public misbehaviour as well as home disturbance.

Socially disruptive behaviour (such as defiance of authority, destructiveness, cruelty) does not alter significantly between 8 and 15 years, but frankly delinquent behaviour (such as theft and serious vandalism) appears. Violent crime peaks in late adolescence; alcohol disinhibits and now appears as a common trigger to aggression and social disorder. Peer-group pressure may have a similar enabling (or disabling) effect.

Conduct disorder is often associated with alienation from parents and a strong identification with antisocial standards. Occasionally, it may represent an adverse reaction to specific life events, for example death of a family member or the psychotic illness of a parent. Physical and sexual abuse has strong links with antisocial behaviour. Impulsive adolescents may have a history of pervasive hyperactivity. 'Sleeper effects', such as the death of a same-sex parent in the preschool period, may be associated with conduct disorders in adolescence.

Case example
A 14-year-old boy presented with long-term faecal soiling. He was pale and below the 3rd centile for height and weight, but with parents of average height and weight. He was in early puberty. His explosive temper led to his exclusion from normal secondary school. His soiling led to taunts which resulted in violence to his tormentors. He also frequently picked on younger children and insulted them about their defects.

He was of at least normal intelligence, and an excellent footballer and snooker player. His non-cooperation at school produced poorer attainments than his IQ would predict, but he had no specific learning disorder. At his best, he was a lovable rogue; on leaving a unit where he was placed, he stole flowers to present to the teacher. He had a wry sense of humour and a sharp tongue.

He lived in an intact family in a rundown area. The family home was reasonably well kept. His parents were united in their concern for him but their discipline was ineffective.

Admission to a child psychiatry unit led to early spontaneous remission of his encopresis. Family work was helpful in indicating his part in his own problems but resulted in only verbal shifts in his parents' disciplinary procedures.

The parents' ineffectual controls, which they showed in the family sessions, were a focus of treatment. They could label their difficulties, but the boy refused to diminish his threatening behaviour, and they found it difficult to be consistent. He saw his behaviour as normal and appropriate. As he was short, he felt that aggression was a reasonable defensive tactic. He agreed that he was the loser in aggressive encounters. He refused to cooperate with social skills training but educational progress was good. He transferred to a school for behaviourally disturbed adolescents and settled well.

Delinquency

This involves breaking laws. The number of offences committed increases fourfold between 10 and 15 years but shows an equally steep fall in the early 20s.

Delinquents may be formally processed through the legal system. Twenty per cent of males and 10% of females will have court records before adulthood. However, most offences remain undetected. Among 13–18-year-olds, 50% admitted to theft, 45% to property destruction, and 35% to assault (Rutter & Giller, 1983). Some offences are defined by age, for example non-attendance at school up to 16 years and driving a car before 17 years.

Sexual offences such as prostitution are found in teenage girls, whereas sexual crimes with a violent content are male activities. Other disorders based on sexual inadequacy such as exhibitionism (flashing) are also the province of the adolescent male.

In spite of this catalogue of difficulties, it is only a hard core of delinquents who go on offending. Such youths often have a long history of conduct problems. During adolescence and later, they may show persistent psychiatric difficulties and antisocial personality disorders.

Stealing

Stealing is the commonest antisocial act at all ages. In adolescence, stealing to have access to money for a variety of pursuits is the most important motive. Stealing for the sheer pleasure of the act is much less common (in contrast to this motive for vandalism). In West's (1982) long-term study of delinquents, boredom and keeping up with peers were also stated as reasons for theft, but much less commonly than material gain and pleasure.

Where it results in psychiatric contact, Rich's (1956) subdivision of stealing into comfort, marauding and proving offences may have some clinical value, even if it remains empirically unproven. Comfort offences are those in which young people begin stealing in response to anger generated by parental rejection and suppression of emotions. Marauding offences are part of socialised conduct disorder in adolescence, with poor material provision and delinquent models. Proving offences are said to have their roots in rebellion against parental overprotection and are bids for a stronger, but antisocial, self-identity.

Truancy

Truancy is voluntary non-attendance at school before the age of 16 years, this being the limit of statutory school attendance in the UK. It is particularly common in the last year of compulsory schooling.

Poor educational achievement and disillusionment with school may be matched by poor school organisation. A lack of school activities, combined with low expectation for work and behaviour by teachers who themselves may have little commitment to the school, may alienate pupils. If such adolescents feel unvalued by staff and are given little responsibility in school, the effect of parents being uninterested in education and peers who have anti-authority and anti-school attitudes will be so much greater.

Solitary truanting (rather than as part of a group) is probably more worrying from a psychiatric point of view as it is associated with later personality and social difficulties, as well as a less stable work pattern (Rutter, 1990).

Truancy may be dealt with by court appearance (or appearing before the Children's Hearing Panel in Scotland) with deferment of disposal until the adolescent has had the opportunity to attend school regularly (Berg *et al*, 1987).

Aggressive behaviour

Aggressive behaviour is one of the most stable patterns of behaviour from childhood through to adult life (Olweus, 1979). It is a learned pattern of responses to internal cues, such as physiological arousal ('going white with rage') and external circumstances, such as perceived threats. Such behaviour is maintained by attention and the sheer relief of inner tension. Obtaining concrete rewards such as money or goods will produce similar conditioning of aggressive responses.

Most aggression in adolescents is unpremeditated and impulsive. Planning violence is associated with greater psychiatric disorder, as is dwelling on its consequences, for example boasting about it.

Abnormal cognitions, such as seeing threats where none exist or mis-perceiving emotionally neutral social approaches as attempts to get 'one up', are often found in aggressive young people. An impulsive style of responding with poor ability to predict the consequences of one's actions is also common. The use of alcohol is frequent before aggressive outbursts.

The family (especially parents and siblings) from which the aggressor comes has often long modelled violent behaviour, both as an appropriate expression of strong emotion and for control over others. The social value of 'macho' behaviour may also favour aggression. In young adult men, individual differences in testosterone levels have been linked to aggression under provocation or threat (Nottelmann *et al*, 1990).

Fire setting

This is seen in two groups of males. The first are younger, often duller, boys who set fires mainly in the home, as a solitary occupation. The other group is older; they set fires outside the home, often in the context of many other types of antisocial behaviour (Stewart & Culver, 1982).

Kolko & Kazdin (1991) have looked at the motives of fire setters. They point out that, traditionally, such motives were split between those who set fires in anger or for revenge and those who were motivated by curiosity about fire. It was hypothesised that the latter group were less psychologically disturbed and required an educational approach to cause them to desist. Those who showed a fascination with fire had longer histories of fire setting, and their parents reported both conduct and emotional problems. The 'angry' fire setters showed more premeditation in their fire raising which was often preceded by other antisocial acts (e.g. vandalism). They seemed to have less widespread behavioural problems. The most recidivist fire setters scored highly on both curiosity about fire and anger. A short-hand description for such boys might be 'fascinated and fiery'.

Both educational and psychotherapeutic interventions need to be combined in the management of those who set fire, as well as close supervision.

Running away from home

This is an increasing problem in both the UK and the USA (White, 1989); it increases in prevalence throughout adolescence. It appears to be related to an increase in family disorder. Homelessness, as a result, is now common-place and compounded by a lowering of financial and social support given to those over 16 by the state.

Family disorder is characterised by parental violence and rejection, often associated with parental alcohol or drug abuse. Sexual abuse, in both sexes, often precipitates running away.

Neglect in the family and poor aftercare for adolescents in the care of local authorities fuel the problem.

The consequences of being a 'runaway' may be personal, such as low self-esteem, or a mistrust of adults. Poor social skills are not helped and, under stress, suicidal impulses and emotional isolation result. Fears about sexuality or even sanity may dominate their thoughts. Many have psychosomatic complaints. The social results exacerbate this personal distress. Homeless young people are vulnerable to exploitation; recruitment into prostitution of both sexes, theft as a means of survival, use in pornography, and involvement in drug use (as users, couriers and 'pushers') may be part of the life of runaways.

Management of conduct disorders

This needs to be collaborative, involving family, social workers (area team, probation, community) and school or college staff (where appropriate). As part of a management package, various treatments may be offered.

Cognitive–behavioural strategies

These may be focused on interpersonal problem solving (Spivack & Shure, 1982), increasing the adolescent's awareness of his or her own and other people's social cues. Anger management strategies are often valuable (Feindler *et al*, 1986).

Family therapy

When these techniques are used with the conduct disordered, they should focus on here-and-now issues. They may involve direct communication training and possibly behavioural contracting (Alexander *et al*, 1976).

Group work and community programmes

In group work particular emphasis should be placed on social-skills and activity-based training and discussion. In community programmes, constructive use of leisure time and work skills should be taught; special family placements may back up such programmes.

Individual exploratory psychotherapy

Such therapy may be useful. It should be short term and focused, addressing specific life events. The case for longer-term, exploratory psychotherapy is more arguable.

Sexual problems

Adolescents become increasingly sexually active during their teenage years (Wyatt, 1990). One-third of them by 16 years and about three-quarters by 19 years have experienced sexual intercourse. Planned sexual activities are rare in early adolescence but increasingly, although not universally, so later.

Pregnancy

Around 10% of girls become pregnant between 15 and 19 years. In an American study of adolescent pregnancy (Zelnick *et al*, 1981), 47% gave birth, 40% had terminations of pregnancy, and the rest miscarried. Each of these outcomes is psychologically stressful. An increasing number of teenagers are delivering and continuing to care for their infants, a high risk for mother and child (Black, 1986). Most teenage pregnancies are unplanned. One in 15 may have been intentional. Motives for this include being accepted as an adult, having an object to nurture, getting one's own back on parents, and escaping from an unrewarding environment. Babies born to these mothers have an excess of low birth weight, neurological deficits, and early childhood illness. Maternal depression is not uncommon.

Support and counselling during and after pregnancy with supported return to education, or work, with shared care of the baby may allow the girl to resume her adolescent development. Early sex education and easy availability of contraception (as in Holland) helps to lower teenage pregnancy rates.

Sexual abuse

Not all sexual experiences of adolescents, and particularly those initiating them into sex, are by their own consent. Sexual abuse does not disappear in adolescence, and much of it is well established before entry into adolescence.

Presentation is often indirect. Mood disturbance is commonly seen; low self-esteem, with guilt and depressive episodes, frequently lead the girl or boy to request help. Self-damaging behaviour (self-injury, self-mutilation, eating disorders or substance abuse) may need exploration to uncover underlying sexual abuse. Interpersonal problems like social withdrawal, major uncertainty about social contacts, continuing discord with parents and teachers, with feelings of social inadequacy, are understandable reactions to abuse.

The adolescent may present with post-traumatic stress symptoms. There may be denial, or obsessive preoccupation with the details of abusive episodes. Unpredictable vivid flashbacks may occur. The victim may alternate between wishing to be alone and a fear of isolation. Somatic, particularly abdominal, complaints are common. Tense watchfulness with severe sleep problems may be present. Panic attacks, provoked by reminders of the abusive scene, may be a presenting feature. The girl may seek, defensively, to restrict the expression of any feeling. Dissociative disorders and Munchausen syndrome may be rooted in sexual abuse. Sexual dysfunction is a well documented consequence. Promiscuity or prostitution may be the end-result of abuse. Disgust and aversion to matters sexual is probably a commoner outcome.

Treatment of sexual abuse

Individual supportive and exploratory therapy seems appropriate. Group psychotherapy is commonly used. Work with the daughter and mother jointly may assist in mitigating the effects of disclosure, and family therapy, involving the perpetrator in cases of intrafamilial abuse, is important, once the victim has been protected from ongoing abuse. Work with the marital couple and any siblings is appropriate as well as with the whole family.

The results of such therapy seem to be variable. The various components of therapy still require careful research validation.

Substance abuse

There is widespread concern about the use of drugs by adolescents. The three commonest drugs in use by adolescents and adults are, however, tobacco, alcohol and cannabis. All of these are drugs sanctioned for use in various societies (Plant, 1987).

Tobacco

This substance has the widest potential for dependence and there is increasing concern about its availability to younger children. Its use (and accelerated damaging effects) is becoming common in females, including teenagers, whereas its use in males is slowly diminishing in Western society.

Alcohol

The use of alcohol is following a similar pattern. Early use is much more widespread. Its acute behavioural effects make it more dangerous than tobacco in the short term. It has an important role in antisocial behaviour and accidents, both of which are common in middle and late adolescence. By late adolescence a small number of people are showing the physical ravages and psychological deficits of dependence – often in the context of conduct disorders and antisocial personality problems.

Cannabis

Cannabis is the focus of media and public attention, but few casual users become dependent. Chronic over-use may result in passivity and self-neglect. Progression to the use of hard drugs is no more common among cannabis users than among cigarette smokers or alcohol users.

Solvents

The regular use of inhaled solvents, glues, cleaning fluids, and hair sprays may be hazardous, causing brain and liver damage, particularly with those containing toluene. Respiratory and cardiac arrest may occur where propellants from aerosols are inhaled, and 1 % of deaths among 10–19-year-old boys are caused by solvent abuse.

Other drugs

Heroin, cocaine, amphetamines, benzodiazepines, and hallucinogens such as phencyclidine and LSD are much more rarely used in adolescence, in spite of media exposure of cases. One needs to look at the context of such drug use in great detail. Those who abuse drugs may have major psychological and personal problems in which drug misuse plays only a part. Delinquent activity may increase to pay for 'a habit' but is usually present before drug abuse becomes established. Most drug use begins for social reasons. Few adolescents become 'hooked' on single doses, even with more powerful drugs like heroin or the 'crack' form of cocaine.

Acute toxic effects

The use of illicit drugs may cause psychological disturbance (e.g. the bad LSD 'trip') but they rarely cause chronic psychological difficulties unless drug taking becomes central to the adolescent's life. Health effects are often secondary to the use of illegally obtained supplies, for example toxicity from additives or impurities, infections such as septicaemia, hepatitis B or HIV (spread by unclean shared needles).

Reasons for drug use

Peer pressure and identification with a drug-using subculture

Where the peer group has an antisocial or a pro-drugs attitude, the adolescent with a strong sense of identification with the group may use drugs as a 'membership' token. A stable use of drugs with little dependence may occur.

Parent–child relationships

Either direct modelling (e.g. alcohol abuse in the parents) or rebellion against neglectful parents may contribute to drug use in the adolescent.

Escape from the pressure of life or boredom

Alcohol is the traditional drug for these purposes and is socially sanctioned in many countries for such use.

Management

Volatile substances such as glues and aerosols are usually used by younger adolescents. Tobacco is also particularly prone to early use, as is alcohol.

Opiates, stimulants and hallucinogens enter the scene in middle and late adolescence. Most drugs are used recreationally. It is only when their use becomes central to the adolescent's life, is associated with physical damage and social dysfunction, or shows evidence of being needed in increasing amounts to prevent severe withdrawal effects, that psychiatric intervention becomes necessary.

Where there is stable use, the options of abstinence or controlled use need to be examined. Substitute drugs may be used for short periods, for example benzodiazepines for alcohol withdrawal; weak nicotine-containing compounds for tobacco; methadone for opiates. Local alcohol or drug-abuse services or voluntary organisations orientated to adult disorder may be consulted, but also social support for the adolescent from the family and peer group should be sought. Hospital admission should be reserved for physical complications or abuse-related psychiatric conditions.

Emotional disorders

These disorders include anxiety states, obsessional disorders, conversion disorders, and depressive conditions.

Depressive disorders

The mood state of depression is hard to assess in younger adolescents who may not possess an adequate vocabulary of emotional *expression* or whose cognitive development may not have reached a stage where the nuances of interpretation of emotional *experience* are possible. Adults are often unaware of the intensity of feeling which adolescents experience (Rutter, 1986).

Feelings of depression

Low mood, of itself, does not imply clinical depression in adolescents. Depressive feelings are markedly more common after puberty. In the Isle of Wight study (Rutter *et al*, 1976), 42% of boys and 48% of girls at 14 years reported appreciable feelings of misery. Nearly 20% of boys and 23% of girls had self-deprecatory feelings. Sadness and a gloomy outlook on the future are likely to be present in normal adolescents.

Depressive syndromes

The pervasiveness of depression, its unresponsiveness to social stimulation, and its prolongation beyond any provoking event mark depressive syndromes off from less significant mood states. Irritability, especially in a previously placid person, especially where guilt over such behaviour is prominent, may mark a shift into a depressive illness. A loss of pleasure in normally enjoyed activities may lead to a giving up, first of pleasures (e.g. visits to friends, hobbies, leisure activities) and then of duties (e.g. homework and school work) as the depression deepens. A feeling of anergy, a loss of vitality, may raise the possibility of physical illness.

Biological symptoms such as loss of appetite with a falling food intake leading to weight loss with sleep disturbance (not necessarily early morning waking until late in the episode) are seen in unipolar and the depressive phase of bipolar illness in adolescence. Cognitive change may also be seen. Feelings of pervasive helplessness and hopelessness about the future and recovery are common in moderate to severe depression. In younger adolescents, the recurrent thought that one is unloved, in spite of evidence to the contrary, is common. Guilt is rare in younger depressives. Tearfulness and misery may be concealed, especially in the early part of the illness, to avoid upsetting parents. Suicidal ideas are common in adolescence. They are discussed in detail below.

In the Isle of Wight study (Rutter *et al*, 1976) such clinically significant depression was found in 0.45% of the 14–15-year-olds. Other studies have shown higher rates of clinical disorder, from 2.1% to 8% (Crisp *et al*, 1981).

Co-morbidity

Although pure depressive disorders can occur, the parallel occurrence of other conditions is far from uncommon. Rutter *et al* (1976) found depression and anxiety occurred together in 1.3% of adolescents.

As many as a third of conduct-disordered patients may have clinically significant depressive feelings.

Separation anxiety disorders with school refusal are commonly accompanied by major depression. Overanxious individuals and those with social phobias may also be depressed.

Significant depression is found both in anorexia nervosa and even more often in bulimic syndromes.

Depressive affect frequently complicates the lives of adolescents with disorders like cystic fibrosis and Duchenne muscular dystrophy. How far these are understandable reactions to life-threatening disorders may depend on careful clinical assessment.

Physical complaints are common in adolescents, who have a high degree of body awareness. After certain viral infections, notably infectious mononucleosis and hepatitis, depressive symptoms may be seen as part of the post-viral fatigue syndrome. Suggestions of cellular abnormalities in muscle and brain after enteroviral infections await elucidation as an associated feature of these symptoms (David *et al*, 1988).

Aetiology of depression

This is no more clear in adolescence than it is in adult syndromes. The family history may incline one to a biological basis for the illness. This is certainly true for bipolar illness in adolescence. The evidence for a biological basis for other depressive syndromes is less sure. Whether the modelling effect of a depressive parent establishes similar responses to stress in adolescent offspring is under investigation. A plausible mechanism is the mediating role of changed parental behaviour in depression. The hormonal changes combined with the strain of acquiring new social roles set in train during adolescence may combine to produce dysthymia of clinical proportions. There is evidence for the role of past loss or recent loss as predisposing and triggering events. Personality traits of perfectionism and pressure to achieve may set the scene for mood disorder in adolescence but how common such traits are in depressed individuals is not yet established.

Investigation

Physical examination should be mandatory in all adolescents presenting with depressive syndromes. Full blood count with an estimation of erythrocyte sedimentation rate will give a simple screen for an underlying physical illness. Tests such as the dexamethasone suppression test, growth hormone secretion studies or studies of sleep architecture using electroencephalography are not sufficiently sensitive for routine use in adolescents.

Treatment

A diagnosis of a depressive illness may be a great relief to the adolescent sufferer and the family. It will allow a treatment programme to be constructed.

Sleep, appetite and energy deficits as prominent features of the illness suggest a more 'biological' disorder. The prescription of a tricyclic antidepressant has some equivocal support from the literature in younger adolescents. With older adolescents the proven response in adults make the ground for medication surer. Relatively higher doses are recommended for older children (up to 5 mg/kg/day, although the higher end of this range should be covered with regular electrocardiographic monitoring). Single night-time dose schedules seem to be effective. The length of treatment necessary will probably be judged by trial and error, often depending on the efficacy of other interventions.

No formal trials of cognitive–behavioural methods have been undertaken in adolescents, but clinical practice indicates their value, even in young adolescents (Start *et al*, 1991). The behavioural aspects of the treatment may be more salient. Assessment will need to be carefully and imaginatively undertaken to 'tune in' to the thinking processes of the adolescent patient. Challenges to dysfunctional thinking should be gentle and in the context of a good working relationship with the therapist. Deficits in social skills may be found to be impeding the implementation of therapy tasks. If such deficits are found, systematic teaching of these skills should be undertaken.

The illness can be explained in family sessions. The family can help in implementing behavioural homework, reinforcing more positive thinking and supporting renewed involvement in activities. Exploratory work into any difficulty in emotional expression or any other communication problems resulting from the depressive state may also be valuable.

Individual or group psychotherapy may be a valuable addition in those cases where there is a more chronic, low-grade depression. Life events may have triggered the episode and their consequences may need to be explored. Chronic grief which has shifted into depressive illness may benefit from such an approach.

Suicide and self-harm

Concept of death

By 10 years all children understand that death is universal and will happen to them at some time. Death may preoccupy some adolescents, and discussions of death-related themes will be found in the school essays and diaries of normal adolescents. In the Isle of Wight study (Rutter *et al*, 1976), 7.6% of 14-year-olds expressed suicidal thoughts at interview. Most adolescents will not be morbidly preoccupied, a few will have made vague plans for self-harm, and even fewer will have carried out those plans (Shaw *et al*, 1987).

The presence of depressive symptoms will set the context for assessing the seriousness of such activities. Heavy weight should be given to such thoughts where there is current family disturbance, a family history of suicide or a history of, or evidence of current, child abuse.

Suicide

The rate of completed suicide doubled in 15–19-year-olds between 1950 and 1980. Between 10 and 14 years, the rate has remained relatively static. Males out-numbered females, 2–3 to 1. In older adolescents it is the third commonest cause of death. Some 'accidental' deaths (e.g. 'accidental' drug overdose, road traffic accidents) may be disguised suicides (Hawton, 1985).

Completed suicide may be a response to anticipated disciplinary action; this is especially likely after previous (recent) threats or attempts. Absence from school may provide an opportunity, and recent psychiatric illness, especially psychosis, in a family member may be the trigger. More remote associations may be high or low intelligence, and height above the 50th centile (possibly because of unrealistic expectations for the taller child). Conduct disorder with or without depressive symptoms may be present (Shaffer, 1974).

No single predictor is always present. Sustained hopelessness seems to be an ominous sign, as is evidence of premeditation (e.g. suicide notes) and planning (e.g. saving pills).

Self-harm

Self-harm is usually impulsive (Hawton *et al*, 1982). It peaks in late adolescence and is more common in females. It may be more life threatening than the adolescent intended. The use of drugs without a true appreciation of their effects, for example, may lead to delayed liver toxicity after ingestion of paracetamol. Failure of discovery may add to the hazards of self-harm. Opportunity may determine the choice of agents used. Thus, younger adolescents may take analgesics, older adolescents psychotropics. Alcohol is frequently involved, adding to medical complications.

The risk of repetition

The highest risk of repetition is seen in older males from large families, especially where there are disturbed family relationships, and particularly where this involves alcohol abuse. They often have long-standing personality and psychiatric problems. Of those who harm themselves once, 15–25% will do so again within a year, and 1–2% of those attempting suicide will eventually succeed (Hawton *et al*, 1982).

In those with mild to moderate conduct disorder, family disturbance or who live away from their families, short-term crises may precipitate self-harm. Such cases are at moderate risk of repetition. More acute instances of self-harm may be in reaction to acute stresses such as arguments with boyfriends or parents, and are less likely to be repeated. The peculiar dysphoric mood associated with self-harm is often relieved by the act of cutting, and such cutting, therefore, is very prone to repetition because of this dysphoria-reducing effect.

Motives for self-harm

Common themes are "I just wanted relief", "I just wanted to get away", "I wanted them to know how bad I felt", "I wanted to make them sorry for what they did to me", "I'll make them change their mind", "I'll make them show they love me", "I'll find out if they really love me", "I'll make them help me". Many adolescents may give a mixture of these reasons for self-harm.

Associated features

Early loss of a parent, particularly if the family is disrupted as a result, may be found in the histories of self-harm patients. A lack of emotional warmth in the family, current poor family relationships, especially with the father, are not uncommon. A history of physical ill-treatment and current sexual abuse are frequent stresses found in such teenagers. There may be a model of self-injurious behaviour in the family or among the peer group. Media models (e.g. soap operas) have a definite influence on such behaviour.

The triggers to self-harm are often disputes with parents or a boy- or girl-friend. School or work problems or sibling conflict also may push the adolescent to act in this way. Current psychiatric problems in a parent may result in teenagers injuring themselves. Such difficulties lead to short-lived anger and misery, followed quickly by self-injuring behaviour (Taylor & Stansfield, 1984).

Management

Assessment may be undertaken by trained junior medical staff, junior psychiatrists, or nurses under psychiatric supervision, depending on local policies.

Adolescents under 16 should always be admitted for assessment, preferably to an adolescent or paediatric ward (Black, 1982). Social work contact may need to be arranged if assistance with social problems is needed. Early review in the psychiatric out-patient department or community service should be offered.

Acute impulsive acts of self-harm require psychiatric assessment on the ward as soon as possible. If no continuing psychiatric disorder is present, a prompt letter or telephone call to the general practitioner will allow early community follow-up. More disturbed self-harming patients should be further assessed; early interviews with family and friends will allow the patient's social supports to be evaluated. Before the patient leaves the ward, the general practitioner should be contacted.

Where chronic disorder is found, with a risk of repetition being high, a short-term psychiatric admission may be advisable. This is usually to an adult ward as in-patient adolescent units, though preferable, are rarely available or sufficiently secure for such patients. This will allow the assessment of any mood disorder and reduce the risk of early repetition of self-harm. A case discussion with all involved agencies may allow a support treatment plan to be developed. In rare instances, admission to an adolescent in-patient unit (for further assessment and treatment) may be negotiated.

Anxiety states

Anxiety states in younger adolescents grow out of the fears which are common at this stage of development. They include: fear of political events (e.g. war), the future and natural phenomena (e.g. thunder). Personal appearance, personal relationships and school performance are common foci for anxiety. Fears for the safety of home and family, for personal safety, and about gender identity are features of anxious adolescents.

Any of these may assume phobic proportions, more commonly in girls. In older adolescents, more adult-style disorders, such as social phobias, agoraphobia, panic disorder and generalised anxiety disorder become established (Gittelman, 1986).

Case example

A 13-year-old girl presented with panic attacks two months after her grandmother died of a ruptured aortic aneurysm. Attacks were mainly nocturnal and caused her mother to spend up to two hours holding and reassuring her. Occasional attacks, during the day, meant she could not go shopping or to the cinema with friends. After six months of attacks and extensive medical tests, she was referred to a psychiatry department.

She presented as a pert, bouncy girl with marked separation anxieties, who was beginning to fail at school because of anxiety. She did, however, also show depressive symptoms such as loss of appetite and weight and general social withdrawal. Marked hyperventilation, with tingling of fingers and dizziness, was observed during one of her attacks. Prescription of a brown paper bag for re-breathing, amitriptyline for her depression and family therapy for the inhibited grieving over the grandmother resulted in a marked improvement in her symptoms and social functioning.

Presentation of anxiety disorders

In separation anxiety disorders, the patient feels secure only in the presence of attachment figures. School refusal is a prominent symptom in younger adolescents, the patient being worried about the health or safety of their parents in their absence. Though sometimes founded on realistic threats to parents (e.g. illness or suicidal gesture), such fears often are extended well beyond what is reasonable. Anger and fear may be experienced together when separation is threatened. In older adolescents, such separation anxieties may shade into panic disorders and agoraphobia.

Particular aspects of school (e.g. fear of crowded assemblies, or undressing for sports, or of particular teachers or subjects) may represent true school phobia. Where more general anxiety is dominant, unrealistic concerns over future events, or excessive fear of personal failure with constant demands for reassurance are often present. Marked self-consciousness and a fear of meeting unfamiliar people are part of a picture of anxious avoidance.

Physical symptoms such as abdominal pain and headache are common and hyperventilation, with shallow, rapid breathing, often contributes to such physical presentation because of the biochemical changes induced.

Aetiology

In about one-third of cases there is a family history of phobic or panic disorder.

Stressful life events are common triggers to anxiety problems and mild neurological impairment in childhood is associated with later anxiety. Social withdrawal as a personality trait is often found in clinically anxious adolescents.

Co-morbidity

Major depression is common, especially in separation anxiety disorders and where there is any degree of generalised anxiety.

Treatment

Exposure to feared situations is recommended, through relaxation training, followed by graduated exposure in imagination. Behavioural rehearsal of feared scenes, with role-playing by the therapist, prepares the patient for *in-vivo* exposure, which is the central plank of treatment.

Treatment of parental anxiety, if appropriate, will allow the patient a better model of anxiety management.

Support for parental firmness in the face of the patient's panic will allow the therapist to help expose the patient to feared situations. Exploration of ambivalence about independence, for both patient and family, will allow any underlying problem to be dealt with.

Group work is useful for training of assertiveness and relationship skills.

Cognitive therapy or psychodynamic exploratory therapy is indicated for abnormal perceptions of threat and specific anxieties.

Imipramine may be useful in school refusal. Short-term, short-acting benzodiazepines allow anxiety confrontation and propranolol or other beta-blockers may reduce disabling physiological symptoms.

Obsessional disorders

Rapoport (1986) has suggested the prevalence of obsessional disorders in adolescents is 1 in 250. Symptoms in younger adolescents centre on grooming and washing rituals, in late adolescence ruminations, doubts and obsessional slowness make their appearance.

Case example

A 17-year-old boy presented with an inability to go into certain buildings because of vague fears of contamination. At interview he sidled through the door, avoiding touching the frame. He reported that he had given up the piano because he feared infection from touching the keys. Study (he was an extremely able pupil) was almost impossible because of inability to begin work for fear of making mistakes. He tyrannised his parents into providing him with a restricted range of 'clean' foods and an endless supply of clean clothes, which he changed several times a day. His illness had begun when his older brother had gone to university. His parents were anxious people and his mother had a history of depression.

Response prevention and thought stopping combined with clomipramine reduced his fears and associated rituals. Family work backed this by re-enforcing parental firmness in the face of his demands. He remains a rather perfectionistic young man with few friends but has since gained a university place. In his new environment he still shows ritualistic behaviour.

Treatment

Clomipramine, the tricyclic antidepressant, and serotonin reuptake inhibitors such as fluoxetine, seem to be moderately effective in alleviating symptoms. Response prevention (Chapter 10), both of thoughts and actions, in alliance with the adolescent's family or partner will assist the ritual aspects of the disorder. Obsessional symptoms may reappear, especially if there is a depressive mood change.

Hysteria (abnormal illness behaviour)

Traditionally, abnormal illness behaviour and hysterical disorders have been separated in psychiatric diagnostic classifications. Abnormal illness behaviour was seen as the prolongation of symptoms after an acute illness or failure to recover, for example after surgery, without demonstrable organic reasons for this. Hysteria was seen as a more active process of symptom production, either conversion or dissociative symptoms, caused by inefficiently repressed anxiety. It is doubtful whether such distinctions are helpful clinically as the two views may represent points on a continuum of severity. In both cases, underlying pathology, either physical or psychological (e.g. depressive disorder, anxiety states), should be sought.

One should always be wary of hysterical disorders – they may be reactions to underlying somatic illness, especially neurological disorder such as metachromatic leucodystrophy, hepatolenticular degeneration (Wilson's disease) or early-onset Huntington's chorea.

Disorders of gait and vision are rare, disorders of speech and consciousness less so. Pain is rarely a conversion symptom but may be part of a depressive disorder. Prolongation of symptoms after an illness is not uncommon, particularly if the illness is not clear cut or is overinvestigated.

Aetiology

Anxiety, perhaps caused by an uncertain diagnosis of illness, may provoke physical symptoms. If there is a family or peer model of illness, the permitted exemption from duties and responsibilities may serve to reinforce illness behaviour.

In closed communities such as barracks for young army recruits, boarding schools for teenage girls or nurses' homes, illness in one or a small group of prominent individuals may provoke symptoms in the group ('epidemic hysteria'). There are still arguments about how much such symptoms are related to viral infections or to behavioural modelling.

Case example

"I've had a stroke doctor", were the opening words of an interview on a neurological ward of a 14-year-old boy who had presented with headache and apparent left hemiparesis. A long history of minor physical complaints was given, with recent deterioration in behaviour at school. Family investigation revealed a rigid-thinking father who found it hard to express emotion. He did not heed his son's emotional signals. The father's business had recently failed because of fraud by a business partner and the family home was under threat because it was part of the business. Early discharge of the boy with a combination of individual sessions centred on the boy's low self-esteem and family sessions which allowed renegotiation of the father–son relationship improved the difficulties. The hemiparesis disappeared within two days of discharge from hospital and no new symptoms appeared.

Tourette's syndrome

Symptoms

Many normal children (5-7%) will have isolated tics in the primary-school years. Most of these disappear spontaneously. In late childhood, motor tics (involving face and neck) are presenting features of multiple tic disorder. At puberty, some of these ticquers will develop vocal tics such as throat clearing, coughing, explosive exhalations. Of these patients, 30-40% will shape these utterances into obscenities. Obscene gestures and echolalia will be found in a minority.

There are strong connections between this more severe form of tic disorder (Tourette's syndrome) and obsessive–compulsive states and attention deficit disorders.

Treatment

Dopamine antagonists (e.g. haloperidol, pimozide, sulpiride) are the main drugs used. Muscle relaxation training is a valuable adjunct to drug therapy, as is repeated voluntary performance of involuntary movements (massed practice) (Robertson, 1989). If major obsessional symptoms are present, the addition of a serotonin reuptake inhibitor (e.g. fluvoxamine) may be needed. The α-adrenergic agonist clonidine has also been used with variable success for the basic tic disorder.

Psychotic disorders

Schizophrenia

Schizophrenia is uncommon before puberty and extremely rare before the age of seven years. As adolescence progresses, classic schizophrenia becomes commoner. In the main, it is a disorder of boys rather than girls.

In children and younger adolescents, the Schneiderian first-rank symptoms are not so obvious and may require careful detailed clinical examination to reveal them. A history of passivity and a short attention span in infancy, with poor emotional control in school, have been found to presage an early onset of psychosis (Parnas *et al*, 1982).

In later childhood and early adolescence, the onset of the illness is characterised by vagueness of thought, circumstantial and tangential thinking, with illogical associations and confusion between categories of ideas. The clinical impression conveyed is one of blunted affect and denial of disorder, with marked evasiveness and suspicion. The mood may be one of intermittent fear and diffuse distress, in contrast to manic patients who are expansive and grandiose but often irritable. The prognosis for early-onset schizophrenia is poor, especially in the presence of neurological impairment (clumsiness, dyspraxias, developmental language abnormalities). Many of these children progress to deficit states, with negative symptoms predominating.

The core symptoms of the disorder are delusions of control, thought insertion, broadcast or withdrawal, auditory hallucinations in the third person and auditory hallucinations addressing the patient but not congruent with the mood state (in the absence of physical illness or clouding of consciousness). Loosening of association between thoughts, bizarre, frequent jumps of thought, flattening of emotional expression and paranoid ideas may occur. Social withdrawal is often seen in schizophrenic adolescents, combined with marked social and educational difficulties.

Case example
A 15-year-old boy presented with auditory hallucinations, especially in the evening. These voices spoke to each other about him. Their comments were usually derogatory. They sometimes told him to do things which he resisted, such as opening the doors or teasing his dog. Sometimes the voices were distinct (when it was quiet), sometimes less clear (when he turned his radio on). He was fearful of the voices.

In early childhood he had complex partial seizures and he had specific learning problems with reading. At nine, he presented with an acute onset of auditory hallucinations at school.

He now had fleeting glimpses of small dark animals who left an odd smell. These were present both at home and in the hospital ward. He believed that (and drew) the animals had a machine in the top corner of the room which forced him to sleep when he did not wish to do so. He had no mood disturbance to account for these perceptions.

On examination he was a quiet, affable young man, having completed his pubertal growth and sexual development early. His parents split up during his first illness, his father having rejected his asocial, 'un-macho' son. He lived with his mother, who was protective of him. A good but partial response to chlorpromazine allowed him to live at home. He was pleasant but had no friends and spent his time out of school listening to music and walking his dog. He attended a school for mildly learning-disabled pupils, where he fitted in well educationally but had made no close friends. The diagnosis made at nine and currently confirmed is schizophrenia.

Diagnostic difficulties

Affective symptoms

Many first episodes of psychoses presenting in adolescence will be diagnosed as schizophrenic when they are, in fact, manic disorders. Formal thought disorder may occur in both disorders in the acute phase. In manic patients there is less likely to be the prodromal loosening of thought structure and poverty of thought and relationships.

As the prognosis is better in manic patients it is important to maintain the distinction. Treatment of the conditions is also different, especially in the long term.

Depressive symptoms in schizophrenia are not uncommon and need to be closely monitored. They are an integral part of the psychosis and often improve with control of the other acute symptoms.

Close observation, with charting of symptoms and recording of mood changes, will elucidate the diagnosis.

Expression of symptoms

In early adolescence, confusion of thought and fluctuating bizarreness with anxiety may dominate. Intense preoccupations with fantasy and outbursts of rage without provocation may also occur. Formed delusions may not be common, though an exaggeration of normal anxieties (e.g. about body parts) may be found.

Confusion with personality features

Where pre-existing features such as social withdrawal or unusual patterns of thought are prominent, the shift into illness may seem like a normal adolescent shift in thinking. The content of thought is usually less understandable, when examined, and has a more ill-structured content than that of a normal adolescent.

Schizoid personality traits are not a frequent precursor of schizophrenia; such adolescents are more likely to remain odd, withdrawn people into adult life.

Aetiology

This is still unsettled. Adult psychiatric texts (e.g. Gelder *et al*, 1989) should be consulted for detail.

Treatment

Physical assessment, especially careful neurological survey, is necessary.

Medication should be prescribed after explanation of the illness to the patient. Chlorpromazine, haloperidol and sulpiride in the initial stages are the commonest drugs used. Dosage should be titrated against clinical response. Anti-Parkinsonian agents may be prescribed, especially in younger patients, as akathisia and restlessness may cause distress – such reactions are said to be more severe in those below 14 years. This should not be done routinely. Anxiolytics may be helpful if sleep disorder or panic is present. Depot preparations for older patients ensure compliance and promote normal routines.

Supportive counselling may reduce distress. Family work with education about the disease, aiming to reduce overprotection and hostility, is a valuable way of reducing the chances of relapse (Vaughn, 1989). Social skills training, either individually or in a small group, can be helpful in rehabilitation.

Prognosis

All of the following features augur well for recovery (Eggers, 1978): higher intelligence, a normal electroencephalogram, acute or relatively late onset, prominent affective symptoms, and a warm, friendly personality.

Manic-depressive disorder

About a fifth to a quarter of adult bipolar illness begins in adolescence, and this presages more frequent episodes, and a higher risk of suicide (Smith & Winokur, 1984). There is often a strong family history of bipolar illness.

The onset of mania is usually acute and there are mood-congruent delusions. Catatonic symptoms may occur. There may have been a previous hypomanic episode in response to antidepressant medication.

The depressive phase of the illness may present with psychomotor retardation and major biological symptoms (e.g. sleep disturbance, appetite and weight loss).

Treatment

Lithium carbonate is an effective treatment, once the acute phase has been controlled by neuroleptic or antidepressant drugs (Carlson, 1990).

Eating disorders

These are the classic disorders of adolescence. Anorexia nervosa and bulimia nervosa are the two central syndromes. Obesity of itself is not a psychiatric disorder but may produce mood and relationship difficulties.

Anorexia nervosa

The peak prevalence of anorexia is around 17 years. Girls are affected up to 10 times more often than boys. The prevalence rate in independent girls' schools is 1 in 100 after 16 years, but only 1 in 300 among girls at comprehensive school. It is rare in males, Afro-Caribbeans and Asians (Crisp, 1983).

Case example

A 14-year-old girl athlete presented with vague physical symptoms. Her height and weight were below the 3rd centile for age. She had a vigorous programme of running which she undertook with her father, but she outlasted him in stamina.

She disliked a wide range of foods but her intake had been even more restricted after a friend had suggested she was fat. She and her mother were dieters, comparing notes on their progress or lack of it. Both were good cooks. She had few teenage friends and, though of only average IQ, she was academically in the top ten of her school group.

On presentation she was a thin, restless girl, resentful of psychiatric intervention, sure that she had a physical disorder. Her parents were equally sceptical. She was prepubertal. The family was a socially isolated one with the traditional social roles of the mining village in which they lived; the father worked and the housewife mother did not challenge her husband's views even when she disagreed with them. The views of the women in the extended family had a major influence on this family's functioning. Neither parent wished their two girls, aged 14 and 16, to be independent; this view was shared by the teenagers.

Anorexia nervosa was diagnosed. The patient herself was able to acknowledge her fears of weight gain and, paradoxically, her anger at her family for failing to help her gain her independence. These insights allowed her to distance herself from her family's 'enmeshment' and to eat more normally with some, but fewer, restrictions.

In-patient admission failed to engage the patient and her family, and though weight gain and eating patterns normalised, psychologically little changed. She was later referred to the local adolescent service with a relapse of her restricted eating, where family work was more successful in acknowledging (and changing) the mutual overdependence of all the family members.

Presentation

There is failure to acknowledge an eating problem, with insistent fear of normal weight and shape. An obsession with size of particular body parts (e.g. thighs, buttocks) and disgust at the thought of fatness are central features. Voluntary starvation, especially of carbohydrate and fat, leads to a preoccupation with food, intense hunger, and a distorted body image. Amenorrhoea, sometimes the first symptom, is inevitable. Emaciation may be disguised by bulky clothing. A high activity level is kept up. Lanugo hair is found on the body, and cold blue or white limbs are evident. Secret vomiting may produce major biochemical upset.

Investigations

The general denial of ill-health makes organic disease unlikely. Normal levels of thyroxine and thyroid stimulating hormone exclude hypothyroidism. Blood counts

may show lymphopenia; levels of luteinising hormone (LH) and follicular stimulating hormone (FSH) in blood are low and non-cyclical. Hypokalaemia needs
to be monitored. Neurological assessment is mandatory.

Aetiology

This is still uncertain. Some adolescents begin their disorder with amenorrhoea,
which may predate other symptoms and may indicate hypothalamic dysfunction.

In our culture of slimness, the ideal female figure is portrayed as having
almost prepubertal characteristics. The rates of anorexia nervosa are increased
in athletes, modelling and ballet students, and may represent exaggerations
of cultural expectations in these groups.

An overemphasis on issues of food as emotional 'currency' and conflicts
over control may be part of the family lifestyle. There may be fear of normal
development. Premorbid perfectionism and histrionic traits are often also
found.

Abnormal family process, as a cause, is much discussed, but rarely
investigated systematically. Overinvolvement and devaluing of individuality,
suppression of emotional expression, associated with promotion of dependence,
and self-sacrifice in the interests of family unity are all suggested family patterns
in relation to this disorder.

Treatment

A structured programme of targeted weight increase (½–1 kg a week), either
as an in-patient or a closely supervised out-patient, is an essential first step.
Monitoring of LH/FSH levels of the blood gives an objective measure of return
to more normal functionings. Skinfold thickness is a more accurate long-term
measure of nutrition than weight alone.

Psychodynamic exploratory therapy to examine autonomy, control and self-
image can be introduced after restoration of weight. Mood disorder may require
careful attention. Cognitive–behavioural therapy, with examination of abnormal
perceptions, attitudes and affects, and behavioural tasks reinforce changes.
Education about nutrition and the effects of starvation is helpful.

Family therapy is particularly effective with younger patients with less
chronic disorders (Russell *et al*, 1987). Early work focusing on parental control
and monitoring of the patient's eating is followed by the exploration of marital
and generational conflicts. Close support of the family by the therapist during
this, often painful, process is necessary. The management of rebellion by the
patient in the family is a later issue in therapy.

Outcome

About half of most series of anorectic patients make a good recovery, at least
as far as weight is concerned (Hsu *et al*, 1979). About a quarter of patients

improve but with persistent diet control and often unstable social relationships. At least 5% become bulimic. Mood disturbance may remain severe. It is a point of argument as to whether early onset indicates a good prognosis or not. Chronicity at presentation and repeated vomiting and purging tend to lead to a poorer long-term outcome.

About 5% will die of suicide, biochemical chaos, inanition or acute gastric dilatation and its effects.

Bulimic disorders

These usually present in late adolescence or early adult life in women. They involve rapid consumption of food in large quantities over short periods of time. This is done in secret, with a mounting sense of guilt. Self-induced vomiting occurs and becomes easier with repetition. Weight is thus regulated, usually within the normal range. Calluses on the fingers from induction of vomiting, damage to tooth enamel (on posterior tooth surfaces) and parotid enlargement are consequences of vomiting. Biochemical disorder may be found coincidentally.

Prominent depression and guilt often cause the patient to present to doctors. The struggle between dietary restriction and loss of control occurs in the context of good social relationships. The patient is aware of the abnormality of her behaviour, unlike anorectics.

Aetiology

Bulimic symptoms can occur as a part of anorexia nervosa or as part of a pattern of normal-weight regulation in those with low self-esteem and insecurity in their gender role. They may also be a manifestation of a depressive condition or an issue in a struggle for impulse control.

Treatment

Cognitive–behavioural treatment and medication with fluoxetine seem to be the most effective treatments for this condition.

Adolescent manifestations of childhood-onset disorders

Infantile autism

In more able, autistic adolescents, language abnormalities may be more subtle but more obvious in social situations than in childhood. Social gaucheness replaces social withdrawal in familiar surroundings. Epilepsy begins in about 15% of patients (and in about one-third of mentally retarded autistic adolescents). Ten per cent may show a major deterioration in language and cognitive functioning, the reason for which is obscure at present (Gillberg, 1984).

Pubertal development is usually normal, and the mismatch between sexual drive and social skills may cause difficulties and embarrassment to adolescents and their families.

Learning disabilities

As with autistic patients, those with learning disabilities (formerly known as the mentally retarded) in adolescence will often show major deficits in social skills, in contrast to their normal sexual and physical development. Mood may be more unstable and aggressive responses to frustration may be more frequent. Education at an appropriate cognitive level, with sexual counselling and occupational guidance, may be needed for the individual. Simple counselling may be appropriate to allow the learning disabled adolescent to form relationships and avoid exploitation. Psychiatric assessment may be necessary for a small number as they are at higher risk of psychoses and other psychiatric disorder than the general population.

Parents are older and may need respite care to help them to go on caring for their disabled child.

Hyperactivity

Attention deficits become less prominent in hyperactive children in adolescence. Activity levels tend to fall but restless impulsivity continues. Major secondary conduct disorders are common, as is family rejection of the untreated. Mood instability seems a frequent difficulty for such adolescents. There are continuing disagreements about whether such sufferers have an excess of alcohol and drug abuse.

Behavioural therapy seems more effective than drug therapy alone (Hechtman *et al*, 1984). Psychotherapy for the patient to deal with low self-esteem and the effects of rejection, with family therapy for the secondary conduct problems, is appropriate. Learning disorders, which are frequently associated, should already be receiving remedial educational help.

Non-medical help

With all of these disabled young people, extended education should be available. Social and vocational, rather than purely academic, aspects should be emphasised. Full use of training facilities and information on social security benefits should be readily available. Social groups and family supports need to be provided to enlarge experience and prevent secondary behavioural difficulties.

G

Conclusion

Psychiatric disorders in adolescence are relatively rare, but most are rewarding to treat. Such treatment will restore the adolescent to the healthy majority who pass through this developmental period with only minor problems and are only transiently a burden to their families and the community at large.

References

Alexander, J. F., Barton, C., Schiavo, R. S., *et al* (1976) Systems behavioral interventions with the families of delinquents. *Journal of Consulting and Clinical Psychology*, **44**, 656-664.

Berg, I., Consterdine, M., Hullin, R., *et al* (1987) A randomly controlled trial of two court procedures in truancy. *British Journal of Criminology*, **18**, 232-244.

Black, D. (1986) Schoolgirl mothers. *British Medical Journal*, **293**, 1047.

Black, M. (1982) The management of parasuicide in young people under sixteen. *Bulletin of the Royal College of Psychiatrists*, **6**, 182-185.

Carlson, G. A. (1990) Child and adolescent mania: diagnostic considerations. *Journal of Child Psychology and Psychiatry*, **31**, 331-342.

Crisp, A. H. (1983) Anorexia nervosa. *British Medical Journal*, **287**, 855-858.

——, Alder, A. G., Isacoff, M., *et al* (1981) Depression: symptoms versus diagnosis in 10,412 hospitalized children and adolescents (1957-1977). *American Journal of Psychotherapy*, **35**, 400-412.

David, S. A., Wessley, S. & Pelosi, A. J. (1988) Postviral fatigue syndrome. Time for a new approach. *British Medical Journal*, **296**, 696-700.

Eggers, C. (1978) Course and prognosis of childhood schizophrenia. *Journal of Autism and Childhood Schizophrenia*, **8**, 21-36.

Feindler, E. L., Elton, R. B., Kingsley, D., *et al* (1986) Group anger control for institutionalized male adolescents. *Behaviour Therapy*, **17**, 109-123.

Gelder, M., Gath, D. & Mayou, R. (1989) Aetiology of schizophrenia. In *Oxford Textbook of Psychiatry*. Oxford: Oxford Medical Publications.

Gillberg, C. (1984) Autistic children grown-up. Problems during puberty and adolescence. *Developmental Medicine and Child Neurology*, **26**, 125-129.

Gittelman, R. (1986) Childhood anxiety disorder, correlates and outcomes. In *Anxiety Disorders of Childhood* (ed. R. Gittelman). New York: Guilford Press.

Hawton, K. (1985) *Suicide and Attempted Suicide Among Children and Adolescents*. Newbury Park: Sage.

——, O'Grady, J., Osborn, M., *et al* (1982) Adolescents who take overdoses. Their characteristics, problems and contact with helping agencies. *British Journal of Psychiatry*, **140**, 124-131.

Hechtman, L., Weiss, G., Perlman, T., *et al* (1984) Hyperactives as young adults. Initial predictors of adult outcomes. *Journal of the American Academy of Child Psychiatry*, **23**, 250-260.

Hsu, L. K. G., Crisp, A. H. & Harding, B. (1979) The outcome of anorexia nervosa. *Lancet*, *i*, 61-65.

Kazdin, A. E. (1987) *Conduct Disorders in Childhood and Adolescence*. Newbury Park: Sage.

Kolko, D. J. & Kazdin, A. W. (1991) Motives of fire-setters: fire setting characteristics and psychological correlates. *Journal of Child Psychology and Psychiatry*, **32**, 535-550.

Nottelmann, E., Inoff-Germain, G., Susman, E. J., *et al* (1990) Hormones and behaviour at puberty. In *Adolescence and Puberty* (eds J. Bancroft & J. M. Reinisch). New York: Oxford University Press.

Olweus, D. (1979) Stability of aggressive reaction patterns in males. A review. *Psychological Bulletin*, **86**, 852-875.

Parnas, J., Schulsinger, F., Teasdale, T. W., *et al* (1982) Perinatal complications and clinical outcome within the schizophrenia spectrum. *British Journal of Psychiatry*, **140**, 416-420.

Plant, M. (1987) *Drugs in Perspective*. London: Hodder and Stoughton.

Rapoport, J. L. (1986) Annotation. Childhood obsessive compulsive disorder. *Journal of Child Psychology and Psychiatry*, **27**, 289-296.

Rich, J. (1956) Types of stealing. *Lancet*, *i*, 496-498.

Robertson, M. M. (1989) The Gilles de la Tourette syndrome. Current status. *British Journal of Psychiatry*, **154**, 147-170.

Russell, G. F. M., Szmukler, G. I., Dare, C., *et al* (1987) An evaluation of family therapy in anorexia nervosa and bulimia nervosa. *Archives of General Psychiatry*, **44**, 1047-1056.

Rutter, M. (1986) The developmental psychopathology of depression: issues and perspectives. In *Depression in Young People* (eds M. Rutter, C. Izard & P. Read). New York: Guilford Press.

—— (1990) Psychiatric disorders during adolescence. In *Adolescence and Puberty* (eds J. Bancroft & J. M. Reinisch). New York: Oxford University Press.

——, Graham, P., Chadwick, O., *et al* (1976) Adolescent turmoil. Fact or fiction? *Journal of Child Psychology and Psychiatry*, **17**, 35-56.

—— & Giller, H. (1983) *Juvenile Delinquency*. Harmondsworth: Penguin Books.

Shaffer, D. (1974) Suicide in childhood and early adolescence. *Journal of Child Psychology and Psychiatry*, **15**, 275-292.

Shaw, K. R., Sheehan, K. H. & Fernandez, R. C. (1987) Suicide in children and adolescents. *Advances in Paediatrics*, **34**, 313-334.

Smith, R. E. & Winokur, G. (1984) Affective disorders - bipolar. In *Adult Psychopathology and Diagnosis* (eds S. M. Turner & M. Herson). New York: Wiley.

Spivack, G. & Shure, M. B. (1982) The cognition of social adjustment. Interpersonal cognitive, problem-solving. In *Advances in Clinical Child Psychology*, vol. 5 (eds B. B. Lahey & A. E. Kazdin). New York: Plenum.

Stark, K. D., Rouse, L. W. & Livingston, R. (1991) Treatment of depression during childhood and adolescence. In *Child and Adolescent Therapy* (ed. P. C. Kendall). New York: Guilford Press.

Stewart, M. A. & Culver, K. W. (1982) Children who set fires. The clinical picture and a follow-up. *British Journal of Psychiatry*, **140**, 357-363.

Taylor, E. A. & Stansfield, S. A. (1984) Children who poison themselves. I Clinical comparison with psychiatric controls. *British Journal of Psychiatry*, **145**, 127-135.

Vaughn, C. E. (1989) Expressed emotion in family relationships. *Journal of Child Psychology and Psychiatry*, **30**, 13-22.

West, D. J. (1982) *Delinquency, Its Roots, Careers and Prospects*. London: Heinemann.

White, J. L. (1989) *The Troubled Adolescent*. New York: Pergamon Press.

Wyatt, G. E. (1990) Changing influences on adolescent sexuality over the past 40 years. In *Adolescence and Puberty* (eds J. Bancroft & J. M. Reinisch). New York: Oxford University Press.

Zelnick, M., Kantner, J. F. & Ford, K. C. (1981) *Sex and Pregnancy in Adolescence.* Beverly Hills: Sage.

Further reading

Hill, P. (1989) *Adolescent Psychiatry.* Current Reviews in Psychiatry no. 3. Edinburgh: Churchill Livingstone.

Mussen, P. H., Conger, J. J., Kagan, J., *et al* (1990) Adolescence. In *Child Development and Personality.* New York: Harper & Row.

10 Treatment in child and adolescent psychiatry

Brian Jacobs

Behaviour therapy ● Cognitive therapy with children ● Individual therapy with children ● Family therapy ● Child and adolescent groups ● Pharmacotherapy ● Day units and residential treatment units ● Non-health settings with a treatment element ● Other treatments ● Ethics of treatment ● Conclusion

---

The range of treatment methods in child and adolescent psychiatry has expanded rapidly over the past 30 years. This has reflected changes elsewhere in psychiatry. In some areas, such as the development of family therapy, treatment methods have provided the bench on which to test underlying theories of change.

This chapter first considers behavioural approaches to treatment in some detail. Methods that have been developed here are often used in other therapy settings as part of a treatment plan. Cognitive–behavioural therapy is the latest therapy to be tried with children in this area.

Psychodynamic methods of treatment are gradually being adapted and their place in the wider range of therapies available today is becoming more accurately defined. They still have a distinctive contribution to make and can inform much other clinical work.

Over the years other family members have been included in treatment plans much more frequently. Family therapy has burgeoned, and now has many different approaches. Many treatments are applicable to individuals or to groups; some work best for groups of young people with similar difficulties.

The development of adult psychopharmacology is mirrored by increasing knowledge of the use of medication in children. As might be expected, there is a lag in this process as psychiatrists are much more cautious in prescribing for children and adolescents. This chapter also briefly considers the use of day units and residential treatment.

In child psychiatry it is very important to remember the sense of failure that is often felt by parents when seeking treatment for their children. They often blame themselves, although they may cover this with a range of responses to professionals. A sense of respect for the parents is vital if they and their children are to be helped. At the same time it is very important that the children feel that their voices are heard and their point of view valued. Whatever therapeutic approach is adopted, successful interventions are based upon skilful interviewing.

Behaviour therapy

Behaviour therapy is based on learning theory as an explanation of human behaviour. As Yule (1985) points out, it is essentially a problem-solving

183

approach to treatment and takes as its starting point the idea that any observed behaviour occurs in a setting and leads to certain reactions from those around the child; such reactions then form the basis for subsequent behaviour. This is a common observation of parents.

Extensive accounts of behavioural approaches are given by Gelfand & Hartmann (1984) and Herbert (1981). This section can only summarise methods that need application with care and skill.

Treatments largely fall into four theoretical groups.

(1) Some treatments are based on stimulus–response theories. An unconditioned stimulus, such as a very loud noise, which is presented with a neutral stimulus, such as a coloured light, will produce a startle reaction. Eventually presentation of the coloured light alone produces the startle response because the loud noise has come to be associated with it. It is now the conditioned stimulus. The main treatment methods are exposure to the avoided stimulus by systematic desensitisation, or flooding.

(2) Operant conditioning techniques use schemes of reinforcement and punishment to modify behaviour. Behaviour modification and contingency management derive from this theoretical approach.

(3) Cognitive theories suggest techniques that seek to alter thought trains to amend behavioural ones.

(4) Social learning theory leads to a group of interventions using modelling, role play and social skills training to expand the repertoire of social interaction skills available to the subject.

Behaviour therapy is applicable to problems of children at home, at school, and elsewhere. It can also offer skill-building approaches for children who are slow learners and can be very useful in helping severely intellectually handicapped youngsters.

Functional analysis

This is a careful process of taking a history and making observations about the problem behaviour. A clear description of how each behaviour is expected to change, as a result of treatment, is necessary. Carers must rank their priorities and realise that their expectations for the child may be unrealistic. For example, the child may not yet be developmentally mature enough to manage certain skills, or intermediate changes in behaviour may be necessary before the parent's goal can be achieved. The history is particularly concerned with developing a clear list of the problems and a detailed description of what happens around each one. This chain is known as the 'ABC' sequence:

Antecedents → Behaviour → Consequences

Antecedents

These events can 'set the scene' – for example the child is expecting to be told off – or they can directly 'trigger' the unwanted behaviour – for example the mother shouts at the child.

The behaviour

A clear description is required of who does what to whom, when and where. One needs to know the frequency, duration and intensity of each of the problem behaviours as well as their meaning for the child, the parents and the therapist.

In general, children are brought because of an excess of undesirable behaviour and deficits in preferred behaviour.

The consequences

It is vital to get a clear idea of what happens after the behaviour has occurred. Are the consequences reinforcing the behaviour in any sense? Is that appropriate? Are they clear cut and predictable? Thus parents may say they are angry with dangerous behaviour but show by their expression that they are proud of their son for his daring. The attention achieved by creating diversions in the classroom may give a child more attention than can be got in any other way from the teacher.

Setting

The ABC occurs within a pattern of variables that do not change but are important to consider. They include the child's age; sex; temperament; cognitive, emotional and motor development; physical health; and self-esteem. Under this heading can also be considered family variables such as parental ill-health and recent major life events.

Baseline observations

It is an essential part of the behavioural approach that the therapist does not rely purely on the initially presented history but obtains baseline structured observations. These can be carried out by parents, teachers or the therapist. For example, with temper tantrums parents may be asked to keep a diary of the target behaviour (temper tantrums), noting each occasion on which they occur, what behaviour of the child and others including themselves preceded the tantrum, what they did about it and the outcome. They would be asked to try to note how long each tantrum actually lasted.

Keeping a diary can thus be therapeutic in itself by helping parents come to a more objective view of the difficulties and their magnitude or otherwise. It helps them begin to observe for themselves the triggers, the antecedents and their own responses. The therapist can test how the carers will be able to help in any intervention. It is important not to discourage potential co-therapists by making unreasonable or over-complex demands on them during this data-collection phase as further collection of data will be needed during the intervention programme.

On other occasions therapists might want to observe for themselves particular events (e.g. around meal times) to obtain a more detailed analysis.

Assets

The child's behavioural and personality assets are important components of developing a successful programme.

Reinforcers

Anything that increases the likelihood of a particular behaviour being repeated is called a reinforcer. They are one of the mainstays of behavioural interventions.

During the functional analysis it is necessary to consider what can be used during the treatment programme to encourage the behaviour that is wanted. The crucial question that needs to be asked here is what will act as reinforcers for this particular child? Broadly, reinforcers fall into four categories: things that the child is given; activities that he or she is allowed to carry out; privileges; and social praise. Often the last has been curiously lacking or become extinct. Adults often expect children to do what they are told without any recognition that they have done well or that it might have been difficult for this particular child to manage. Reinforcers are frequently seen as bribes rather than a legitimate means to help the young person change behaviour. The adults often fear that it is a slippery road and that other siblings or class members will be jealous.

In behavioural programmes with children it is usually necessary to have material reinforcers initially. These should be coupled with social praise.

Gelfand & Hartmann (1984) suggest that useful reinforcers should be immediate, practical, resistant to satiation, administered in small amounts, compatible with the overall treatment programme, and under the therapist's control.

Treatment interventions

Generally, interventions can: (1) be designed to increase behaviour that is absent or occurring too infrequently – *deficit behaviour*; or (2) be constructed to decrease unwanted behaviour that is occurring too frequently or in inappropriate settings – *excess behaviour*. Other classes of interventions such as relaxation techniques and social skills training are discussed later.

Figure 10.1 gives a summary of the process of behaviour modification, and Fig. 10.2 summarises the types of treatment.

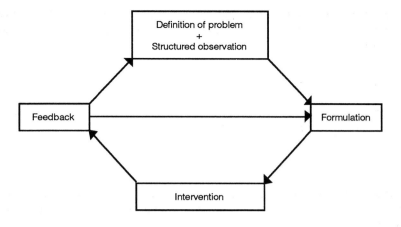

Fig. 10.1. The process of behaviour modification.

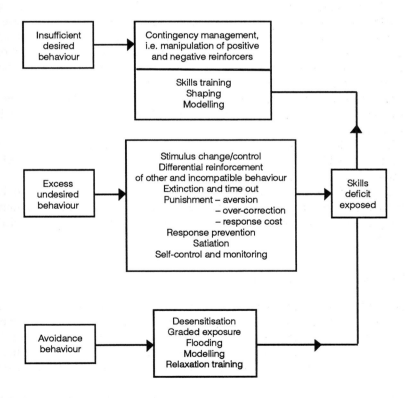

Fig. 10.2. Types of behavioural therapy.

Procedures to increase deficit behaviour

(1) *Positive reinforcement*   This is the preferred approach to intervention. Children should be working to goals that they can easily achieve from the outset and be getting rewards that they want. *Children must succeed early.* Otherwise, they can become rapidly discouraged. For example, a child may be disruptive in class, leaving his seat and distracting other children. It might be that leaving his seat might have to be the first target behaviour. It is best to label this as the desired behaviour rather than the problem; here it could be called 'staying in your seat'. The teacher would have to praise the child every two minutes or even more frequently initially for remaining in his seat. This praise need not be lengthy. At the end of the target time the child should be immediately rewarded with one of the pre-agreed material reinforcers. The aim of this intervention is to stabilise him remaining in his seat and then gradually to increase the time between each episode of reward. In general it is thought that achievement of the desired behaviour with an 80% success rate is necessary before moving to the next stage.

(2) *Shaping behaviour*   This refers to the steady approximation of the child's behaviour towards that which is desired. In the example above the child is first rewarded for learning to stay in his seat regularly rather than wandering about the class. One would then want to shape his behaviour by setting him work targets that gradually increased towards a normal work output by using positive reinforcement for defined amounts of work produced. Reinforcement programmes can be rewarding both to the child and to the adults carrying out the programme, though it often involves the latter apparently giving the child extra attention. Often this is more apparent than real as considerable time and effort has been spent by the adult until this point in confrontation with the child but none the less giving him attention.

(3) *Negative reinforcement*   This involves the removal of an aversive stimulus if the child complies with the desired behaviour. On the whole it is a less effective method, although it has its place. It can form part of a contingency management programme such as a token economy (see below).

(4) *Modelling*   These techniques can be helpful in overcoming fears and phobias. Models, sometimes other children, that are credible for the child and that are not perceived by the child as being so much more successful than he or she is in other areas are most helpful. Fears of, for example, heights or dental examinations can be overcome by these means. In *guided participation*, the child first watches the model and then gradually imitates him or her.

(5) *Cueing*   The provision of ambiguous or incorrect cues by others may lead to the child not producing desired behaviour even when the child has such behaviour within his repertoire. The father who encourages his son to enter the water while appearing very fearful himself cannot be surprised at his lack of success.

(6) *Social skills training*   (see below).

Procedures to decrease excess behaviour

There are a range of methods that can be applied to decrease or remove unwanted behaviour. It is essential to have informed parental consent before any of these methods are used. It is also important in most cases to have explained the programme to the child.

(1) *Punishment* Unpleasant consequences are often used by parents and teachers to try to prevent unwanted behaviour. Although effective in the short term, it quickly tends to fade because the child becomes habituated, inviting an unhelpful escalation. It is easy to get into a cycle whereby the child is receiving a great deal of attention through punishment without much effect.

(2) *Satiation* If it is not dangerous, allow or even encourage the child to perform the behaviour until he or she is thoroughly bored with it. In a variant of this sometimes used for tics or mannerisms, the child is asked to repeat the behaviour in a rehearsed form for some minutes and to carry out this procedure each hour initially (*massed practice*).

(3) *Extinction* If the response that the child usually obtains from the behaviour is not forthcoming then it may be expected to decrease and disappear. Often this means ignoring the behaviour so that the social reinforcement of any adult response is removed. Frequently there is a time during which the frequency and intensity of the behaviour increases first. This may not be tolerable or safe to ignore. One danger is that reinforcement is maximal when irregular – if the adults' nerve cracks and they do respond then they have set themselves a harder task still.

(4) *Stimulus change* Here the preceding stimulus that is thought to be triggering the behaviour is either removed, where possible, or altered. Parents often do this when they arrange for two siblings to play in different parts of the house.

(5) *Differential reinforcement of other behaviour (DRO)* This, for example, would be rewarding the child for set periods of time that are free of the unwanted behaviour.

(6) *Differential reinforcement of incompatible behaviour (DRI)* For example, prosocial behaviour and responsibility in the classroom tends to be incompatible with playing the role of the disruptive clown.

There is a group of techniques that are used in conjunction with the above that require a price to be paid for carrying out the unwanted behaviour:

(7) *Response cost* This method gives the child tokens or points for desired behaviour and fines the child if he or she shows the unwanted behaviour. The tokens can be exchanged for reinforcers at set intervals.

(8) *Overcorrection* Essentially, this requires the child to correct and then make additional restitution for the results of the bad behaviour. If possible, the corrective task should relate very directly to the damage done.

(9) *Time out* (from positive reinforcement)   This requires removing the child from the situation where he or she is getting reinforced for adverse behaviour to a setting which is unrewarding. It can be a very effective technique if carefully applied but, like other 'negative' techniques, it should only be used in conjunction with positive programmes to encourage wanted behaviour. Difficulties in implementing time out include: a child being too large to be easily removed to the time-out room; the child's removal becoming an overexcited struggle; a lack of suitable space. Parents have often sent children to their rooms and then complain that this does not work. Often the child has been sent for an indeterminate time in a framework of contingencies that is muddled and inconsistent. The child may have played or been destructive and the effort abandoned. Clarity and consistency are vital. This can mean repeatedly having to place the child in the time-out situation on the first occasion it is tried, before the child is convinced of the inevitable consequence of a particular behaviour.

(10) *Desensitisation*   The simplest example of this technique is the treatment of simple phobias. The child is gradually given increasing exposure to the phobic stimulus (e.g. spiders). It is accompanied by muscle relaxation training to help the child in anxiety management (other anxiety management techniques include cognitive restructuring, social skills training and hypnosis – see below). More complex programmes of exposure to a hierarchy of feared situations can be used. There are indications that actual exposure is better than using a hierarchy in imagination with children. This method has been used very successfully in the treatment of school refusal.

(11) *Flooding*   Here children are held in the most feared situation of their phobic hierarchy and not allowed to leave it until their anxiety has fallen and remained down. It extinguishes the fear.

(12) *Response prevention*   This technique has been successfully applied in obsessional–compulsive disorder (Bolton *et al*, 1983). The rituals are regarded as attempts by the child to manage anxiety. Parents are taught to intervene and stop the usual ritualistic responses the child uses to cope with the feelings of anxiety until desensitisation occurs. It works less well if the obsessional symptoms are accompanied by conduct disorder.

(13) *Relaxation training*   Children are taught a programme of tensing and then relaxing various muscle groups while using mental imagery of quiet, tranquil scenes to give them an increased ability to counteract the sensations and dysphoria of anxiety states and to help them regain a sense of control.

Contracts

Many therapists like to work in the framework of a verbal or written contract. These specify for the child, the parents or teacher, and the therapist:

(1) what the expected behaviour will be
(2) what the child can expect if the set targets are achieved
(3) what the consequences will be if the child fails to achieve the target
(4) what the consequences will be of certain unacceptable behaviour
(5) the expectations of the parents are also spelt out clearly so that it is clear if they have not kept to their part of the bargain
(6) some contracts also specify what the therapist will do as their contribution

Cognitive therapy with children

The application of cognitive–behavioural techniques to child psychiatric problems is relatively new and is still evolving rapidly (Kendall, 1991). These techniques are related to the behaviour therapies; they arise specifically from social learning theories (Rotter *et al*, 1972; Bandura, 1977) in which it is seen that the likelihood of a particular behaviour being performed is related to situationally specific reinforcement, and the anticipation that the behaviour will result in the expected reinforcement. Bandura's theory pointed to additional cognitive factors such as: how effectively a person feels he or she is able to perform the behaviour; what behaviour confirms the person's self-image; and the person's selective attention to certain role models.

The central idea is that much child and adult psychiatric disorder arises from difficulties in two areas: firstly, patients show *cognitive deficiencies* – an absence of careful information processing that would help in the situation; secondly, they have *cognitive distortions* – a tendency to misconstrue and distort the situation that faces them, usually in various negative ways.

Kendall (1991) reviews the approach. The techniques have been applied with enthusiasm to a wide variety of child psychiatric disorder with some success, although it seems rather too early to say where these methods will finally best be applied. Thus they have been used with conduct disordered youngsters with modest success, with anxiety-related difficulties, and with depressed children. They have also been tried in helping children with serious physical illness improve their sense of limited mastery.

Lochman *et al* (1991) quote research on three areas of cognitive deficiencies and distortions in aggressive children.

(1) *Social cognitive products.* Aggressive children have a bias to being overly sensitive to other's hostile intentions and underestimate their own aggressiveness. They have deficiencies in their social problem-solving skills, with more solutions involving actions than words. They are poor at correctly labelling their own emotions, especially in tending to mis-label other forms of arousal as anger. In addition they are poor at empathising.

(2) *Cognitive operations.* Attention span is poor. They make mistakes in their short-term memory. The automatic scripts that they tend to retrieve for instant reactions from long-term memory are aggressive.

(3) *Beliefs and expectations*. These children wish to dominate others and revenge is to the fore in their thinking. They are not very bothered by the possible reactions of the victim or other consequences of their actions. They expect aggression to produce tangible rewards. They have poor self-esteem.

This leads to a therapeutic approach which requires careful assessment of cognitions in each area before a treatment package is designed. Often small-group treatment allows for brainstorming and the use of role play. In their anger-coping programme, Lochman *et al* developed an 18-session intervention that takes place in schools. Children are taught self-management/monitoring skills. Essentially this means that they are taught to recognise internal emotional states and their precipitants, with the accompanying thoughts and the autonomic physiological cues. They are taught to use these bodily and emotional cues as signals. Cognitive self-control strategies are taught through 'self-talk' – what can the children say to themselves that will increase or decrease their anger?

'Social perspective taking' is taught through role plays, modelling, group discussion and structured exercises. Everyday situations of potential conflict at home and at school are used to generate scripts and discussion. Children are encouraged to develop alternative understandings about other's thoughts and their intentions. Exercises are used to increase social problem-solving skills. Essentially this includes problem identification; generation of several possible solutions; and evaluation and prediction of the consequences of whatever action they choose. A key element is to help children spot potential problems early, so that they have time to think and to implement their new strategies. Back-up solutions are important, as is the development of other social skills where these are deficient. Practice in the treatment sessions, with peer comment and homework projects, are an essential part of this treatment.

Interestingly, there has been relatively little application of these techniques to the family as yet, but one of the more successful programmes resulting in longer-term change included a booster series for each child and family one year after the original treatment of groups of children (Lochman *et al*, 1991). This is likely to be an important area for development as there is also research showing that adults in these families show some of the cognitive deficits and distortions that are seen in their children and also have limited strategies that they apply in the home in their child management.

Cognitive–behavioural approaches for depression have to contend with the poor motivation of depressed youngsters and the boredom induced by their anhedonic state.

Social skills training

Social skills training has concentrated either on developing 'micro-social' skills (e.g. amount and timing of eye contact, body position) or more 'macro-skills' (e.g. introducing yourself to somebody). The latter approach has been generally found to be more helpful in work with children and adolescents. Social skills training is now often used as a part of packages of treatment such as cognitive-behavioural therapy, and anxiety management programmes.

Individual therapy with children

In contrast to the behaviour therapies, psychodynamic approaches focus on the child's inner experience and, to a varying degree, elements of this of which the child is unaware. Various forms of psychotherapy can be delivered to an individual. These differ in their conceptual frameworks but share the particular interactions and sense of being special that tend to be emphasised when a child is given individual attention by an adult. Individual therapies can be directive and educative in their style, such as cognitive–behavioural approaches, or very non-directive, such as some forms of psychodynamic psychotherapy. Most involve playing with the children or young people for a purpose, or helping children to move to a point where they can begin to allow themselves to play literally or metaphorically. Therapies with young people use different media for communication of emotionally laden material. This varies with the developmental stage that the child has reached as well as the particular channels of communication to which the child responds. The most frequent approaches are to use play with younger children and, with adolescents, to move towards talking therapies. However, use of art materials, drama and music have all been adapted to specific experiential therapies.

The therapy environment

As with adult patients, therapists have learned that a number of issues need attention to foster the trust that is needed during therapy (Wilson & Hersov, 1985). These include:

(1) *The treatment setting*. This is the boundary of a regular meeting place and time with respect for confidentiality and safety of the child and the room.

(2) *The therapist's personal style*. This includes the degree of activity and intervention during the sessions on the part of the therapist, any tendency to use humour, to be parental in style or appear very restrained and perhaps a bit remote. Psychological containment and safety should be conveyed to the child. Therapists must be able to be in contact with very powerful emotions that surface unpredictably from the child. These can elicit powerful responding or reactive emotions in the therapist. As Wilson & Hersov (1985) state there can be dangers in the therapist becoming "excited or frightened by the child's powerful sexual or destructive fantasies, reacting either impulsively or provocatively or in a defensive manner by avoiding painful feelings or trying to control them".

(3) *The working alliance*. Children contribute to this with their readiness to work or otherwise: the degree to which they can acknowledge that they have a problem and to which they can be aware of their thoughts and actions.

Therapists contribute their attention – to the setting, to the child, and by their attitudes. They have the task of stimulating a sense of enquiry in children about their difficulties and a sense of self-observation. Adolescents need to keep an emotional distance because of their need to move towards independence and their fears of dependency. Difficulties often arise in stabilising a working alliance because of the perceived dependence.

(4) *The transference*. In psychodynamic therapies the tendency to repeat with the therapist relationships from elsewhere in the child's life is known as transference and is thought to be centrally important. It affects and distorts the working alliance; this can be material for consideration in therapy. In other forms of individual therapy the therapist will want to minimise this process, regarding it as a potential interference in a rational consideration of the problems under discussion.

(5) *Countertransference*. This is the presence of similar feelings to those described above but in the therapist and directed towards the child. These reactions tend to be stirred up particularly strongly in individual therapists working with children and adolescents. They can lead to very strong feelings of wishing to protect the child inappropriately, or less commonly of distaste towards the child.

(6) *Connecting with the child*. Young children naturally use play. The therapist will encourage them to use expressive materials and small dolls to communicate. Through attention the therapist conveys to the child an idea that there is a joint task to understand what the child is trying to impart. This attention is an important element in the process of showing respect for the child's thoughts and feelings and through that of establishing a connection with the child. Some therapists structure the child's play by suggesting themes of making particular materials more readily available, such as water, clay or puppets. With adolescents, regard to their interests in the outside world conveys respect and often provides a safe means to communicate about personal dilemmas through seemingly more distant and safer metaphors.

Types of psychodynamic psychotherapy with children

Approaches vary from brief psychotherapy through prolonged but non-intensive psychotherapy to intensive psychotherapy/child psychoanalysis.

Brief psychotherapy

The therapist here is working with a clear aim for an increase in understanding by the child and other family members of a specific difficulty or crisis that has arisen. The intention is to achieve this in ten sessions or less over a few months only, using a variety of interpretive and management techniques to encourage rapid change. The child and parents are encouraged to use their resources for increased mutual understanding and to change behaviour. The therapist will help them to arrange appropriate environmental changes.

Sometimes therapists hold separate sessions with the parents as well as the child, or conjoint sessions. Transference interpretations are used infrequently. Clinically, brief psychotherapy has been found to be useful in overcoming specific crises, such as after an impulsive overdose, minor emotional disorders, unresolved grief, and the less severe mixed emotional and conduct disorders. It requires strong motivation on the part of the child and parents.

Non-intensive psychotherapy

This is usually once a week, and uses more clarification of internal feeling states and some interpretations. It may actively work on the transference that the child or adolescent comes to feel towards the therapist. However, the therapist actively encourages a positive alliance rather than ambivalence, and will work to achieve this.

Intensive psychodynamic psychotherapy with children

Children are seen three to five times weekly. The therapy is non-directive. Some schools of therapy based initially on the work of Klein (1932) and Anna Freud (1946) regard a child's play as the equivalent of an adult's attempts to free associate lying on the psychoanalytic couch. Through the child's play or adolescent's verbal and non-verbal communications, a detailed exploration of feeling states and their appropriateness to specific situations is undertaken. This involves interpreting unconscious psychological themes, particularly emotionally laden material and misconstructions that have been laid down as affect-laden memory traces. The therapist works on the premise that these are inappropriately acted upon as if they were occurring in the present and cause distress for the child.

For such therapy to be possible, the young person must have considerable practical support. All too frequently the therapy ends abruptly because of changes that are affecting the parents that have little to do with the child. Further, the disruption to the child's life entailed by such therapy must not be underestimated.

Supportive psychotherapy (counselling)

This differs from the above therapies in that it may last a long time; it aims to help the young person cope with the reality of the difficulties that he or she faces in the external environment. It is most appropriate for those cases where the child is very vulnerable psychologically and where the therapist decides that the child or adolescent could not tolerate a more detailed and perhaps confronting approach (Campion, 1991).

Other experiential therapies

All children and adolescents should be given opportunities for creative work. Beyond that, the creative arts have been adapted for specific therapeutic work with young people and adults. Consideration should be given to music therapy and art therapy, which are often practised in an individual setting, and drama therapy which is carried out as a group activity. There is a further distinction.

Music and the visual arts allow a choice by therapists as to whether they are using the chosen medium as a staging post for the child to put ideas, thoughts and feelings into words, or whether they are using it to allow expression and communication with the therapist without speech. Therapists who take the first stance will interpret unconscious material and also the transference on occasion. Others regard this as non-therapeutic and constraining on the medium as therapy. They take the view that sharing the making of the artefact or music acts as a therapeutic experience; it encourages self-esteem and bypasses language.

Kramer (1971) gives a helpful account of the use of art therapy with children. She sets the therapy in the context of other artistic experience and societal expectations that the children will have experienced. She gives many clinical examples which illustrate the need for the therapist to comprehend the meanings for the child that are attached to the production or inhibition in production of his or her work. The importance of allowing children to experience their interactions with the medium and the therapist can help them to know and modify their sense of themselves in the outside world. This may never be dealt with through words in the therapy.

Kramer sees the use of art therapy as mainly applying to those children who have developed the capacity for symbolisation as opposed to the playful exploration of arts materials. This, she states, is acquired between the ages of three and five years. She is also cautious about children who are functioning in a very obsessional manner and others for whom the threat of the unstructured medium may prove too frightening.

Music therapy has been used with handicapped children, (e.g. with Down's syndrome and language difficulties; Nordoff & Robbins, 1971, 1977), but has only recently been applied to the practice of child psychiatric problems in the UK.

J. Eisler (unpublished) has written of how the musical dialogue of improvisation becomes a powerful language not bound by words in the communication between therapist and patient: "The improvisation should be based on the sounds and activities offered by the child, to which the therapist responds in musical terms, acknowledging their validity whilst also offering support, encouragement and developmental challenges." In the multidisciplinary team, music therapy can offer a specific opportunity for children who are difficult to engage in treatment. It is non-verbal yet it "offers a strongly self-expressive form of treatment so that even the young emotionally withdrawn and older disturbed child can respond to it without feeling threatened. The inherent structures and forms of music, on the one hand are capable of expressing the child's feelings but at the same time can offer a sense of security and familiarity that helps to satisfy, stabilise, integrate, and stimulate".

One advantage is thought to be that the child can function musically as a very young child without embarrassment in this setting. As with other experiential therapies the aim is to improve self-esteem and to increase the child's capacity to tolerate variable success.

Research into the psychodynamic and experiential therapies

Levitt (1957, 1963) reviewed the area of psychodynamic psychotherapy with children and concluded that there was no evidence that child psychotherapy was more effective than not treating the child. Barrnett *et al* (1991) reviewed research into child psychotherapy since 1963. They point to the criticisms that have been raised against Levitt's views:

(1) that they were based on old studies and that techniques of therapy have changed
(2) two of the studies had estimated the improvement in untreated, unrepresentative samples
(3) diagnostic assessments may themselves be therapeutic
(4) those who do not proceed to therapy may be an unrepresentative group and might be the most healthy
(5) all of the studies had significant methodological flaws.

Barrnett *et al* then reviewed the 43 studies of child psychotherapy that had since been published which met the criteria of including a group that had individual psychodynamic treatment; that also had a comparison group; and that did not focus entirely on other treatment methods. They excluded those studies where there was a mixed adolescent and adult group. Few studies that meet even these criteria have been published since the early 1970s. Unfortunately, they found that there continued to be major methodological flaws in almost all of the studies. They argue that this makes interpretation of the results well nigh impossible. There were 12 studies claiming that children given individual psychotherapy did better than untreated children, although nine studies found no difference. No direct comparisons of different treatments showed more improvement in those getting individual psychotherapy.

Barrnett *et al* concluded that there have been advances in individual therapies for adults which have arisen out of individual psychodynamic therapies. They suggest that these have arisen in part because of more careful characterisation of appropriate patients, therapies, and therapists. This has led to better research, with valuable information appearing about which treatments are appropriate and about the process of therapy. The implications for future child psychotherapy research and clinical work are important.

Ricks (1974) compared the adult outcome of therapy by two experienced therapists working with adolescents suffering from severe psychiatric disorders. He found that the better outcome was associated with the therapist who adopted a directive, educative approach to the youngsters rather than the therapist who was primarily concerned with material of psychodynamic interest. The former therapist tried to foster autonomy in the adolescents, encouraged them to use a variety of community resources, and used the therapy to help them to make sense of their functioning and feelings in these settings.

There is little empirical work examining the efficacy of other experiential therapies as yet.

In summary, there is still much work to be done in specifying more clearly what are the indications for psychodynamically based individual work with children. The mass of individual case reports indicate a belief that these forms of therapy can give relief to children but firmer evidence will be required as resources become more scarce.

Counselling and case work with parents

Kraemer (1987) has drawn attention to the widespread use of case work and parent counselling in child guidance clinics, often by highly skilled psychiatric social workers. To some extent the increase in the use of family therapy has reduced the amount of direct work with one or both parents excluding the children, but there are still many occasions when it is useful. In case work, there is often a shift in the subtle balance between advice on parenting and behavioural management, and allowing the parent or parental couple to explore the patterns that are repeating across generations from how they were treated as children. He also points to the dearth of empirical work in this area.

Family therapy

Family therapy has developed rapidly over the past 40 years. It has resulted in a major change in child psychiatry, with a move from treating the individual child with individual psychotherapy and the mother being given social case work separately, to a model in which whole families are commonly seen from the outset. Children are seen in their context. The central tenet of the various family therapy models is that members of the family exert influences and pressures on each other that are more than the sum of the individual relationships between them. The theory and approaches to practice are reviewed by Gorrell Barnes (1985) and by Dare (1985). A variety of treatment approaches has evolved and continues to do so.

Brief therapy

Watzlawick, Weakland and others of their group have developed a therapy at the Mental Research Institute, Palo Alto, which aims to help families make goal-directed changes (Watzlawick *et al*, 1974). They have described the important concepts of *first-order change*, in which there is an alteration in the balance of activity in a system but no fundamental change, and *second-order change*, where the pattern in the system can no longer return to its previous set of interactions.

These ideas have been further developed by de Shazer (1988) into specific techniques which aim to encourage change that is already thought to have begun by the time the family presents for therapy. It is a therapy that is specifically looking for 'solutions' rather than further descriptions of the problem. The therapist wants the family to notice behaviour that they wish to continue, and is also concerned to help the family look for occasions on which the symptoms do not occur – 'the exceptions' – and then to ask what has enabled the cycle to be interrupted. The therapist wants the client families to notice change, and he or she firmly continues to work for further change.

Structural family therapy

Minuchin & Fishman (1981) have developed a therapy which is concerned with establishing an appropriate hierarchy and structure in families, with clear intergenerational boundaries and coherent supportive subsystems. Structural family therapy is very much concerned with the functioning of the family in the present rather than its developmental history. This group has written about psychosomatic families (Minuchin *et al*, 1978). They suggested that families with a young person with anorexia nervosa show characteristic patterns of interaction, namely enmeshment, overprotection, rigidity and failure of conflict resolution. These families are not the only ones to demonstrate such patterns. In this model, the therapist is firmly in control of the process of therapy and has a clear picture of 'the shape' of the healthy family.

Strategic family therapy

Here, the therapist takes a similar position to that above. The method derives from the work of Jay Haley (1973), who developed an interest in the waking hypnotic techniques of Milton Erickson and adapted these through his later work with Minuchin. In *Problem Solving Therapy* (Haley, 1976) he sees any presenting problem "as a type of behaviour that is part of a sequence of acts between several people. The repeating sequence of behaviour is the focus of therapy. A symptom is a label for a crystallisation of a sequence in a social organisation. Thinking of such symptoms as 'depression' or 'phobia' as a contract between people and therefore as adaptive to relationships leads to a new way of thinking about therapy". Interventions aim to change the social context so that the symptom is no longer able to serve its function. The therapist does this by prescribing particular rituals and tasks.

Systemic family therapy

In *Paradox and Counterparadox* (Palazzoli *et al*, 1978) the Milan group described their method of circular questioning around an evolving hypothesis to describe the function of the symptom in the family. They also delineate their work as a team with peer supervision and their view of the importance of neutrality in their questioning style and their interventions. The latter are aimed at preventing the family's 'games', that is, their habitual verbal and non-verbal recursive, cyclical patterns of interchange.

The team prescribes the symptom, positively connoting the way it helps the family with other relationship difficulties. This process is referred to as counterparadox.

One of the hallmarks of this style of work is the concept of 'neutrality' (Palazzoli *et al*, 1980). The therapist strives to avoid invitations to alliances with family members, avoids moral judgements of behaviour, and does whatever is necessary to maintain him- or herself at a different level of thinking from the family. It means that the solutions brought by the family are often quite unpredictable and are often rather creative. This is very different from the style of the structural family therapist who has a proposed family solution.

Other methods, and research

In the UK there have been exponents of each treatment approach but in addition there has been an eclectic melding of techniques from different schools. A multigenerational framework of thinking, which acknowledges its psychoanalytical roots but which allows interventions in different styles, has been developed by Bentovim & Kinston (1987).

Jenkins (1990) reviews the interface between research and family therapy and developments in the past ten years. He points to the considerable difficulties in carrying out scientific studies, in that the intervening mechanisms of change are difficult to dissect. There is ample evidence that the introduction of additional people into the family produces discontinuous change in the observed interactions (e.g. Dunn & Kendrick, 1980). However, effective studies of family therapy that do operationalise the treatment interventions are now becoming available in the work of Leff & Vaughn (1985) and that of Russell *et al* (1987), who carried out a detailed comparison of family therapy and individual treatment in the management of anorexia nervosa.

Family therapy - the practicalities

The decision as to whether family therapy is suitable is difficult before a diagnostic assessment. However, it is often appropriate to convene all the family members living at home for the diagnostic interview because they will have important points of view about the nature of the problem.

Family therapists have developed a variety of techniques for 'joining' the family; essentially, all family members must feel that their view has been attended to with respect and interest. This can be an unusual experience for children.

In making a diagnostic assessment the therapist will want to elicit and evaluate:

(1) a detailed description of the problems as seen by the family members
(2) the family interactional patterns – their hierarchical patterns and boundaries; their communication styles; coalitions – are these cross-generational?
(3) the family atmosphere – what is its general nature, in what way is it affected by the symptomatic child, what might be the nature of the atmosphere if this problem were not present, etc?
(4) where the family is on its 'lifecycle' – is the presenting problem one of a difficulty with a transition between lifecycle stages for the symptomatic child or another family member?
(5) what the real external constraints on this family's functioning are – socio-economic and cultural
(6) whether there are unresolved issues from the parents' own families of origin or a clash between their previous experiences that is preventing them from finding an appropriate solution to the problem
(7) what the parents' problem-solving skills and style are, and how the therapy can help them adapt this creatively.

Therapeutic interventions will depend to a large extent on the nature of the therapy that is being practised. If a pragmatic approach is adopted, then behavioural intervention techniques that can be taught to parents can be successful as a first approach. They often provide an effective remedy, and if they are unsuccessful then much further information is gained about how the family has approached the task.

Often a detailed family tree can provide a task involving all family members and give a useful vehicle for exploring the parents' families of origin and interactional styles across the generations. This can free the present parents from the rules of behaviour and family myths that may have been appropriate in the families in which they grew up but are now dysfunctional. Sometimes it is necessary to convene a meeting of the extended family with key participants from the grandparental generation to give permission for change. The importance of myth in shaping families and in enabling change has been well explored by Byng-Hall (1973). Occasionally paradoxical injunction is necessary to circumvent the needs of the family to maintain the symptom.

Outcome

There are numerous case studies indicating the efficacy of family therapy. Jenkins (1990) cites several pieces of research that point to the efficacy of these approaches.

Child and adolescent groups

Group treatments have been widely used in adult psychiatry and related fields but less commonly in child and adolescent psychiatry. Treating young people in groups has certain advantages. It can be an economic use of therapeutic time, with several patients being seen at once. The contact with other children of similar age allows feedback from peers which is often respected more than that from therapists, particularly in adolescence. Rubbing up against each other's difficulties can provide a graphic illustration for children of the problems they are having and their maladaptive ways of solving them. It allows for neutral sharing and generation of new solutions.

From the therapist's viewpoint it gives advantages by providing a richer, wider range of material, whatever specific theoretical framework is being used. For example, in social skills training (see above), role play of certain situations between peers and with other youngsters commenting tends to be a strong reinforcer to observing adult modelling.

Difficulties of treating young people in groups include a coherent attack on the group's function which can be initiated by one member and prove just too exciting to resist by the rest of the group. If one child's difficulties are too different from the group norm then the flexibility offered by an individual therapeutic approach may be preferable.

Research by the Newcastle group (Kolvin *et al*, 1988) suggests that group treatments can be effective for children with emotional and behaviour problems.

Groups have been used for the application of a variety of other treatment techniques to obtain peer models and allow discussion. They have been used for children or adults who have had similar experiences (e.g. the victims of child sexual abuse and for the survivors of disasters suffering from the post-traumatic stress disorder).

Parent groups

Parent groups can again be run in a variety of styles. They can be professionally led or organised on a self-help basis. Examples of the latter include groups where the parents have a child with a specific physical disorder. Professionally led groups for parents may be around a specific issue, for example child sexual abuse in the family, or where parents find themselves in a similar situation, for example for isolated parents or those with children who are psychiatric in-patients. Approaches used in such groups may focus on one theoretical stance such as a reflective Rogerian approach or may be more eclectic. Counselling and the teaching of specific behavioural approaches to use with their children have been used. In groups where there is a more behavioural focus it can be shown that attitudinal changes also occur. Groups can be used to enhance or re-establish a sense of self-esteem and competency, particularly in parents who feel a terrible sense of failure in having to seek help at all with their children.

Pharmacotherapy

Drug treatments are sparingly used in child and adolescent psychiatry, and then mostly only as an adjunct to psychological treatments. The best account of the use of psychoactive drugs in child psychiatry remains that of Werry (1978). Reviews that are pertinent for clinicians are provided by Taylor (1985) and by Campbell & Spencer (1988). There is general agreement that there are still many unanswered questions concerning the effectiveness and safety of various psychoactive medications for use with children.

Pharmacotherapy is used rather sparingly in the UK and more liberally in the US. This means that much of the recent research emanates from the USA. Most authors emphasise that drug treatment should be used as an adjunct to other therapies, most often behavioural therapy.

Antipsychotic drugs

These drugs have been used for the treatment of schizophrenia, control of mania, the treatment of childhood movement disorders, and experimentally in the treatment of aggressive, overactive and antisocial behaviour. The phenothiazines, butyrophenones and thioxanthines are widely used in adult psychiatry for the control of the positive symptoms of schizophrenia such as agitation, hallucinations and delusions.

There is little specific information available on the body's handling of these drugs in children. Attention should be paid to the possible side-effects including:

movement disorders hypotension obesity photosensitivity	common
impaired hearing corneal opacities retinopathy	occasional, depending on drug used
agranulocytosis cholestatic jaundice	rare but dangerous

Acute dystonic reactions can be particularly troublesome in young people. Periodic blood counts and liver function tests are necessary.

Schizophrenic disorders

Clinical evidence suggests that antipsychotics are less effective in prepubertal schizophrenics than in adulthood. A trial of medication is indicated in children where the diagnosis is established. It is less clear whether the major tranquillisers are effective in the longer term in children.

The choice of which is the appropriate drug should be made on similar lines to that in adulthood. It is first sensible to try drugs with which there is most clinical experience (e.g. haloperidol and chlorpromazine). A trial of medication over one month should guide the clinician. The drug treatment should be reduced and stopped after a maximum of six months to assess whether further drug therapy is justifiable. It is important to allow a long enough break from the medication to ascertain whether any deterioration is due to the rebound phenomenon or whether it represents a stable state.

Drug treatment should be used in combination with other approaches to help the child. Particularly important in this respect is the attention to the family and whether their style of interaction shows high levels of expressed emotion.

Movement disorders

Iatrogenic, drug-induced movement disorders are of great concern to psychiatrists. The phenothiazines cause acute dystonic reactions, including oculogyric crisis, spasm in muscle groups causing torticollis, inability to speak and posturing, which can be frightening. Unfortunately, children are particularly prone to these reactions. Akathisia can also occur early. The neuroleptic malignant syndrome described by Caroff (1980) is rare but can be fatal.

Tardive dyskinesia is a particular worry with young people because it can be irreversible. It tends to appear on stopping long-term phenothiazine treatment and can be confused with withdrawal dyskinesias, which should disappear within four months. Symptomatically they are similar to dystonias, facial movements such as grimacing and torticollis, athetoid movements and chorea affecting any part of the body. Campbell & Spencer (1988) suggest that periodic discontinuation of phenothiazine treatment should be considered every four to six months for four to six weeks, although they suggest that this will increase the rate of withdrawal dyskinesias. Taylor (1985) warns that the appearance of a withdrawal dyskinesia should be an indication to stop drug treatment except in the most severe and disabling psychiatric conditions.

There is no recent study on the effect of medication on tics. By contrast, there has been much interest in the treatment of Tourette's syndrome with medication. Dopamine antagonists, such as haloperidol in low doses and pimozide, are effective in reducing the symptoms, while drugs that have a dopamine agonist action (e.g. methylphenidate, and l-dopa) make them worse. Clonidine also has a place in the treatment. It seems to have most effect on the compulsive, aggressive and attentional difficulties experienced in Tourette's syndrome. Thioridazine has been found to be an effective drug in the treatment of stereotypies.

Infantile autism

Haloperidol may reduce the stereotypies seen in this condition and increase discriminant learning in a laboratory situation. The 29% risk of drug-induced dyskinesias suggests that it should be used with great caution in this chronic condition.

There was much interest in fenfluramine, a potent antiserotonergic agent, as a possible treatment in infantile autism. However, that it reduces symptoms and increases IQ has not been borne out by subsequent studies (Stern *et al*, 1990).

Psychostimulant medication

Methylphenidate, dextroamphetamine and the longer-acting amphetamine pemoline are centrally acting stimulant drugs. They have a marked effect on inattentive restlessness. They increase sustained attention on psychometric tests of attention and vigilance. They also decrease absolute levels of activity, although not through sedation. These drugs frequently produce misery and dysphoria when started rather than the euphoria found in adults.

The brain mechanisms responsible for these actions are still unclear. Various sites in the brain have been suggested but their role remains unproven. The most likely mediation seems to be through catecholamine discharge.

Side-effects include:

transient dysphoria, headache, abdominal pain, insomnia
interference with learning in higher doses
tics and stereotypies
hypertension and tachycardia
hypersensitivity (rare)
paranoid psychosis (rare in children).

With use over many months there is significant growth retardation but catch-up growth seems to occur on cessation of treatment so that final height is not significantly affected if relatively low doses are used.

Taylor (1985, 1988) discusses the role of psychostimulants in the treatment of hyperactivity. He stresses the inappropriate overuse of these drugs by primary-care physicians in the USA in the treatment of children who are said to have attention deficit disorder with hyperactivity (ADDH) but who probably have oppositional behaviour and conduct disorder. Children with pervasive restlessness and inattentive behaviour are helped, with an improvement in their ability to concentrate on their class work. Psychostimulants do not improve overall intellectual ability. Further, the medication can interrupt the negative cycle of family interactions often found in these families. Parental warmth increases towards the affected child and coercion decreases. This gives the opportunity for behavioural interventions. It may increase the receptiveness of the child to efforts to help with peer interactions.

Antidepressant medication

There is very much less experience of the use of tricyclic antidepressants for depression in children than in adults. They have been used for persistent enuresis and for hyperkinetic disorder. One group (Gittleman-Klein & Klein, 1971) has used imipramine in high dosage for the successful treatment of school phobias. This may well be unjustifiable given its dangerous side-effects. In particular, children are particularly prone to develop hypotension or occasionally hypertension and cardiac dysrhythmias on tricyclic anti-depressants. Imipramine has a role in low dosage (0.5–1.5 mg/kg) in the treatment of enuresis to produce a temporary suppression of the symptoms on occasions when bedwetting would particularly embarrass the child. When the medication is stopped the wetting promptly restarts. The drug probably has an action on the central nervous system, but this must be different from its antidepressant effect because of its rapid onset.

Imipramine has a limited use in the treatment of hyperactivity because of its side-effects. In the presence of affective symptoms it may act as a second-line drug.

Depression

Depression in childhood and adolescence is treated by various psychotherapies with some effect. Family therapy, individual counselling and group work each have a place. More recently, the cognitive therapies developed for adults have been applied successfully with young people.

Depression has proven difficult to treat by medication in childhood and adolescence. Puig-Antich *et al* (1987) found no superiority of antidepressants over placebo in prepubertal children, nor were there significant improvements in the adolescents studied by Kramer & Feiguine (1981). High plasma levels of imipramine in prepubertal children may be associated with a good clinical response.

It is suggested that antidepressants should be prescribed only if other psychotherapeutic interventions have failed and then only under carefully controlled conditions; the electrocardiogram pulse and blood pressure must be monitored and plasma levels of the drug should be taken regularly. There are newer antidepressants which claim to have much reduced cardiotoxicity in adults. At present, there is no research evidence for their side-effects or efficacy in children, so they cannot be recommended.

Lithium

Clinically, this is a useful prophylactic treatment in the rare cases of bipolar affective disorder seen in childhood and early adolescence. There are few controlled trials as yet. The unwanted drug reactions and side-effects are those seen in adults. Combining the drug with haloperidol should be avoided because high doses of lithium with haloperidol have given rise to an acute encephalopathy in adults. Renal and thyroid function must be monitored alongside drug plasma levels. Neurological examination should be repeated at intervals.

Aggression

There have been a few drug trials (Campbell *et al*, 1984; DeLong & Aldershof, 1987) that have suggested that lithium may have a role in the treatment of severe aggressive conduct disorder.

Other drugs that have been tried with aggression include haloperidol, other phenothiazines, and benzodiazepines. The latter are ineffective and can disinhibit aggressive behaviour. Phenothiazines run the risks of the dyskinesias. If the aggression is associated with epileptic seizures, it is usually an interictal phenomenon, although occasionally a postictal automatism. Here, the anticonvulsant medication should be reviewed. There is a suggestion that a subgroup of aggressive youngsters are primarily depressed. Puig-Antich (1982) found that an antidepressant improved conduct in a group of teenage boys with severe conduct disorder. This awaits confirmation.

Anticonvulsants

As well as their effects on epilepsy, these drugs have been used for their sedative effects. Carbamazepine was shown by Remschmidt (1976) to be an effective treatment for overactive and aggressive children. However, Taylor (1985) cautions against the use of this and other drugs in this class because of their side-effects and the lack of evidence that they provide sufficient improvement to outweigh their toxicity.

Minor tranquillisers

There are few indications for the use of benzodiazepines and other minor tranquillisers in child psychiatry. The treatment of night terrors and other parasomnias by lorazepam or diazepam in low dosage can be effective in the short term. They act by reducing the amount of time spent in stage 4 sleep.

Anxiety

There is no consistent evidence to suggest that minor tranquillisers are better than beta blockers or major tranquillisers in low dosage in the support of a behavioural desensitisation programme where the levels of anxiety are too high initially to be controlled without medication as an adjunct to the therapy. There is a suggestion from one study that diazepam can increase anxiety (Aman & Werry, 1982).

Desamino-D-arginine vasopressin (desmopressin)

This drug has been used recently in the treatment of enuresis, with some success. However, there is a high relapse rate. It can be useful to help a youngster through a crisis or short-term event such as a school trip away from home but is not a first-line treatment. Usually, enuresis is best treated with behavioural therapy programmes (Dische, 1971).

The use of psychotropic medication with the cognitively impaired

Taylor (1988) refers to the development of drugs to help learning in some groups of cognitively impaired young people. Piracetam is not yet available in the UK although there is some experience with it elsewhere in Europe. It is claimed to have a small but significant effect on the reading performance of dyslexic children.

The treatment of other psychiatric disorders in the mentally impaired should be that of the underlying disorder. Aggressive and self-injurious behaviour can be a particular problem. In general, behavioural and psychosocial measures are effective but occasionally drug therapy has to be used in addition. Many drugs have been tried. Most clinical experience seems to be with haloperidol. All the cautions about dyskinesias described above apply. Other drugs have been tried and described in small, open studies, and often without controls. These include carbamazepine, which has been suggested for the episodic dyscontrol syndrome, beta blockers, and opiate antagonists.

Day units and residential treatment units

Day and residential units allow treatment or assessment of more intensity than can be provided in a community or out-patient setting. A variety of patterns of day facilities cater for the needs of young children with severely disturbing behaviour and for children who are at risk of abuse or neglect. Particular service patterns vary according to the area, and many such facilities are run by local-authority social services departments with consultative input from child psychiatry, clinical psychology, etc.

Day units

These units aim to try to keep children living with their parents by providing a treatment facility that shares the burden with the parents. Such programmes bring together several disciplines and skills to work with a particular child, siblings and parents. Depending on the age of the child this may include specialist teaching in small groups, or a nursery school in which age-appropriate behaviour is encouraged and the parents are helped to practise consistent, firm but positive handling of their children. Many of the parents attending such units have never experienced or learnt these parenting skills. The setting provides a focus for conjoint work with the whole family and an environment in which newly acquired skills can be practised.

There are some advantages of a day hospital over in-patient units. They allow assessment and treatment of serious and complex problems to occur when the child is too young to consider separation from their parents. They may prevent the need for in-patient treatment by partially relieving the parents of the sense that they are the only people trying to grapple with the serious mental health difficulties of an adolescent. They may provide a particular focus for a specialist treatment package aimed at one group of youngsters. Finally they may provide the opportunity for supervision of, and therapy for, families where there is a concern about abuse.

In-patient units

These cater for a small minority of patients where the child psychiatric pathology is too severe to be treated or managed in the community. Generally, there are different units for adolescents (often 13 years and older) from those provided for younger children. This is justified because there is more frank adult-type psychiatric illness in adolescence and because the developmental issues are very different. In some districts child and adolescent psychiatrists admit children and adolescents to paediatric wards for treatment of psychiatric disorder. This may be advantageous for short-term admissions but usually the paediatric ward cannot offer the same therapeutic milieu nor the wide range of therapies that are available on specialist in-patient units.

Usually, there has already been an attempt at out-patient treatment that has been unsuccessful, although occasionally the difficulties are acutely so severe that emergency admission is necessary (e.g. of a suicidally depressed youngster). Life-threatening disorders such as severe anorexia nervosa may force an in-patient admission. Children have often shown bizarre behaviour that has excluded them from schooling. They may be a severe danger to themselves or less frequently to others.

In-patient units are useful for assessing complex diagnostic problems with a mixed physical and psychiatric aetiology. Thus the child who has uncontrolled diabetes mellitus and recurrent hypoglycaemic attacks may be surreptitiously injecting him- or herself with extra insulin. Treatment plans giving appropriate weight to these interactions can be devised in such settings.

In-patient treatment carries the risks of separating sometimes difficult and unpleasant children from their parents. Home life can be much more pleasant without the 'problem' child so that it becomes difficult to return the youngster. To minimise this, much careful attention is paid to involving the family fully in the admission; this can include several out-patient meetings to consider the purpose of the admission. During the admission family work is one tactic used to counter the notion that all the difficulties lie in the identified child alone. Sometimes siblings at home continue their misbehaviour, highlighting the previous tendency to scapegoat the identified patient. There is an expectation that children spend weekends at home unless there are over-riding therapeutic reasons. Such visits act as a probe for the progress of the admission.

Parents frequently feel deskilled and blamed at the time of a psychiatric admission of their child. An unhelpful sense of competition occurs between staff and the parents over who is the more competent parent. Careful attention must be paid to finding ways of helping parents make a positive contribution to the ambience of the unit and to the treatment of their children.

Like day units, in-patient units provide the opportunity to bring together a number of different disciplines to work together for the child and family's benefit. It is important to produce a clear, shared description of the young person's difficulties. This allows a problem-orientated approach to treatment. However, it is often difficult to be certain which aspects of the therapeutic opportunities offered in such settings have been the most important for which types of difficulties.

The therapeutic milieu of the in-patient ward is important. A few adolescent units adopt the model of the therapeutic community, but for the most part they use a more eclectic model. For children's psychiatric wards, the therapeutic community is an inappropriate model. Behavioural treatments, social skills training, counselling and an opportunity to talk about particular fears in a safe setting are important. Sometimes individual psychodynamic psychotherapy can help particular children, but for many, therapies that directly address changes in the child's behaviour are apparently more helpful. In addition the creative therapies provide many child patients an opportunity to gain self-confidence so they can begin to tolerate more positive relationships with others.

The in-patient unit can provide an important and safe setting in which to start and monitor a trial of psychotropic medication.

The school facility

A school attached to child and adolescent in-patient units has a crucial role in that it provides a setting for careful and detailed assessment of the child's functioning and educational difficulties. There is opportunity for remedial work, for the child to succeed and begin to enjoy school, often for the first time. It can give guidance for education authorities in deciding what is appropriate educationally for these children after discharge.

Physiotherapy and occupational therapy

Both these activities have important roles to play in in-patient treatment units and elsewhere. Physiotherapy is used to help to mobilise children who have been confined to bed or a wheelchair because of myalgic encephalomyelitis or because of hysteric conversion. It provides the child with necessary mobilisation of stiff joints but also a rationale to change behaviour without loss of face. Occupational therapists can provide skill-building work, trust group work and other activities to help children improve their self-esteem.

Outcome of in-patient treatment

Unfortunately, the research in this area is limited and not yet of high quality, so that only limited conclusions can be drawn. There is a problem of defining an appropriate control population and of defining the treated group sufficiently narrowly. As in the field of mental handicap, studies that fail to delineate a narrow group diagnostically are flawed. There are indications that florid antisocial features, severity of psychopathology and a high degree of organicity and of family pathology all predict a poor outcome (Pfeiffer & Stzelecki, 1990).

Non-health settings with a treatment element

Boarding schools

Sometimes, young people need a particular type of environment consistently for the whole day rather than just the time they spend in school. This may be a rather structured setting or one with special opportunities or experience of managing complex difficulties. Such children may include those with frequent epileptic fits that could not be managed in a day school or some children with extremely impulsive behaviour who need a consistent and reliable setting.

In recent years there have been moves to reduce the numbers of such children in special boarding schools because it isolates them from their peers and can institutionalise them. Nevertheless, there remain some children for whom this is still the least unfavourable option.

Intermediate treatment units

These units aim to work with disaffected teenagers who are often already delinquent. Such units have been created jointly by social services departments and education authorities, often with child psychiatric consultation to aid their work. They provide a mixture of remedial or appropriate academic work tailored to the particular youngster, with practical work experience and opportunities to develop the more positive aspects of their personalities.

Other treatments

Electroconvulsive therapy

This is used extremely rarely for children and adolescents. The indications are limited to life-threatening depressive withdrawal and refusal to eat or drink that can be managed in no other way. If electroconvulsive therapy is to be used in an adolescent it is wise to first seek a second opinion. Most frequently with adolescents, it is possible to sustain them while other medication and psychological treatments take effect.

Diet therapy

Reducing diets are used together with behavioural approaches in the treatment of obesity. Diet has also been widely popularised as a treatment of hyperkinetic syndrome. Until recently, there has been little evidence that such diets were effective or that removal of certain additives such as tartrazine would help calm young children. It has been thought that the alterations of behaviour might be explained by the greatly increased attention required to implement such diets.

However, there is now some preliminary evidence that removal of certain dietary components can alter children's behaviour (Egger *et al*, 1985). This awaits confirmation but is likely to prove yet again that parents are accurate observers of their children.

Holding therapy

This is an unproven therapy for infantile autism. It is based on the idea that a central difficulty in autism is held to be a profound ambivalence by such children towards allowing themselves to be in comfortable proximity to others. The parent is guided through prolonged holding and cuddling of the child despite their protests and struggles to free themselves.

Hypnosis

This has been used, mainly by clinical psychologists, to help children facing frightening treatments such as surgery or major dental treatment. It has been found to improve the child's acceptance of the treatment. It is thought to work by helping the child to feel in partial control of what is happening. It has also been used with youngsters facing painful chemotherapy for malignancies (Zeltzer & Le Baron, 1983).

Ethics of treatment

As in every other branch of medicine, the usual ethical standards apply. However, there are particular issues that arise because of the age of the patients and because children are presented or fail to be brought to treatment by the adults responsible for them. They are not free agents.

Parental responsibilities

In recent years there has been a considerable clarification of the nature of parental rights and responsibilities. It has become much clearer that parents exert their rights over the care and control of their children by the proper exercising of their responsibilities to them. Borzormenyi-Nagy (1985) gives some principles in his 'relational ethical' model:

(1) Adults are ethically and legally responsible for their actions.
(2) Prospects for the young and even for as yet unborn children represent the highest ethical priority for their parents.
(3) "The chain of consequences points towards the interests of posterity", that is, the principle suggested in (2) above should apply to other responsible adults in relation to children.

These principles help when the interests of the child have to be given priority over that of the parents. It means that doctors have a duty to break the principle of confidentiality by informing the social services department when they think that a child is at risk of physical, sexual or emotional abuse or of neglect. The over-riding nature of this principle was recognised by the General Medical Council's ethical code drawn up in the 1980s.

The Children Act 1989 is very concerned with the concept of parental responsibilities and how the proper exercising of these can be recognised (see Chapter 12).

Compulsory treatment

Parents have the legal right to say where their children should live. Elsewhere in medicine, they are responsible for giving consent to treatment on behalf of their children. However, increasingly, there is the recognition that children can give informed consent at differing ages, mostly from early teenage years. The Mental Health Act 1983 specifically differentiates assessment from treatment and requires an order under the act except in life-threatening emergency. It can be argued that if a child is able to give or refuse informed consent, then refusal must not be over-ridden by accepting parental consent but should lead to the use of the Mental Health Act if appropriate.

If parental consent for necessary treatment is refused for a younger child, then the clinician has to decide whether the treatment is so imperative that the advice of the local-authority social services department, and if necessary a care order, should be sought. Under the Children Act 1989 the court might direct treatment to occur without removing the child from the parents' care.

Breaking the child's confidentiality

On occasion, children will tell professionals worrying information that refers to serious threats to the child. In such circumstances the professional will have to decide whether the parent or other adults have to be informed. This can seriously impede a therapeutic relationship, particularly if the child is misled into believing that the relationship can be completely confidential. It is therefore unwise to promise children absolute confidentiality.

Treatment methods

Some treatments use techniques of punishment or of isolating the child (e.g. 'time out'). It is important that this is carefully monitored and consent obtained where appropriate. Approaches that use positive reinforcement are preferable and should be emphasised in treatment programmes.

Similarly, it is both common sense and ethically correct to try simple, often brief, psychological interventions before more complex methods are tried. Some very effective methods of treatment can be construed as manipulative. Here, supervision and consultation will aid the therapist in selecting the appropriate treatment.

Conclusion

This chapter has indicated the breadth of treatments in child psychiatry today. As will be apparent, the empirical evidence favouring one approach over another is still woefully inadequate. However, understanding of the developmental aspects of psychopathology and its relationship to adult psychiatric difficulties is gradually becoming clearer. Understanding of psychopharmacology, psychological and medical treatments is becoming more refined. The specific indications for particular treatments are often complex because there are several elements to the disorder that are maintaining the problems. This may necessitate more than one treatment being used.

References

Aman, M. G. & Werry, J. S. (1982) Methylphenidate and diazepam in severe reading retardation. *Journal of the American Academy of Child and Adolescent Psychiatry*, **21**, 31–37.

Bandura, A. (1977) *Social Learning Theory*. New Jersey: Prentice-Hall.

Barrnett, R. J., Docherty, J. P. & Frommelt, G. M. (1991) A review of child psychotherapy research since 1963. *Journal of the American Academy of Child and Adolescent Psychiatry*, **30**, 1–14.

Bentovim, A. & Kinston, W. (1987) Focal family therapy. In *Handbook of Family Therapy* (eds A. Gurman & D. P. Kniskern). New York: Brunner/Mazel.

Bolton, D., Collins, S. & Steinberg, D. (1983) The treatment of obsessive–compulsive disorder in adolescence: a report of fifteen cases. *British Journal of Psychiatry*, **142**, 456–464.

Borzormenyi-Nagy, I. (1985) Commentary. Transgenerational solidarity – therapy's mandate and ethics. *Family Process*, **24**, 454–456.

Byng-Hall, J. (1973) Family myths used as a defence in conjoint family therapy. *British Journal of Medical Psychology*, **131**, 433–447.

Campbell, M., Small, A. M., Green, W. H., *et al* (1984) Behavioural efficacy of haloperidol and lithium carbonate: a comparison in hospitalised aggressive children with conduct disorder. *Archives of General Psychiatry*, **41**, 650-656.

—— & Spencer, E. K. (1988) Psychopharmacology in child and adolescent psychiatry: a review of the past five years. *Journal of the American Academy of Child and Adolescent Psychiatry*, **27**, 269-279.

Campion, J. (1991) *Counselling Children*. London: Whiting & Birch.

Caroff, S. N. (1980) The neuroleptic malignant syndrome. *Journal of Clinical Psychiatry*, **41**, 79-83.

Dare, C. (1985) Family therapy. In *Child and Adolescent Psychiatry: Modern Approaches* (eds M. Rutter & L. Hersov). Oxford: Blackwell.

DeLong, G. R. & Aldershof, A. L. (1987) Long-term clinical experience with lithium treatment in childhood: correlation with clinical diagnosis. *Journal of the American Academy of Child and Adolescent Psychiatry*, **26**, 389-394.

De Shazer, S. (1988) *Clues: Invesitgating Solutions in Brief Therapy*. London: Norton.

Dische, S. (1971) Management of enuresis. *British Medical Journal*, *i*, 33-36.

Dunn, J. F. & Kendrick, C. (1980) The arrival of a sibling: changes in patterns of interaction between mother and first-born child. *Journal of Child Psychology and Psychiatry*, **21**, 71-89.

Egger, J., Carter, C. M., Graham, P. J., *et al* (1985) Controlled trial of oligoantigenic treatment of hyperkinetic syndrome. *Lancet*, *i*, 540-544.

Freud, A. (1946) *The Psychoanalytical Treatment of Children* (published articles 1926-1945). London: Imago.

Gelfand, D. M. & Hartmann, D. P. (1984) *Child Behaviour Analysis and Therapy* (2nd edn). Oxford: Pergamon.

Gittelman-Klein, R. & Klein, D. F. (1971) Controlled imipramine treatment of school phobia. *Archives of General Psychiatry*, **25**, 204-207.

Gorell Barnes, G. (1985) Systems theory and family therapy. In *Child and Adolescent Psychiatry: Modern Approaches* (eds M. Rutter & L. Hersov). Oxford: Blackwell.

Haley, J. (1973) *Uncommon Therapy: The Psychiatric Techniques of Milton H. Erickson*. New York: Norton.

—— (1976) *Problem Solving Therapy*. San Francisco: Jossey-Bass.

Herbert, M. (1981) *Behavioural Treatment of Problem Children – A Practice Manual* (1st edn). London: Academic Press.

Jenkins, H. (1990) Family therapy – developments in thinking and practice. *Journal of Child Psychology and Psychiatry*, **31**, 1015-1026.

Kendall, P. C. (1991) *Child and Adolescent Therapy: Cognitive-Behavioural Procedures*. New York: Guilford Press.

Klein, M. (1932) *The Psychoanalysis of Children*. London: Hogarth Press.

Kolvin, I., MacMillan, A., Nicol, A. R., *et al* (1988) Psychotherapy is effective. *Journal of the Royal Society of Medicine*, **81**, 261-266.

Kraemer, S. (1987) Working with parents: casework or psychotherapy? *Journal of Child Psychology and Psychiatry*, **28**, 207-214.

Kramer, A. D. & Feiguine, R. J. (1981) Clinical effects of amitriptyline in adolescent depression: a pilot study. *Journal of the American Academy of Child and Adolescent Psychiatry*, **20**, 636-644.

Kramer, E. (1971) *Art as Therapy with Children*. New York: Schocken Books.

Leff, J. & Vaughn, C. (1985) *Expressed Emotions in Families*. New York: Guilford Press.

Levitt, E. E. (1957) The results of psychotherapy with children: an evaluation. *Journal of Consulting Psychology*, **21**, 186-189.

—— (1963) Psychotherapy with children: a further evaluation. *Behaviour Research and Therapy*, **60**, 326–329.

Lochman, J. E., White, K. J. & Wayland, K. K. (1991) Cognitive behavioural assessment and treatment with aggressive children. In *Child and Adolescent Therapy: Cognitive-Behavioural Procedures* (ed. P. C. Kendall). New York: Guilford Press.

Minuchin, S., Rosman, B. L. & Baker, L. (1978) *Psychosomatic Families: Anorexia Nervosa in Context*. Cambridge: Harvard University Press.

—— & Fishman, H. C. (1981) *Family Therapy Techniques*. Cambridge: Harvard University Press.

Nordoff, P. & Robbins, C. (1971) *Therapy in Music for Handicapped Children*. London: Gollancz.

—— & —— (1977) *Creative Music Therapy*. New York: Harper and Row.

Palazzoli, M. S., Boscolo, L., Cecchin, G., *et al* (1978) *Paradox and Counterparadox*. London: Jason Aronsen.

——, Cecchin, G., Prata, G., *et al* (1980) Hypothesising – circularity – neutrality. *Family Process*, **19**, 3–12.

Pfeiffer, S. I. & Stzelecki, S. C. (1990) Inpatient psychiatric treatment of children and adolescents: a review of outcome studies. *Journal of the American Academy of Child and Adolescent Psychiatry*, **29**, 847–853.

Puig-Antich, J. (1982) Major depression and conduct disorder in prepuberty. *Journal of the American Academy of Child and Adolescent Psychiatry*, **21**, 118–128.

——, Perel, J. M., Lupatkin, W., *et al* (1987) Imipramine in major prepubertal depressive disorders. *Journal of the American Academy of Child and Adolescent Psychiatry*, **44**, 81–89.

Remschmidt, H. (1976) The psychotropic effects of carbamazepine in non-epileptic patients. In *Epileptic Seizures – Behaviour – Pain* (ed. W. Birkmayer). Berne: Hans Huber.

Ricks, D. F. (1974) Supershrink. Methods of a therapist judged successful on the basis of adult outcomes of adolescent patients. In *Life History Research in Psychopathology, vol. 3* (eds D. F. Ricks, A. Thomas & M. Roff). Minneapolis: University of Minnesota Press.

Rotter, J. B., Chance, J. E. & Phares, E. J. (1972) *Applications of a Social Learning Theory of Personality*. New York: Holt Reinhardt and Winston.

Russell, G. F. M., Szmuckler, G. I., Dare, C., *et al* (1987) An evaluation of family therapy in anorexia nervosa and bulimia nervosa. *Archives of General Psychiatry*, **44**, 1047–1056.

Stern, L. M., Walker, M. K., Sawyer, M. G., *et al* (1990) A controlled crossover trial of fenfluramine in autism. *Journal of Child Psychology and Psychiatry*, **31**, 569–585.

Taylor, E. (1985) Drug treatment. In *Child and Adolescent Psychiatry: Modern Approaches* (eds M. Rutter & L. Hersov). Oxford: Blackwell Scientific.

—— (1988) Psychopharmacology in childhood. *Association for Child Psychology and Psychiatry Newsletter*, **10**, 3–6.

Watzlawick, P., Weakland, J. & Fisch, R. (1974) *Change: The Principles of Problem Formation and Problem Resolution*. New York: Norton.

Werry, J. S. (1978) *Pediatric Psychopharmacology – The Use of Behaviour Modifying Drugs in Children*. New York: Brunner/Mazel.

Wilson, P. & Hersov, L. (1985) Individual and group psychotherapy. In *Child and Adolescent Psychiatry: Modern Approaches* (eds M. Rutter & L. Hersov). Oxford: Blackwell Scientific.

Yule, W. (1985) Behavioural approaches. In *Child and Adolescent Psychiatry: Modern Approaches* (eds M. Rutter & L. Hersov). Oxford: Blackwell Scientific.

Zeltzer, L. & Le Baron, S. (1983) Behavioural intervention for children and adolescents with cancer. *Behavioural Medicine Update*, **5**, 17–22.

11 Child abuse and disorders of parenting

Christopher Phillips

Physical abuse (non-accidental injury) ● *Sexual abuse* ● *Emotional abuse and neglect* ● *Munchausen's syndrome by proxy* ● *Child protection* ● *The role of the child and adolescent psychiatrist*

Parenting consists of meeting the needs of children in an effort to ensure their optimal development and to prepare them eventually for life outside the family home. No parent can meet all of their children's needs all of the time, but all parents may reasonably be expected to provide parenting which does not hamper or seriously damage a child's development.

Every child needs continuity of care and the opportunity to form attachments. Other basic needs are for physical nurture and protection, affection and approval, stimulation and education, discipline and control, and the opportunity and encouragement gradually to become autonomous, all provided in an age-appropriate way, and in a manner appropriate for the particular child.

In addition, parents must provide a range of models of behaviour and relationships for their children to imitate, identify with, or react against; in particular those of gender identity, adult partnership and, of course, parenting itself.

A child is abused if he or she is treated in an unacceptable way by an adult in a given culture at a given time. Cultural and temporal relativity are important in defining abuse, but even when these are taken into account, abuse may be seen to occur in all times and across all cultures.

Parents or other carers (i.e. those who while not parents have actual responsibility for a child) may harm children either by direct acts (abuse) or by a failure to provide proper care (neglect), or both. Abuses may be physical, sexual or emotional, and may occur singly or in combination.

Provisional figures obtained from the Department of Health at March 1990 indicate that 43 900 children and young people were on child-protection registers (Department of Health, 1990).

Physical abuse (non-accidental injury)

Physical abuse may be defined (for the purposes of inclusion on a child-protection register) as any form of physical injury (including deliberate poisoning) where there is definite knowledge, or a reasonable suspicion, that the injury was inflicted or knowingly not prevented by a person having custody of a child.

Injuries include bruises, cuts, burns, scalds, fractures, head injuries, and the sequelae of poisoning. It is important to realise that non-accidental injury (NAI) occurs in all walks of life and family types, and is inflicted on boys and girls of all ages. However, known risk factors include:

(1) socially deprived parents
(2) parental youth and immaturity
(3) a parent figure or co-habitee who is biologically unrelated to the child
(4) a parent who was abused as a child
(5) first-born children

Young children are most at risk because they are more vulnerable and cannot seek help. Children under two years old are most at risk of death or serious injury from severe physical abuse. Death from NAI is rare after one year of age, but four children a week die in Britain from abuse or neglect (Meadow, 1989). It is common for only one child in a family to be abused, while the others escape such treatment (scapegoating).

The diagnosis of NAI on the basis of the injury is the province of the paediatrician, but everyone dealing with children needs to be on the alert. The history is important and the following should arouse suspicion and careful further investigation:

(1) a direct report by a child or a witness that an injury was inflicted
(2) an injury for which the parent can give no explanation or only an implausible account
(3) the suggestion that an injury was self-inflicted or perpetrated by a sibling
(4) delay in presenting the child for treatment
(5) lack of appropriate concern about the child or the injury
(6) defensive rebuttal of unmade accusations
(7) a wish to take the child home before adequate examination has been completed.

Emotional and behavioural characteristics shown by children who have been physically abused vary, and depend to some extent on the age of the child but common features are: a failure to enjoy usually pleasurable things, low self-esteem, withdrawal and apathy, hypervigilance and 'frozen watchfulness', oppositional behaviour, poor social interaction, and pseudo-adult behaviour.

Case example 1

A single mother referred her seven-year-old child on the advice of the school because of enuresis and an episode when the child had urinated in the playground. At the initial assessment interview a burn on the child's wrist was noticed and the mother admitted to deliberately inflicting it with a hot iron in a moment of exasperation with her daughter a few days earlier.

Social services were informed by telephone in the mother's presence and arrangements made for an immediate physical examination by a community paediatrician. As there were no other emotional or behavioural difficulties, the injury was consistent with the mother's story and she was willing to cooperate with agencies, the child-protection case conference decided that registration was not required. The mother and child attended for treatment of the enuresis, which improved but did not clear. It subsequently emerged that conflicts between the mother and her parents underlay her uncharacteristic exasperation and assault on her child.

Case example 2

A court report was requested by social services because a mother was contesting the adoption of her two-year-old son, Steven. Steven had been placed on the child-protection register at birth, but in spite of a comprehensive protection plan and extensive social-work support, he had sustained facial bruising and a head injury when a few months old for which the mother could give no adequate explanation.

He was placed with foster-parents with a view to him being adopted, and when he was seen with them by the child and adolescent psychiatrist, he proved to be very happy, with a secure attachment, and developing normally.

The natural mother's own mother had left her when she was a baby and she had been raised first by her paternal grandmother and then by her father after he remarried.

Steven's mother had three children by her first husband, who now had sole care of them. He no longer allowed her to have access to them. Her fourth child, a daughter, had been placed on the child-protection register when four years old because of grave concern at the child's overactivity, aggression towards other children, poor speech and cognitive development, and indiscriminate attachment behaviour. While on the register she had sustained a considerable number of minor injuries, including a cigarette burn on her hand. Eventually a care order was obtained and the child placed with foster-parents. Although rehabilitation was considered, the mother had not wanted to participate and the child was adopted.

When interviewed, the mother subtly distorted the facts about this daughter's removal into care, defined her disturbance as 'wicked naughtiness', could not acknowledge any connection between the child's behaviour and the erratic care she had provided, and criticised social services for failing to help her properly.

She had no capacity to place Steven's needs before her own, did not believe he would be upset at being removed from the people he had come to view as his parents, and could not accept that it was her own behaviour that was responsible for him being in the care of others. She still could not account satisfactorily for his head injury.

A recommendation was made to the court that Steven should be adopted by his foster-parents and no access be given to the natural mother. The judge ruled that the mother's consent was being unreasonably withheld and Steven was freed for adoption.

Sexual abuse

Sexual abuse may be defined as "the involvement of dependent, developmentally immature children and adolescents in sexual activities they do not truly comprehend, to which they are unable to give informed consent; or which violate social taboos of family roles" (Standing Medical Advisory Committee, 1988). A simpler and more pragmatic definition is that it is the use of children by an adult for sexual gratification.

Children may be involved in sexual activity of all kinds – being enticed into watching sexual acts, pornography or exhibitionism; fondling and masturbation of the child by the adult or vice versa; sexual intercourse – oral, anal and genital; and rape – heterosexual and homosexual. Involvement in various perverse and ritualistic practices is also reported.

The exact incidence and prevalence of sexual abuse is unknown: widely differing definitions of child sexual abuse and non-random samples of the general population account for the unreliability of quoted figures. Baker & Duncan (1985) report the results of interviewing a sample of 2000 people representative of the population. Ten per cent of respondents reported sexual abuse before the age of 16 years. The definition of abuse was broad, but 51 % of those reporting abuse said that it involved physical contact and 5 % (0.5 % of the total sample) reported sexual intercourse.

Sexual abuse tends to present in one of five ways:

(1) an account by the child
(2) an allegation by parent, relative or other adult
(3) disturbed behaviour or obvious changes in behaviour
(4) physical symptoms and signs (e.g. perineal soreness, vaginal discharge, or anal bleeding)
(5) in association with other forms of abuse, especially physical abuse.

Disclosure of abuse may occur quickly when the perpetrator is a stranger, but where it is perpetrated by family, friends or acquaintances it may not be revealed for many years. Although specific signs and symptoms do not exist, some have a definite association with the sexual abuse of children of different ages: sexualised behaviour and play in children under six years; anxiety-related symptoms coupled with sexual preoccupations in the 7–12-year-old; and in teenagers, acting out, deliberate self-harm, anorexia nervosa, drug and alcohol abuse, and prostitution.

Young children do not usually falsely report sexual abuse, initiate sexual activity with adults, or tell of their experiences easily. This latter is because they are told not to, or threatened with rejection or violence to themselves or those they love. They fear the activity is wrong, feel guilt, and fear punishment, or do not want the family to break up if they do tell. They fear no one will believe or support them, and very young children may just not have the language to speak of what is happening.

Children of all ages and both sexes are sexually abused. The abuser is usually a male known to the child, but women do, on occasion, sexually abuse children. Risk factors in the family for abuse to occur include previous sexual abuse of either of the parents, loss of inhibition due to alcohol abuse, and sexual disinterest in or rejection of the father/male partner by the mother. Where the man has a history of sexual offences or a definite paedophilic orientation the risks are also increased.

Suspicions of child sexual abuse (CSA) may arise during the assessment of children referred initially for unrelated problems, or in relation to those already in treatment for some psychiatric disorder. However, child and adolescent psychiatrists may become involved in other ways where there is pre-existing suspicion of CSA on the part of the referrer. Psychiatric assessment of the child in such situations includes an assessment of the parents and their marital functioning and parenting capacity. The child should be seen with the parents, but also on his or her own.

Initially general evidence of traumatisation, attachment problems, behavioural difficulties and problems with peer and adult relationships, unusual knowledge of sexuality or of sexual patterns within the family is sought. If sufficient basis for continued suspicion of CSA emerges, then a more facilitative approach may be adopted with the child on his or her own. This requires considerable skill and training, and includes the use of different types of facilitative questions and the use of 'anatomically correct' dolls. (These are four large cloth dolls representing a man, woman, boy and girl which include oral, anal and vaginal orifices, breasts, pubic hair, and male genitalia.) They can be undressed and used by the child to illustrate specifically sexual matters. Children who have been sexually abused play with them in a different way to non-abused children, the play being much more sexualised (White *et al*, 1986).

Case example

Nadine, a five-year-old, was referred by social services for assessment following the allegation by her mother that she had been sexually abused by a maternal uncle living in another town. Social services and the police were already involved and Nadine's name was on the child-protection register. After initial discussion it was felt that an interview employing anatomically correct dolls, with the police watching from behind the screen, was the appropriate next step. This was arranged with the mother's consent and Nadine was brought by her mother.

Nadine was upset and clingy on separating from her mother, but once parted from her became inappropriately friendly and intimate with the male psychiatrist, easily snuggling up to him. During the interview she showed abnormal and disinhibited interest in the male doll's penis, and demonstrated explicitly on the female doll how her uncle had inserted a finger in her vagina. The interview was terminated abruptly, however, by her mother (who had been left with her other younger child in the waiting-room) barging into the room and wanting to take Nadine home, an unexpected turnabout of her previously cooperative stance.

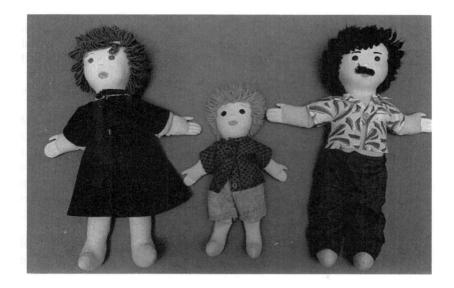

(a)

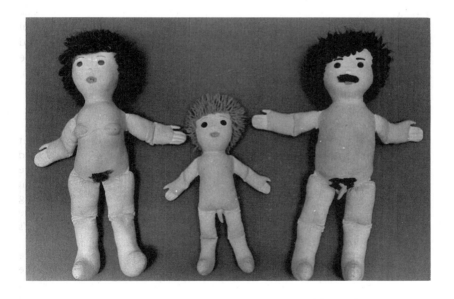

(b)

Plate VI(a,b). Three members of a family of anatomically correct dolls used as part of the assessment and treatment of child sexual abuse

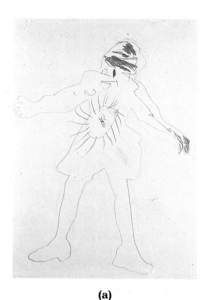

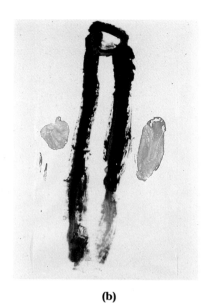

(a)

(b)

Plate VII(a). A self-portrait by a five-and-a-half-year-old girl who had been sexually abused by her older brother. She drew her body outline and then filled this in with colour and detail. The picture shows her experience of impregnation – the girl felt she was pregnant. She had blotted out her face and the hand with which she was forced to masturbate her abuser.

(b) Her image/portrait of her brother, consisting wholly of a penis

Following this, concern began to mount about the mother and her boyfriend's behaviour. Nadine was admitted from home to hospital because of vulval inflammation and suspicion by a locum general practitioner of sexual abuse. She was seen by a junior and inexperienced house officer and, before a more senior paediatrician could see her, was removed from hospital by her mother. After discussions between psychiatrist, paediatrician and social worker, admission to a paediatric ward was arranged and the cooperation of the mother was once more obtained. A case conference was called and during it the mother attempted to remove the child again. An emergency protection order was obtained and subsequently an interim care order. Nadine was placed in foster-care and an extended psychiatric assessment was undertaken.

In care Nadine proved to be very disturbed. She had a voracious appetite, was preoccupied with food, and would eat other children's food if given a chance. On one occasion she gorged to the extent of making herself sick. She would forage at night, steal from the refrigerator, and hide food under the bed. She would spontaneously assert that her mummy and daddy slapped her and that her mummy would hang her over the balcony. When an access visit was observed Nadine showed abnormal attachment behaviour towards her mother, clinging to her incessantly and whimpering, but being indifferent to her leaving and showing no signs of the usual protest on separation. Her mother interacted very little with her. Careful exploration of Nadine's medical history via the general practitioner, paediatrician and health visitor revealed a history of temper tantrums, nose bleeds, 'easy bruising', vomiting after eating, and thinning and loss of hair.

Psychiatric assessment of her mother showed her to have a personality disorder. She had been sexually abused herself by the brother now suspected of abusing Nadine, and had a history of overdosing, self-inflicted injuries and prostitution. Exploration of her relationship with her boyfriend revealed considerable discord between them.

The conclusion of the assessment was that Nadine showed signs of severe emotional deprivation, and physical and sexual abuse. Attempts to work with the family proved impossible and prospects for change and rehabilitation seemed negligible. Nadine's mother lied persistently and while Nadine was in care became pregnant again, making it even more unlikely that she could devote the necessary attention to Nadine, meet her emotional needs, or protect her from further abuse.

The court agreed with the child psychiatrist's recommendation and ruled that Nadine be placed for adoption, and access to her mother terminated. Once adopted, Nadine received individual therapy and her disturbance diminished considerably in her new home.

Emotional abuse and neglect

Neglect may be defined as the persistent failure to protect a child from dangers and may usefully be divided into neglect of physical care, medical care and education, and emotional deprivation. While the first of these is concrete and can be easily observed, the last is not, yet is more far reaching and pervasive in its effect. The omissions of neglect and emotional deprivation shade imperceptibly into the comissions of emotional abuse, which is defined as the severe adverse effect on the behaviour and development of a child caused by persistent or severe emotional ill-treatment or rejection. Such ill-treatment may take the form of habitual harrassment of the child through criticism, ridicule, threats, derogatory remarks, and withdrawal of affection.

Emotional abuse may be witnessed directly in the way a parent treats a child, but usually it is signs in the child that lead one indirectly to suspect abuse or neglect. These signs vary with the age of the child.

In very young infants neglect quickly becomes apparent because of the infant's high level of dependency. Babies need to be fed, kept warm, clean and dry, and handled sensitively and responsively. Recurrent infections, rashes and failure to thrive (defined as a poor rate of growth increasingly divergent from standard values) may all indicate neglect. Serious neglect may result in developmental delay – milestones for sitting, crawling, walking and talking falling far behind the normal because of understimulation and a lack of encouragement to learn these skills. Understimulated infants may try and stimulate themselves with persistent rocking or head banging.

In the emotionally deprived or abused child, attachment behaviour may be abnormal in one of two ways:

(1) the child does not show attachment, roaming away from the mother, not seeking her out for security and comfort, and possibly distancing him- or herself and watching frozenly from some corner of the room, or

(2) the attachment seems anxious and insecure, the child clinging to the mother, whining, whimpering, without any confidence to explore things away from her, and the mother responding to this with irritation or anger.

In preschool children the main indicators of emotional abuse tend to be behavioural, especially in social settings with other children. A short attention span with failure to settle to any task for more than a few seconds and general overactivity is often seen, as is poor social interaction, with aggression and swearing and an inability to play cooperatively. Indiscriminate attachment and friendliness, which may manifest as a craving for physical contact and intimacy even with complete strangers, is an important indicator of deprivation and abuse in this age group, as is short stature with a small head circumference.

In school-aged children, severe long-term emotional abuse may give rise to deprivation dwarfism. The children are short in stature, below the 3rd centile, with appropriate weight for height and below average head circumference. Behaviour towards food is highly characteristic with food being stolen, foraged for at night, and hoarded in the bedroom. Pica is a feature, and left to eat as much as he or she likes, the child gorges until sick.

Pathognomonic of the condition is that once the child is removed from home up to a tenfold increase in the rate of growth occurs in a few months (Skuse, 1989).

Such a dramatic picture is not often seen and indicators of emotional abuse tend usually to be emotional problems, behavioural difficulties, poor social adjustment, and learning difficulties. Such children have low self-esteem and feel guilty. They fail to make friends, lacking the social skills to do so, or may make friends only with adults. They may identify with their abusive parent, abusing others and handing it on or in some cases behaving in bizarre or inexplicable ways, injuring themselves or urinating and defaecating in their clothes or other inappropriate places.

Case example 1
Luke, a four-year-old, was referred by his general practitioner for persistent head banging. During the course of the initial assessment it emerged that his mother was locking him and his six-year-old brother in their bedroom from 5 p.m. in the evening until 7 a.m. the next day. Social services and

a home visit revealed appalling conditions. The boys' bedroom was little more than a cell, and the single light bulb had been removed, the boys being locked in the dark at night. There was no appropriate food for them in the house, and they had virtually no toys. A case conference was convened and the children's names placed on the register on the grounds of actual neglect. A comprehensive protection plan involving financial assistance, consultation/liaison with the nursery and social worker, and individual help for the mother was organised, with the result that the home circumstances improved greatly, Luke's aggression in the nursery diminished, and his head banging ceased.

Case example 2

A court report for care proceedings was requested by social services on Anne, a 15-year-old schoolgirl. Five child-protection case conferences had been called in the preceding nine months because of Anne being punched in the face or hit with objects thrown by her mother. Her mother had severe learning difficulties and had spent most of her life, until she married, in institutional care. She suffered from temporal lobe epilepsy, and on numerous occasions had been admitted to psychiatric hospital, often on a section of the Mental Health Act.

In the family interview Anne's mother persistently disqualified her daughter's comments, vilified her, and accused her of lying, encouraging the psychiatrist not to believe anything her daughter said. In an individual interview Anne was despondent, tearful and had very low self-esteem. She could not think of anything good about herself and had no real aspirations. She had no friends to speak of, and spent most of her time in the garden with her pet rabbits. She had few social graces, no dress sense, looked dishevelled, and lacked any real interests. Her mother and she could prevent arguments and possible violence between them only by avoiding one another. She was however adamant that she wanted to stay with her family, that she would run away if taken into care, and there seemed a good relationship between her and her father. A supervision order and family therapy was therefore recommended to the court, but the court decided to make no order. The family failed to keep appointments and within weeks of the hearing Anne was again seriously assaulted by her mother.

This was a case of physical and emotional abuse. The failure of the family to attend for treatment, and the recurrence of further violence indicated that the family really could not remain together for the time being. The case returned to court, a care order was made, and Anne went to a foster-family.

Munchausen's syndrome by proxy

This syndrome is said to exist when false evidence of an illness is deliberately fabricated by a child's carer (invariably the mother) in order to mislead the medical profession into offering treatment. A medical history is invented, clinical signs are fabricated, and the deception may be carried to fatal lengths.

The incidence and prevalence are unknown and although rare it has become a well recognised syndrome since Meadow (1977) first described two cases, and subsequently presented details of a further 19 children that he and other paediatricians had encountered (Meadow, 1982). Since then the boundaries of the syndrome have been extended and found to blur with other forms of abuse. Meadow (1989) describes the syndrome as presenting in four ways:

(1) fabricated illness
(2) perceived illness
(3) 'doctor shopping'
(4) enforced invalidism

Case example

Hugo, aged seven months, was admitted under the paediatricians with dehydration, diarrhoea and vomiting. He was found to have a high serum sodium for which no explanation could be found, despite extensive investigation. He gradually improved but relapsed several times when he returned home. Eventually Munchausen's by proxy was suspected and, with some reluctance on the part of the ward staff, very close observation of his mother was instituted. Shortly thereafter the mother was observed introducing salt into his feeds. When confronted she initially denied this, but after her visits were temporarily stopped there were no further episodes and the baby thrived.

A care order was made and after six months' work with a talented social worker, the mother was finally able to acknowledge her role in administering salt to the baby in order to keep him in hospital. She had been finding it increasingly difficult to cope with her three other children with little support from her partner.

Fabricated illness will usually present first to the general practitioner or paediatrician. Warning signs are: a persistent, recurrent yet inexplicable illness; investigation results that are not consistent with the general health of the child; prescribed treatment that is unexpectedly ineffective or is not tolerated; an excessively attentive mother who refuses ever to leave the child alone on the ward; symptoms and signs that do not occur in the mother's absence; and lack of maternal concern in spite of serious symptoms and signs.

Seizures, haematuria, haematemesis, fever, diarrhoea, vomiting and rashes have all been fabricated. Measures to achieve such signs include suffocation, pressure on the carotid sinus, administration of warfarin, insulin, laxatives, allergens by injection, emetics and poisons, mixing blood obtained from meat or tampons with a child's specimens, falsifying temperature charts or warming thermometers and so on.

The mother usually fabricates the illness while the child is under the age of two years. Often the mothers have been nurses or in some way connected with health services and about a fifth have a history of presenting unexplained illnesses themselves. The consequences of the syndrome are several and serious. Children receive needless and harmful investigations and treatments, as well as suffering all the disadvantages that chronic illness brings. Some die as a result of a miscalculation on the mother's part as to the degree of insult to inflict, others have a genuine disease induced either by the mother or iatrogenically, as with a steroid-induced Cushing's syndrome.

Child protection

When a child is being abused it is necessary that steps are taken to protect him or her. The safety and welfare of any child is of paramount importance and over-rides all other considerations. The following section refers to practice in England and Wales. It is encumbent upon all practitioners working with children and their families to familiarise themselves with the relevant local procedures and with the legislation. Statutory responsibility to protect children rests with local-authority social services, the National Society for the Prevention of Cruelty to Children (NSPCC), and the police, but all professionals coming into contact with children have an obligation to familiarise themselves with their local child-protection procedures.

When abuse is suspected social services must be informed. They have a statutory duty to investigate such reports. They should hold a preliminary strategy meeting to decide whether an investigation is necessary and, if so, how to go about it. An initial investigation will usually entail them consulting all other relevant agencies including the police, checking the child-protection register, seeing and interviewing the child's parents/carers, and other members of the household or other carers if this seems appropriate, seeing and listening to the child, and ensuring the child is examined by a doctor when necessary. If it is decided that there is a child-protection issue to be resolved, a child-protection case conference will be convened. If immediate protection is needed an emergency protection order will be applied for.

The emergency protection order is one of five orders in the Children Act 1989 of particular importance in the protection of children; the others are the child assessment order, supervision order, care order, and recovery order.

The emergency protection order replaces the old, much criticised, place of safety order. The purpose of the new order is to enable children in a genuine emergency to be removed from where they are, or to be kept where they are (e.g. in hospital), if, and only if, this is what is needed to provide immediate protection. Anyone may apply for an emergency protection order, but it will be granted only if the court is satisfied that there is reasonable cause to believe the child is likely to suffer significant harm if either: (1) the child is not removed to accommodation provided by or on behalf of the applicant, or (2) the child does not remain in the place in which he or she is then being accommodated.

Significant harm includes ill-treatment (physical, sexual and emotional abuse) and the impairment of health (physical or mental) and development (physical, intellectual, emotional or social). The order lasts for as long as the court specifies, up to a maximum of eight days. It may be extended for a further seven days in some special circumstances. Parents may apply to have it discharged after 72 hours, and numerous directions may be attached to the order by the court at the time it is granted.

When the situation is not an emergency a child assessment order may be granted by the court if it is satisfied that the applicant (which must be a local authority or an 'authorised person') has reasonable cause to suspect that a child is suffering or is likely to suffer significant harm, and that an assessment is needed and that it is unlikely to take place or be satisfactory if an order is not granted. The order lasts for seven days from a specified date. Children can refuse assessment if they have sufficient understanding to make an informed decision.

Child-protection case conferences bring together everyone with relevant information, and enable them to participate in planning and decision making. Invitations to attend the conference may be extended to numerous professionals such as an educational welfare officer, health visitor, school nurse, general practitioner, paediatrician, local-authority solicitor, community paediatrician, child psychiatrist, etc., and to the parents. Any professional may request a child-protection case conference, but the decision to hold one is usually taken by the chair of the child-protection team (one or two people in a district usually chair and convene all such conferences).

The tasks of the conference include examination of the evidence of abuse or risk of abuse to the child, considering the child's name for inclusion on the child-protection register, considering whether legal action is necessary to protect the child, considering whether the family will cooperate with agencies and making plans for further work with the family, follow-up and review. Roles and responsibilities in relation to the child and family are delineated and clarified, and a multi-agency plan formulated.

The role of the child and adolescent psychiatrist

Child psychiatrists offer assessment, treatment and consultation/liaison with other professionals involved in child abuse, and can make important contributions to the management of cases. Their broad training and special expertise in child development, individual psychopathology and family dynamics make their contribution especially relevant when children show emotional problems, behavioural difficulties, or developmental delay, and where parental mental illness and personality disorder is present or suspected.

Their contribution at case conferences includes taking part in decisions about whether a child should be registered, removed from or returned to their family, and recommendations about specific management and treatment. They are able to speak authoritatively as to whether emotional abuse is occurring, and comment on to what degree a child's mental state and emotional development is being affected by it.

The assessment of parenting capacity, the quality of family relationships, the parents' emotional responsiveness and child-rearing skills, and the likelihood of any necessary changes being made in time for the child are all evaluations in which child and adolescent psychiatrists have a part to play because of their knowledge and skills. Their independence from other agencies enables them to be an advocate for the individual child's emotional needs and to speak for basic principles of child care such as speedy and clear decision making, planning for the long-term future of a child, and paying due consideration to the child's attachments. Preparation of court reports and giving evidence in court as an expert witness is another contribution of the child and adolescent psychiatrist in cases of child abuse. There is also a significant role under the new Children Act in ascertaining the wishes of children and commenting on their capacity to give informed consent.

Finally, all forms of abuse and neglect may damage a child's emotional development, and psychiatrists and other members of the child psychiatric team have the skills to offer treatment to abused children, individually, in groups, or within the family, in an effort to help the child recover from the abusive experiences and prevent their repetition in the next generation.

References

Baker, A. & Duncan, S. (1985) Child sexual abuse: a study of prevalence in Great Britain. *Child Abuse and Neglect*, **9**, 457–467.

Department of Health (1990) Children and young persons on child protection registers, year ending 31 March 1990 - provisional feedback. *Department of Health, Personal Social Services, Local Authority Statistics*. London: DOH.

Meadow, R. (1977) Munchausen's syndrome by proxy – the hinterland of child abuse. *Lancet*, *ii*, 343–345.

—— (1982) Munchausen's syndrome by proxy. *Archives of Disease in Childhood*, **57**, 92–98.

—— (1989) Epidemiology. In *ABC of Child Abuse* (ed. R. Meadow). London: British Medical Association.

Skuse, D. (1989) Emotional abuse and delay in growth. In *ABC of Child Abuse* (ed. R. Meadow). London: British Medical Association.

Standing Medical Advisory Committee (1988) *Diagnosis of Child Sexual Abuse: Guidance for Doctors*. London: HMSO.

White, S., Strom, G., Santilli, G., *et al* (1986) Interviewing young sexual abuse victims with anatomically correct dolls. *Child Abuse and Neglect*, **10**, 519–529.

Further reading

Adcock, M. & White, R. (eds) (1985) *Good Enough Parenting. A Framework for Assessment*. London: British Agency for Adoption and Fostering.

Department of Health (1991) *An Introduction to the Children Act 1989*. London: HMSO.

—— (1991) *The Children Act 1989. An Introductory Guide for the NHS*. London: HMSO.

—— (1991) *Working Together under the Children Act 1989. A Guide to Arrangements for Inter-Agency Co-operation for the Protection of Children from Abuse.* London: HMSO.

Independent Second Opinion Panel (Chair I. Kolvin) (1988) Child sexual abuse: principles of good practice. Report submitted to the Cleveland Child Abuse Judicial Enquiry. *British Journal of Hospital Medicine,* 54–62.

Jones, D. H. (1992) *Interviewing the Sexually Abused Child. Investigation of Suspected Abuse* (4th edn). London: Gaskell.

Royal College of Psychiatrists (1988) Child psychiatric perspectives on the assessment and management of sexually mistreated children. Report of a working group of the Child and Adolescent Psychiatry Specialist Section. *Bulletin of the Royal College of Psychiatrists,* **12**, 534–540.

12 Forensic child and adolescent psychiatry

Jean Harris Hendriks

Current law ● Courts for children ● Support services for a family jurisdiction ● The knowledge base for a forensic service ● Liaison in child and adolescent psychiatry ● Areas for research ● How to do the work ● Conclusion ● Appendix: assessing children for forensic reports

---

During the last two decades child and adolescent psychiatrists have moved into medicolegal work, and without this expertise it is not now possible to provide a comprehensive service. During a period when the rights and needs of children have become prominent within our society, psychiatrists work alongside social workers, lawyers, judges, magistrates and law makers, and they must become familiar with the civil and criminal law related to children.

Stewart & Tutt (1988), supported by a panel of academic and practitioner social workers, lawyers, psychologists and psychiatrists, examined legislation concerning mental health, education, social services and criminal justice in respect of children within the three jurisdictions of the UK together with that in the Republic of Ireland. (The word 'jurisdiction' refers to the territory within which is constructed a framework of courts, court staff, judges, magistrates, lawyers and the laws and regulations which they uphold.)

The above study, the only one of its kind to date, focused on the custodial care of children, but it still provides a useful introduction and reference list to this complex field. A more extensive study is necessary but has yet to be undertaken.

Laws concerning child protection and placement, domestic violence, adoption, education and all other aspects of welfare provision are as important to child and adolescent psychiatrists as the law on mental health to the general psychiatrist or that on criminal justice to the forensic psychiatrist. It is recommended that all practitioners study and critically evaluate the law concerning children in the jurisdiction within which they practise.

Irrespective of that jurisdiction, it is appropriate to develop and adhere to principles for practice which comply with but transcend it. High standards of ethics, clinical practice and research are of the essence within any legal framework, and child psychiatrists may do more than practise such standards – they may work to improve them.

Case example

When Thomas was 18 months old his mother, a single parent, developed a florid schizophrenic illness. He was taken into care under emergency legislation and placed with 'temporary' foster-parents. As his mother became less ill she moved between hospital and the care of her own mother, a widow who denied her daughter's illness and constantly exhorted the girl to "make an effort" so that Thomas could be returned to them. At contact visits the young mother was remote from Thomas, while his grandmother was extremely strident and talked incessantly. Thomas tended to play at a distance from each of them and his foster-mother reported that the child was very difficult to settle, crying and clinging to her at bedtime for days after each encounter with his mother and grandmother.

A year later there had been no decision about Thomas's future. His foster-parents were most concerned that he looked to them as though they would be there always; his mother's psychiatrist said it was too early to give an opinion as to whether his patient ever could care for her child, but he hoped that "in a few months" she might be well enough to do so. The mother now planned to marry a fellow patient who had a history of alcohol abuse. The social services thought Thomas had waited long enough already and that the risks in returning to his mother were far too high, both in respect of her illness and because her new boyfriend was an additional source of concern. They thought that the little boy should be placed in an adoptive home where he could grow up in security, and sought the advice of a child psychiatrist about this and about the genetic risk of Thomas developing mental illness.

Child mental health services should contribute to a family jurisdiction concerned with children like Thomas, and indeed to all situations where a child's safety, behaviour and well-being require assessment within a legal framework. For example, a child and adolescent psychiatrist advised a court concerned with Thomas's adoption regarding genetic risk, the risks if he were parented by an ill, insightless mother, his attachment needs and his prognosis; the court's decisions depended upon this advice.

Current law

Children Act 1989

In England and Wales the cases of Thomas and many children like him are heard within the framework of the Children Act 1989, which has reviewed and consolidated the law concerning children, hitherto in a state of disorganisation and fragmentation unparalleled in the history of legislation. The main aims of the new act are to bring together 'private' law concerning disputes between individuals, and 'public' law concerning disputes between parents, children and the state. It aims to identify the rights of children in law and to achieve a better balance between adult duties to protect children and the need to allow parents to challenge state authority fairly and quickly. The new legislation also aims to encourage greater partnership between state and parents and to promote the use of voluntary arrangements. Key changes and principles embodied in the act include the following.

(1) The welfare of children must be the paramount consideration of courts in making decisions.

(2) The act provides a check-list of factors to be considered as a matter of principle by the courts before reaching decisions. These include issues concerning the wishes of the child, and the racial origin, colour and linguistic background of the child.

(3) A court should not make an order unless this is shown to be better for the child than not making an order. This involves theoretical and practice issues concerning parental competence, the needs and rights of the child, and the availability of resources.

(4) Any delay in deciding questions concerning the upbringing of a child is identified as likely to prejudice that child's welfare. (The act does not define 'delay' – the opinion of child psychiatrists regarding the effects of delay in relation to the child's age and developmental needs is likely to be of crucial importance in many cases.)

(5) The concept of 'parental responsibility' is introduced to replace that of 'parental rights' (the emphasis is on the duties and obligations of the parent, not on their 'possession' of the child concerned).

(6) The law increases the opportunities for children to be parties, separate from their parents, to legal proceedings concerning them. (There is concern among lawyers and social workers about the resource implications of this important legal right.)

(7) The law confirms certain duties and responsibilities of local authorities to provide services to children and their families. (Again there are important resource issues here: it may be possible, although undesirable, for a local authority to recommend that no order be made because resources are not available for the child or children concerned.)

(8) Local authorities are charged with a duty to safeguard and promote the welfare of children in need. (From the point of view of child mental health services, 'need' is identified in broad terms and includes children suffering from mental and physical handicap or from psychiatric illness.) The orders relevant to child protection and child assessment are described briefly in Chapter 11 (pp. 229, 230).

(9) The concepts of juvenile justice and welfare are differentiated.

The Royal College of Psychiatrists has produced a concise guide to the Children Act (Williams, 1992) which provides accurate summaries of this legislation and should be available for ready reference to all child and adolescent psychiatrists in current practice. The Department of Health (1991a) has produced its own guide.

The Children and Young Persons Act 1969 (CYPA 1969) England & Wales

Those parts of this law which relate to child protection were repealed when the Children Act became law, but portions of this act dealing with juvenile justice remain in force. Delinquent behaviour by children is now dealt with separately from child protection. The CYPA did not discriminate between welfare and justice, concerning itself with the 'needs' of the child. This led to a debate as to whether abused and neglected children were being stigmatised by association with the penal system, whereas offenders might find themselves involved, in an overintrusive way, with welfare assistance to them and their families. A Criminal Justice Bill, concerning 'delinquent' behaviour in young people, may create an appropriate pathway whereby children who have committed criminal offences, and admitted them or been found guilty, and who also are in need of protection within a civil framework, may be referred to the appropriate court.

Juvenile justice

Children who commit crimes are accessible to the law in the four separate jurisdictions of England and Wales, Scotland and Northern Ireland, and the Republic of Ireland but the age at which children are considered answerable to legal proceedings varies according to the framework in which they find themselves. In England and Wales children above the age of 10 years are considered answerable to a court if they have committed an offence, being labelled as 'children' until the age of 14 and as 'young persons' until they reach 17 years.

Children above the age of criminal responsibility may, after finding of guilt, be subject to a range of provisions, from adjournment via conditional discharge through fines to a range of orders affecting children and their parents, which may include custodial sentences. Children between 10 and 13 years are now dealt with in more flexible ways, including the greater use of cautioning by police (with a consequent fall in numbers dealt with by courts) and a range of provisions for those found guilty (for detailed discussion see Black *et al* (1991), Chapter 12). One-third of offenders sentenced for indictable offences in England and Wales are aged between 10 and 20 years, and of these many would benefit from assessment by mental health services.

For a discussion of the concept of criminal responsibility in the four jurisdictions see Stewart & Tutt (1988). The duties of the child and adolescent psychiatrist in relation to juvenile crime are outlined later in this chapter.

The Education Act 1981 and Education Reform Act 1988

These acts provide a framework in which the rights of children, including those with special educational needs, are defined. In the UK children have an obligation to attend school from the age of five years until they have completed one full term after their 16th birthday and the failure to attend school – truancy – is a status offence (that is, an act which can only be an offence in law between the ages specified).

The Mental Health Acts (England and Wales 1983, Scotland 1984 and the Mental Health Order (Northern Ireland) 1986)

These acts are enacted without lower age limits and in a number of respects are relevant for children and adolescents. Handbooks provided by the Royal College of Psychiatrists (1983, 1984) are convenient for reference (see also Hoggett, 1984; Stewart & Tutt, 1988).

Other relevant legislation

In England and Wales, adoption law and the law on divorce are currently under review with particular reference to the needs of children. Readers in all jurisdictions are advised to inform themselves about developments in legislation. Departments of child and adolescent psychiatry should obtain subscriptions to legal and social work journals appropriate to the jurisdiction within which they practise.

Consent to treatment and access to health records

Where a patient is receiving particular treatment, consent has been defined as voluntary and continuing permission for it. This must be based on knowledge of its nature, likely effects, aims, and risks. The patient must be able to consider the likelihood of success and be appraised of any alternative forms of treatment (see Department of Health and Welsh Office, 1990, for more detailed discussion). These rules, that consent must be fully informed and freely given, apply to children as well as to adults (Jones, 1991). Hitherto, rules and practice regarding consent have been the subject of case law or common law, but in respect of children, in England and Wales, these are brought on to statute via the Children Act and this is likely to create a framework for practice of which account will be taken in other jurisdictions.

The Family Law Reform Act 1969 England and Wales (section 8) has stated that a young person over the age of 16 years may give or withhold consent to treatment as though he or she had reached the age of full majority. In Northern Ireland, the Age of Majority Act 1969 allows that the consent of a young person who has attained 16 years, to any treatment, is sufficient in itself except when he/she is not deemed competent to give valid consent, in which circumstance, up to the age of 18, the consent of the parent or guardian must be sought.

The ability of children under 16 to give consent remained unclear until scrutinised in the Gillick case (*Gillick* v. *West Norfolk Wisbech Health Authority and the DHSS 1985* (3WLR830), which clarified that such children were capable of giving full consent "if of sufficient understanding to make an informed decision"). Thus the Children Act gives statutory force to the Gillick judgement, using comparable terminology. Where children are not competent it is envisaged that consent of a parent or guardian is appropriate.

Emergencies and controversies

Section 3(5) of the Children Act provides that "a person who a) does not have parental responsibility for a particular child; but b) has care of the child, may, subject to the provisions of this Act, do what is reasonable in all the circumstances of the case for the purpose of safeguarding or promoting the child's welfare". Thus, adults not holding parental responsibility may give consent for emergency medical procedures and, where care is shared between parents, or between parents and a local authority, responsible adults may act in the best interests of the child. What is not clear, and will require case law to clarify, is the position where a competent child does not give consent for treatment but an adult acting in a parental capacity considers the treatment to be needed. It will be necessary to seek legal advice, perhaps through the inherent jurisdiction of the High Court, regarding controversy over medical or surgical treatments. It may be appropriate to use the mental health legislation where young people under 16 years of age are seen as requiring psychiatric treatment rather than to rely on parental consent or the consent of a local authority in *loco parentis*.

The Access to Health Records Act (England and Wales) 1990

This legislation has been enforced since November 1991 and creates a framework in which patients may obtain access to their health records. The principles regarding children are similar to those concerning consent to treatment: if a child is competent to give or withhold consent to treatment he or she is also competent to decide about access to records. If there is conflict in this respect between the wishes of a parent or guardian and that of the child, the best interests of the child are paramount.

Good practice

In summary, the law has created a workable situation in which young people should be consulted and involved with every aspect of their health care. It is good practice to include in such consultations parents or guardians and, where there is conflict between the wishes of the child and those of a parent, to attempt to resolve these by mediation. Parents or guardians may act on behalf of younger children but the borderline to be decided in respect of consent to health care by older children is a matter of clinical judgement. In an emergency, a responsible adult may give consent. In case of dispute, legal advice or the use of mental health legislation will be appropriate. Doctors in doubt are advised to consult colleagues, to keep detailed signed notes of decisions made, and to consider consultation with defence unions.

Good record keeping with overarching attention to the best interests of the child will enable practitioners to regard the involvement of children and parents in decision making as a necessary and continuing aspect of good practice (see Black *et al*, 1991).

The law in Scotland, by Les Scarth

In Scotland the legal situation *vis-à-vis* child protection and juvenile justice is somewhat different from that in England and Wales. Scotland has a unique system of children's hearings, which were established after the Kilbrandon report in the late 1960s. Children's hearing panels consist of three lay members advised by an official, called the reporter to the children's hearing, who is qualified in either law or social work. Their role is purely advisory, although they also act as filters to referrals, which may come from anyone.

In relation to child protection work, if a child is to be detained under a place of safety order, this order extends for 72 hours and during that time an emergency children's hearing must be called to hear whether in fact there are "grounds for referral", namely that the child in fact has been or is at risk of abuse. The child can then be detained for up to 28 days before a full children's hearing is convened, where the evidence of abuse can be heard at greater length.

If there is a police investigation then the police will report any evidence of criminal activity on the part of an adult against the child to the Procurator Fiscal, a law officer who has discretion to prosecute. Where the child is young, for example an infant, or legally incompetent, certainly below the age of seven years, the children's hearing will almost automatically refer the case to the Sheriff Court for proof, that is for establishing whether in fact there are valid legal grounds for the children's hearing system dealing with the child protection issues. This will also occur at the initial children's hearing. Anyone involved, including the child if older, can object to the grounds of referral to the children's hearing.

The Sheriff Court is a much more formal procedure in its hearing than the relatively informal children's hearing. The children's hearing has the ability to detain the child in his or her own home under a supervision order or to remove the child to another place, under a supervision order with a residential requirement. Where there is a supervision order on the child, then a named social worker is appointed by the local social work office to supervise the child and his or her family. All supervision requirements must be reviewed via the children's hearing system at least once a year, although emergency children's hearings may be called at the request of families, children, or professionals at any time.

Northern Ireland, by Noel McCune

The relevant statute is the Children and Young Persons Act 1968, which is broadly similar in scope and powers as was the CYPA 1969 (England & Wales). The parts of the law relating to the protection of children are in the process of being reviewed, and a new Children Order (Northern Ireland) is to be prepared. This will be similar to the Children Act 1989.

The Republic of Ireland, by Anthony Carroll

From the Act of Union 1801 to the establishment of the Irish Free State in 1922, the 26 counties comprising the Republic of Ireland were in the United Kingdom. Legislation was therefore enacted by the Westminster Parliament. Following the establishment of the Irish Free State, this legislation, unless specifically repealed by the new government, continued in operation. In fact, up to the enactment of the Child Care Act 1991, whose various sections are being gradually brought into force, the principal legislation enabling statutory provisions regarding children and their welfare was the Children Act 1908. The fact that it could operate reasonably satisfactorily for so long is an indication of how enlightened and comprehensive it was at the time. Of course, other legislation was enacted by the new government, including the Children Acts 1934, 1941, the Health Act 1953, various School Attendance Acts, and so on.

A significant difference between legislation, and therefore practice, stems from the enactment in 1937 of the Constitution of Ireland. Articles 41 and 42 of the constitution recognise the family as the most important social unit within the state, which guarantees its protection and pledges itself to defend the institution of marriage. Social changes, particularly over the last two decades, have led to the constitution itself having to be altered by referendum with increasing frequency. This will have to be faced by the government that came into office in January 1993, and which is committed to introducing divorce legislation, as paragraph 3.2 of Article 41 states, "no law shall be enacted providing for the grant of dissolution of marriage."

In addition to different legislation in relation to children and the family, the Republic also of course has its own legislation, for example on mental health, juvenile justice, adoption and consent to treatment. To a child psychiatrist trained in the UK, and considering practice in the Irish Republic, all this might seem to be a formidable hurdle. In fact this is not the case. The underlying principles guiding child practice are the same everywhere. Even in the absence of divorce, there are many families who are legally separated, and child psychiatrists give evidence in court in relation to custody, access, and so on. Just as practitioners in England and Wales have had to modify their practice after the enactment of the Children Act 1989, so too those in

Ireland are facing the implications of the Child Care Act 1991. The main provisions of the act are as follows:

(1) the placing of a statutory duty on health boards to promote welfare of children who are not receiving adequate care and protection
(2) strengthening of the powers of health boards to provide child care and family support services
(3) improved procedures to facilitate immediate intervention by health boards and the Gardai where children are in serious danger
(4) revised provisions to enable the courts to place children who have been assaulted, ill treated, seriously neglected or sexually abused or who are at risk in the care of or under the supervision of health boards
(5) the introduction of arrangements for the inspection and supervision of pre-school services
(6) revised provision in relation to the inspection and approval of residential centres for children.

These provisions are laid out in ten parts, each with a number of sections, and they are being brought into force in phases. The new act raises the age at which a care order remains in force to 18 years. Another enlightened feature is section 25, which empowers a court to make a child a party to all or part of care proceedings, and to appoint a solicitor to represent the child in any case where the court is satisfied that this is necessary in the interests of the child.

In addition to a new Child Care Act, practitioners in the Irish Republic expect new mental health legislation in the near future, which will also modify clinical practice.

Courts for children

In England and Wales there is a three-tiered system comprising the High Court, county courts and magistrates' courts. The Children Act 1989 legislates for important judicial and procedural changes in the court structure: the purpose is to enable children's hearings to take place at the most appropriate level of court, according to their length and complexity. The act enables the creation of family proceedings courts at magistrates' level, staffed by a family court panel. It is intended that magistrates and judges on such a panel will have made a special study, and be experienced, in the practice of family law. A family courts consortium has been established comprising the major professional bodies of law, social work and medicine, together with a range of voluntary bodies concerned with children and their families; it will monitor the process of the law and the framework within which it is practised (Family Courts Consortium, 1991).

Support services for a family jurisdiction

It will be necessary also for child psychiatrists to understand the network of support services for the family jurisdiction within which they practise. Currently, the most important of these are child protection services and family placement services funded, supported and staffed by local authorities and, to a limited extent, by voluntary associations such as the National Society for the Prevention of Cruelty to Children, National Children's Homes, charitable adoption societies and others. The welfare and conciliation services of the divorce court vary considerably in their organisation, the range being from those staffed almost entirely by the civil arm of the probation service to those subsisting outside the formal court system and manned by volunteers. Panels of guardians ad litem or reporting officers (social workers independent of any local authority with legal duties in respect of a particular child, whose task is to represent children in the relevant court proceedings) are established, funded and maintained by a variety of mechanisms. It is proposed, but has not yet been achieved, that guardians ad litem should be linked directly with the office of the Lord Chancellor.

White *et al* (1990) provide a comprehensive text and commentary upon the Children Act. Hunt & Murch (1990) and Murch & Hooper (1992) provide critical commentary on current and prospective support services for the family jurisdiction.

The knowledge base for a forensic service

This comprises the whole of child psychiatry. In particular, it is essential to have detailed knowledge of attachment theory and current related research (Bowlby, 1977; Parkes & Stevenson-Hinde, 1982). It is important to have an up-to-date knowledge of the literature on child abuse and neglect, and a good working knowledge, not just of the genetic disorders of childhood, but of the genetic risk to children whose parents suffer a major psychiatric disorder (Robins & Rutter, 1990).

Assessment of parental competence requires knowledge of these fields of practice and also effective liaison with general psychiatrists (Oates, 1984; Reder & Lucey, 1991). This area of work includes the prediction of dangerousness – a difficult and uncertain field (Scott, 1977). Practitioners must bear in mind complex ethical and legal considerations, being aware always of the law and guidelines on confidentiality in respect of legal minors, their ability or otherwise to consent to treatment, and the issue of access to records, a matter of particular relevance where complex assessments include children, families and a range of external agencies (Harris Hendriks *et al*, 1990).

Liaison in child and adolescent psychiatry

Case example
Angela, aged 14, had lived alone with her mother since her father deserted the family when Angela was eight years old. Mother and daughter were

said to be "very close". When she moved to upper school at 13 years old, Angela began to refuse to go to school, being "panicky" and tearful, and repeatedly going to her general practitioner, backed by her mother, with complaints of abdominal pain. When Angela's mother invited a new man-friend to join the household, the school teachers at first thought things were better, since Angela began to attend regularly. Within six months, however, Angela was truanting, staying out late and on one occasion was found drunk with a group of friends in the shopping precinct near her home. Soon afterwards, the police were called to the home by neighbours when Angela's mother was heard screaming. Angela's mother had a black eye but insisted she had no problems requiring the police and did not need any help. Angela's general practitioner asked for help and advice from the local child psychiatric service, and on the same day the education welfare officer for Angela's school telephoned to ask whether it would be possible to make a referral. Both were concerned that Angela's risk-taking behaviour reflected severe stress about her relationship with her mother's man-friend. The general practitioner was unsure whether Angela could be described as being in need of care and protection which she would not receive unless legal protection was offered to her.

The child mental health service responded in two ways. Firstly, consultation was offered both to the education welfare officer and to the general practitioner regarding the decision which each of them must make as to whether to refer Angela to child protection services. The general practitioner decided to do this when, after discussion of Angela's problems again with her mother, referral to any assessment service was refused.

The child psychiatrist was involved subsequently at the request of the guardian ad litem who represented Angela's interests in care proceedings. This enabled an assessment of Angela's mental health, developmental needs and her prognosis with and without child protection services.

Child psychiatrists can and should contribute to support services for a family jurisdiction capable of offering effective help, to children like Thomas and Angela, and indeed in all situations where a child's safety, behaviour and well-being require assessment within a legal framework. Services may be offered in the form of direct clinical assessment, the writing of reports, consultation and the offering of advice informally or to case conferences, and the presentation of evidence in court. Liaison with child protection services is dealt with in Chapters 11 and 13.

Child mental health expertise may be offered to social services and voluntary child-placement agencies concerned with fostering, adoption and, to a limited but important extent, to social services providing institutional care for adolescents.

The welfare and conciliation services of the divorce court make use of child mental health services for advice, consultation, direct clinical assessment and the writing of reports. In particular they look for help in reducing the impact on children of parental divorce, for example by working to improve contact with non-resident parents, in ascertaining the wishes of the young people concerned and in reducing conflict.

J

Guardians ad litem and reporting officers acting in care proceedings or in disputed adoptions and freeing for adoption hearings regularly make use of expert opinion and evidence. It is part of their duty to consider whether the arrangements recommended by a department of social services, or by any other party, are the best for the child under the circumstances. They may wish for help in assessing genetic or environmental risk to the child, in considering the value and stability of affectional relationships available to the child, and in making choices between various placement plans.

Solicitors are instructed by the guardian or reporting officer representing the children concerned and it is good practice for a psychiatrist to link with each component of this team. Liaison is valuable also when conducted with solicitors who act on behalf of local authorities and those who may represent any of the parties to cases concerning children and adolescents such as parents, foster-parents, grandparents and others. The office of the Official Solicitor, answerable to the Lord Chancellor, is an invaluable source of independent evaluation, advice and evidence in respect of the most complex and controversial cases concerning legal minors in England and Wales.

Where children are offenders, child mental health specialists may be called upon to provide reports directly to courts regarding the mental health of the offender and advice concerning court decisions, placement and possible therapy of a juvenile concerned. They may find it a duty also to point out to the court the welfare and child protection issues which may be relevant to the circumstances in which the offence occurred. Liaison with the probation service is an essential component of a comprehensive psychiatric service.

Children who have been victims of violent crime, either directly through assault, abuse or neglect, or indirectly, through injury or death to those caring for them, are eligible for compensation from the Criminal Injuries Compensation Board. Many are also eligible for civil claims concerning accident or injury. Presentation of these claims requires both direct psychiatric assessment and effective liaison with other medical and surgical services, with social workers concerned with welfare issues, and with lawyers who prepare and present the case on behalf of the child.

A child psychiatrist on occasion may recognise a duty to initiate, or to identify the need to initiate, legal action on behalf of an abused or neglected child, to identify the child's need for reliable parenting or the right to compensation. Effective 'advocacy' is an important skill in clinical and liaison work.

A duty may be to emphasise, when giving advice about children and adolescents 'in need', the resource implication of the services to be provided and the effects of delay in decision making (which must be balanced against the need for comprehensive assessment). The child psychiatrist must be aware of the potential gap between the (considerable) advantages to children of the revised law and the reality of a partially reformed court system with severely underfunded support services available to it.

Areas for research

These, with potential for liaison between legal, health and social work practitioners, include:

(1) the outcome of adoption when compared with that for children contained in disadvantaged families, foster-children, and a comparison group of children reared in their families of origin

(2) research into the maintenance of links with natural parents when children are placed for adoption, with non-resident parents after divorce, and with wider families under both sets of circumstances

(3) the assessment of non-family-based care such as hostels, small group homes, secure accommodation and landlady schemes for adolescents in relation to the mental and physical welfare of the children concerned

(4) the aims and outcome of custodial and non-custodial sentences on children convicted of crime, with particular reference to the regime provided

(5) the relevance of race, skin colour, culture, religion and social class to child mental health requires extensive research (e.g. see Tizard & Phoenix, 1990); the Department of Health (1991*b*) provides valuable guidelines to current practice and future research

(6) forensic liaison work, both clinical and research, requires consideration of the effects of social and economic policy on the mental health of children

(7) the effectiveness of legislation and the legal infrastructure (courts, judges, magistrates, lawyers) must be evaluated in relation to child health and welfare

(8) the instigation of outcome research on the effects of legal decisions on the lives of the children who receive them is a high priority.

How to do the work

Standard good practice applies regarding the taking of a history, classification, formulation and the making of a prognosis with recommendations for further investigations and actions.

An additional framework, as required for forensic work, is appended. Today, all child mental health specialists must be aware that they may be required to appear in court, as witnesses of fact if they have knowledge, professional or otherwise, relevant to a legal decision concerning a child, as professional witnesses if they have information culled from their routine clinical work, and as expert witnesses if they have extensive specialist knowledge. All reports, at any time, are best written as though they may have to be made available in a court of law and read and discussed by any of the parties to the case. The preparation of such reports, the clear presentation of evidence, and the costing of the work involved (time, manpower, fees) are skills to be acquired in clinical practice and which should be included in higher specialist training.

Conclusion

It is not now possible to provide a comprehensive child mental health service without acquiring clinical, liaison, research and audit skills in forensic child and adolescent psychiatry. It behoves child psychiatrists to do this on behalf of all children in need within our society.

Appendix. Assessing children for forensic reports

When taking a referral ask:

Why this child?
  at this time?
  at this agency?
  by this referrer?
  for what purpose? (public, private, or criminal law?)

When is the report needed? Is a hearing date fixed? Can I do the work in time? Can I be available for court? Is the assessment requested:

 on behalf of the child?
 on behalf of a local authority?
 on behalf of a parent?
 on behalf of other parties (grandparents, prospective adopters, others)?
 other?

Who is making the request:

 solicitor in general practice?
 guardian ad litem?
 reporting officer (Scotland)?
 divorce court welfare officer?
 local-authority solicitor?
 local-authority social worker?
 department of the Official Solicitor?
 Criminal Injuries Compensation Board?
 other?

Has permission been given by those holding parental responsibility or the court for:

 interviewing the child?
 reading relevant documentation?

Have the parties agreed to be interviewed and to the preparation of the report? Has agreement been reached that the report may be read by all the parties? Will my report stand alone or is it to be read in conjunction with others (e.g. of the guardian ad litem or divorce court welfare officer)?

If I accept the referral will I work alone or with colleagues? Will I use videos, one-way screen, audio tapes?

Who will pay for the report?

legal aid?
local authority?
private fee paid by a party?
Criminal Injuries Compensation Board?
civil authority involved in compensation hearing?
Department of the Official Solicitor?
other?

Will the report have secondary aims? –

guidance to local authority?
basis for negotiation of therapeutic work?
if used for civil case, may it also be used in a compensation claim?
teaching?
peer review?
clinical audit?
research?
other?

Where will it be filed? Who has access to the file? Must I store an audio- or videotape record?

References

Black, D., Wolkind, S. & Harris Hendriks, J. (eds) (1991) *Child Psychiatry and the Law* (2nd edn). London: Gaskell.

Bowlby, J. (1977) The making and breaking of affectional bonds. *British Journal of Psychiatry*, **130**, 201–210, 421–431.

Department of Health (1991*a*) *An Introduction to the Children Act 1989*. London: HMSO.
—— (1991*b*) *Working Together: A Guide to Interagency Cooperation for the Protection of Children from Abuse*. London: HMSO.

Department of Health and Welsh Office (1990) *Code of Practice. Mental Health Act 1983*. London: HMSO.

Family Courts Consortium (1991) *Bulletin*. London: FCC.

Harris Hendriks, J., Richardson, G. & Williams, R. (1990) Ethical and legal issues. In *Child and Adolescent Psychiatry into the 1990s* (eds J. Harris Hendriks & M. Black). Occasional paper no. 8. London: Royal College of Psychiatrists.

Hoggett, B. (1984) *Mental Health Law* (2nd edn). London: Sweet and Maxwell.

Hunt, J. & Murch, M. (1990) *Speaking Out for Children*. London: Children's Society.

Jones, D. P. H. (1991) *Working with the Children Act. Tasks and Responsibilities of the Child and Adolescent Psychiatrist* (ed. C. Lindsey). Occasional paper no. 12. London: Royal College of Psychiatrists.

Murch, M. & Hooper, D. (1992) *The Lineaments of Family Justice*. Centre for Socio-Legal Studies, University of Bristol.

Oates, M. (1984) Assessing fitness to parent. In *Taking a Stand* (ed. M. Oxtoby). London: British Agencies for Adoption and Fostering.

Parkes, C. M. & Stevenson-Hinde, J. (1982) *The Place of Attachment in Human Behaviour*. London: Tavistock.

Reder, P. & Lucey, C. (1991) The assessment of parenting: some interactional considerations. *Bulletin of the Royal College of Psychiatrists*, **15**, 347–349.

Robins, L. & Rutter, M. (eds) (1990) *Straight and Devious Pathways from Childhood to Adulthood*. Cambridge: Cambridge University Press.

Royal College of Psychiatrists (1983) *The Mental Health Act 1983. England and Wales. Summary of the Main Provisions*. London: Royal College of Psychiatrists.

—— (1984) *The Mental Health Act Scotland 1984. Summary of the Main Provisions*. London: Royal College of Psychiatrists.

Scott, P. D. (1977) Assessing dangerousness in criminals. *British Journal of Psychiatry*, **131**, 127–142.

Stewart, G. & Tutt, N. (1988) *Children in Custody*. Aldershot: Avebury.

Tizard, J. & Phoenix A. (1990) Black identity and trans-racial adoption. *New Community*, **15**, 427–437.

White, R., Carr, P. & Lowe, N. (1990) *A Guide to the Children Act (1989)*. London: Butterworth.

Williams, R. (ed.) (1992) *A Concise Guide to the Children Act 1989*. London: Gaskell.

Further reading

Bluglass, R. & Bowden, P. (1989) *Forensic Psychiatry*. London: Churchill Livingstone.

Martin, F. M., Murray, K. & Fox, S. J. (1981) *Children Out of Court*. Edinburgh: Scottish Academic Press.

13 Liaison child and adolescent psychiatry

Dora Black, David Cottrell, Tony Kaplan & Robert Jezzard

Liaison with health services ● The child with a handicap ● Liaison with education services ● Liaison with social services

Liaison child and adolescent psychiatry refers to the partnership of child psychiatry, paediatrics and other specialties and agencies concerned with children to provide integrated medical and psychological care for children and adolescents. The development of liaison services in this field is comparatively recent and there are different models of functioning as well as ways of overcoming obstacles (Bingley *et al*, 1980; Black *et al*, 1990). In this chapter liaison with health services (with a separate section for mental handicap) and with education and social services is considered.

Liaison with health services, by Dora Black

In this section we discuss liaison services in hospitals to departments of paediatrics, neonatology, general psychiatry, oncology, haematology, surgery, accident and emergency, and other specialties, and in the community to primary-care teams and community child health services including child development teams.

Hospital liaison services

General psychiatry developed specialised general hospital liaison services in the UK earlier than child psychiatry (see Lloyd, 1980, for summary) as the greater number of general psychiatrists enabled subspecialisation. Liaison child psychiatry as a subspecialty hardly exists even today in the UK except in a few of the better-staffed hospitals. Most child psychiatrists are struggling to offer comprehensive services to a district and have to spread themselves thinly. Often the hospital liaison is done by only one member of the multidisciplinary team – perhaps a clinical psychologist, social worker or psychotherapist – and consequently only partial services can be offered – usually staff consultation and advice, referred cases being taken back to the child psychiatric service, which might be at some distance from the hospital. Yet in those services where the child psychiatrist can be a presence in the hospital for a substantial period of the week (or ideally full-time), the scope of psychiatric help is widened considerably.

In order to change attitudes and demonstrate that the specialty has something useful to offer medical and nursing colleagues, a rapid response to requests for help is needed and the psychiatrist and team must be proactive rather than only waiting for referrals. The majority of referrals are of children and adolescents with behavioural or emotional symptoms associated with physical illness or with a physical complaint that might be non-organic (McFadyen *et al*, 1991).

The components of a hospital liaison service

(1) Joint rounds

A good hospital liaison service would include joint ward rounds with the paediatric teams and with other specialties caring for children, as well as less frequent but regular meetings with specialties in which parents might have serious illnesses affecting their parenting capabilities – certainly general psychiatry, obstetrics and gynaecology, haematology and oncology, but also medicine and surgery more sporadically.

These rounds offer the opportunity both for the two teams to review all child in-patients and selected out-patients where there are concerns, and for two-way informal advice and consultation. This may lead to the child or family being seen by a member of the psychiatric team for assessment or some kind of therapeutic input or for guidance about management to the referring team.

(2) Routine assessment

Assessment by the child psychiatrist alongside the paediatrician could occur in conditions known to have a high psychiatric morbidity. These include chronic serious and life-threatening illnesses and those where the treatments are painful, mutilating or distressing, such as chemotherapy and radiotherapy, bone-marrrow transplant and dialysis, and other transplants. The advantages of routine assessment are that the patient and family become familiar with the psychiatrist at the outset and if these services are later needed, the family do not feel singled out. Otherwise, a referral to the psychiatrist may cause parents to feel that, in addition to the burden of a serious physical illness, their child is being stigmatised by being labelled as 'mad'. A routine meeting with the psychiatrist can allay these fears.

(3) Rapid response

The ability of the liaison team to respond rapidly to a request for assessment or help should be similar to that of acute medical and surgical teams, who would expect to see cases within a few hours of the request. A response should certainly be made as promptly, although after discussion it might be possible or even desirable to postpone the assessment until the parents may be available or the child has recovered from acute toxicity (e.g. in the case of an admission for an overdose).

(4) Staff support and education

Staff support is an important role for the liaison psychiatrist. This might involve regular meetings for the student nurses to help them cope with the behavioural problems of patients and the anxieties of parents and children, as well as supporting them in coping with life-threatening illness and death. Support for other members of staff might be less formal, and much of the work of a joint round is implicit staff support. Regular workshops on specific issues, such as alleviating anxiety or dealing with life-threatening illness, can be multidisciplinary and include play leaders, hospital school teachers, nurses, junior doctors and others. Such occasions combine education with an opportunity to talk about feelings, which is rarely otherwise available to staff on children's wards.

(5) Prevention of psychiatric disorder and promotion of mental health

Liaison meetings in a special-care baby unit or an obstetric unit offer the liaison team a unique opportunity to do preventive work with new parents under stress, and to identify potential high-risk family groups so that more intensive help can be organised. The treatment of post-partum psychiatric disorders will generally be the remit of the liaison general psychiatrist, but these disorders are more likely to be detected if a familiar and accepted member of the child psychiatric team meets regularly with the staff of the unit.

Liaison work involves having a general regard for the psychological well-being of patients, their families and the staff who care for them. It should enable the consultant child and adolescent psychiatrist and the psychiatric team to influence and enhance the psychological environment in which all of them function. The Department of Health (1991*a*) has published useful guidelines concerning the welfare of young people in hospital. Ward meetings at, say, termly intervals which include all the staff of the ward that can be spared and which focus not on individual patients but on improving the ward functioning are a useful preventive activity. It is essential that the consultants are present for them to be effective.

(6) Access to other psychiatric services

Finally, the full range of child psychiatric treatments as outlined in Chapter 10 should be available to in-patients in a good liaison service. This means that there should be enough professionals trained in a wide variety of therapeutic techniques, able to make brief interventions, and familiar with the range of provisions available in the community and further afield.

Conditions seen in liaison work

(1) Physical illnesses with psychological causes

Some physical illnesses are brought about by an abnormal state of mind. Overdosing is a common example of this, as are the medical sequelae of substance abuse and anorexia nervosa.

Illness in a child brought about by an abnormal parental state of mind can be either physical (child physical and sexual abuse, including factitious illness) or psychological. Children who present with somatic symptoms for which no organic illness can be identified may either be showing physical signs of anxiety – including separation anxiety and school refusal (of which abdominal and limb pains and headaches are the commonest) – or manifesting abnormal illness behaviour (hysteria). Often a minor physical illness may be prolonged because of the rewards that the child obtained while ill. On the whole, the disorders of this kind which present to a liaison team will be quite complex and require a joint assessment by the paediatrician and psychiatrist from the beginning if an optimal diagnosis and management plan is to be achieved.

Case example
Donald, aged 15, was transferred from another hospital, after consultation. An initial diagnosis of myalgic encephalomyelitis (ME) had not been sustained on investigation and abnormal family interaction had been noted. On admission, Donald could not walk or speak above a whisper. He seemed content to be in hospital and was indifferent to his symptoms. He was physically well grown, although functioning in the range of moderate learning difficulty. His parents rarely visited and the marital relationship seemed poor. His mother had had a miscarriage recently and Donald's symptoms had developed soon after. The parents were wedded to a diagnosis of ME and were reluctant to allow psychological exploration.

An approach which gave Donald a feeling of mastery was decided upon. A programme of physiotherapy gradually mobilised him and he began to speak during school lessons at the hospital school. Arrangements were made for extra help at his mainstream comprehensive school with the aid of state-menting procedures (see p. 265) and he was discharged after 12 weeks, walking, talking and able to return to school. In this case a combined approach using the facilities of a general hospital (investigations to exclude organic illness, psychiatric assessment and advice, physiotherapy and speech therapy, educational assessment and provision) were well used and coordinated to achieve a limited improvement and an expectation that the adolescent's improved self-image, coupled with his physical maturity, could enable him to resist family pressures. The inability to work with the whole family meant that our goals had to be limited, but improvement of symptoms in this case seemed helpful, at least in the short term.

(2) Physical illnesses exacerbated by psychological factors

Many common childhood disorders fall into this category. Asthma, for example, occurs in those with a labile bronchial mucosa, which reacts to allergens, infectious agents and emotional triggers alike, with bronchoconstriction. An approach to treatment which combines paediatric management with family therapy has been found to improve conventional management (Lask & Matthew, 1979). Similary many diabetics become out of control at adolescence. This results from a combination of rapid growth and psychological factors which make compliance with treatment less likely. A combination of psychological and physical management can enhance compliance and reduce complications (see Rapoff & Christophersen, 1982, for a discussion of non-compliance with medical regimes). Family factors such as good parental communication, cohesiveness and lack of conflict have been found to be associated with good diabetic control in children (Marteau *et al*, 1987) and these findings hold generally for good outcome in chronic illness (Eiser, 1990).

(3) Psychiatric disorder caused or exacerbated by physical illness

Repeated admissions to hospital, the experience of traumatic treatments, especially in the young, and fear of the unknown or of the future can all increase psychiatric morbidity in the physically ill child. About 20% of the child population suffer from chronic disease and the incidence of psychiatric disorders in this group is approximately twice that in the general population. In disabled children the incidence is three times that in the general population and if the disease affects the central nervous system this rises to about four times (Rutter *et al*, 1970). About one-third to one-half of children with chronic illness therefore suffer from a recognised psychiatric syndrome.

Chronic illness and disability also affect learning, not only because of the disease, but because of interrupted schooling. The effects on the children of parental distress, depression, anxiety and financial difficulties, as well as the reactions of siblings and peers, can also enhance psychological dysfunction. Siblings often feel neglected when parents have to attend to a sick brother or sister and may scapegoat the ill child. Any intervention by the liaison team must address all these family members and their functioning for optimum therapeutic effectiveness.

(4) Serious and life-threatening illness, terminal illness, death and bereavement

Children and adolescents with serious and life-threatening illnesses, especially those which require repeated, or lengthy hospital admissions or those which involve disfiguring, painful or frightening treatments, have a higher risk of developing psychiatric disorders than less seriously ill children. For example, the incidence of behavioural problems in leukaemic children is about 40% (Maguire *et al*, 1979). Many of the procedures that children have to undergo are painful and bewildering. Young children may find it difficult to understand why their parents appear to condone these 'assaults' rather than protecting them, and this may lead to withdrawal and a loss of trust in parents and adults generally. Children, especially older ones, also recognise the need to protect their parents and do not always let them know of their distress. Repeated traumatic experiences may lead to anxiety, depression and the symptoms of post-traumatic stress disorder. The child may express a wish for there to be an end to treatment which there may be pressure to accede to by parents or paediatrician. Careful assessment by a child psychiatrist may reveal a psychiatric disorder which when treated enables the child to be supported through such traumatic times.

Childhood cancer commonly has significant psychological sequelae, even if there is no further life threat (Koocher *et al*, 1980). Siblings and parents of children with serious illness have raised levels of psychological dysfunction, and marriages are put under stress by the demands of the sick child and by his or her treatment needs, which often separate parents and increase work and financial strains. Good liaison services include the whole family in the treatment remit.

Sick children may die and their death brings grief and mourning to their family and friends, and sometimes psychological morbidity. One study found that over 70% of parents had severe and troubling grief reactions after the death of a child and only a minority of them received adequate support (Sumner *et al*, 1991). Pathological grief reactions include absence of grief, prolonged grief, delayed grief, and distorted and deviant grief reactions (see Black, 1994, for a fuller account of parental and sibling grief). Since there is evidence that pathological grief reactions can be reduced in frequency and intensity by bereavement counselling, it is important for a liaison team to provide counselling before and after bereavement.

(5) Children caught up in trauma and disaster

Children have been shown to suffer psychological sequelae after trauma, particularly if there has been injury to themselves or to their parents. If children witness violence or an accident involving injury to one of their parents, the incidence of post-traumatic stress disorder is high. There is some evidence that this disorder can be prevented by emergency 'psychological debriefing'. This involves giving the child the opportunity to describe, using non-verbal techniques if necessary (drawing, doll play, etc.), the experience in detail soon after the occurrence (Pynoos, 1986). The role of the psychiatrist in mass disaster is outlined in a recent publication (Disasters Working Party, 1991).

(6) Children affected by parental illness and death

The morbidity among the children of sick parents is considerable (Black, 1978). Whether the parent is physically or mentally ill, the effect on the children depends on the quality of child care and the maintenance of good affectional relations between sick parent and child. Young children who lose their chief carer to hospital require good substitute care from someone with whom they are familiar and who knows them. The child psychiatrist can be helpful in aiding the staff of the psychiatric service and those responsible for the psychosocial care of adults (usually the social services department) to think about the needs of the children of their patients. If there is a mother-and-baby unit for parents with puerperal mental illness, there is a specific role for the child psychiatric team in monitoring the well-being of the child and offering consultation about the child's needs. The child may need his or her own advocate in a service which is primarily focused on the adult as patient.

Case example

A 21-year-old woman was delivered of a normal full-term baby. She had a history of mental illness and personality disorder. It was noted on the postnatal ward that she was holding the baby dangerously, balancing him on her knees without support so that without the intervention of a nurse he would have fallen. The mother seemed unperturbed by the danger. Assessment by a general liaison psychiatrist ruled out postnatal depression or other psychiatric illness. The child psychiatrist who was also consulted advised that the parenting abilities of the mother were poor and the child would be in danger if she cared for him single handedly.

The father of the baby was unknown and the grandparents felt unable to care for him. With the mother's agreement, mother and baby were admitted to a family assessment unit run by the local authority social services department. The mother used the opportunity to leave the baby in the care of the staff while she resumed her hectic lifestyle, and after many unsuccessful efforts by a social worker, staff of the home and child psychiatry department to help the mother assume responsibility for the baby, the local authority applied for and obtained a care order. When the baby was three months old he was placed for adoption.

Up to half of bereaved children may have psychological symptoms one year after the death of a parent and there is evidence that this high morbidity can be reduced by bereavement counselling (Black & Urbanowicz, 1985). The long-term effects of loss of a parent seem to be related to difficulties that children have in mourning and to the difficulties in caring for them by a single parent who is grief stricken and who may develop depression. Probably, if there are the resources, all the children of parents who die should have some brief counselling and surveillance thereafter.

Liaison in the community

Some child guidance clinics share premises with a group of general practitioners and informal contact is facilitated by this arrangement. For most districts, contact between the primary and secondary services is by referral. There may be possibilities for child psychiatrists to do a clinic in a health centre. Most of the liaison work outlined above is applicable to primary care also. In addition, there is scope for work with health visitors (Stevenson, 1989), community paediatricians, school nurses, district handicap teams, community psychiatric

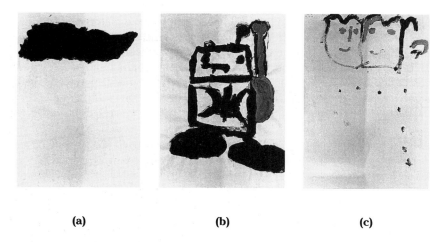

(a)   (b)   (c)

Plate VIII(a). A painting by a six-year-old shortly after a diagnosis of leukaemia. The cloud was painted with thick black paint. **(b)** A painting by the same child two weeks later. The child was painted all in black, the drip (to the right) in a vivid green. **(c)** A painting by the same six-year-old four months into treatment. The faces are painted in blues and yellows

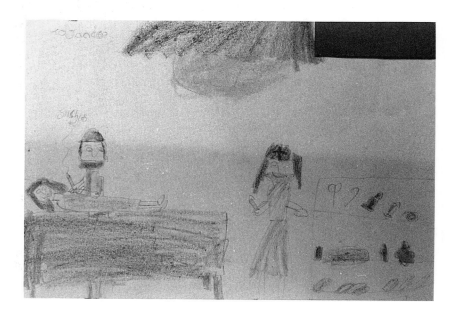

Plate IX. A painting by an eight-year-old girl admitted to hospital for a minor operation

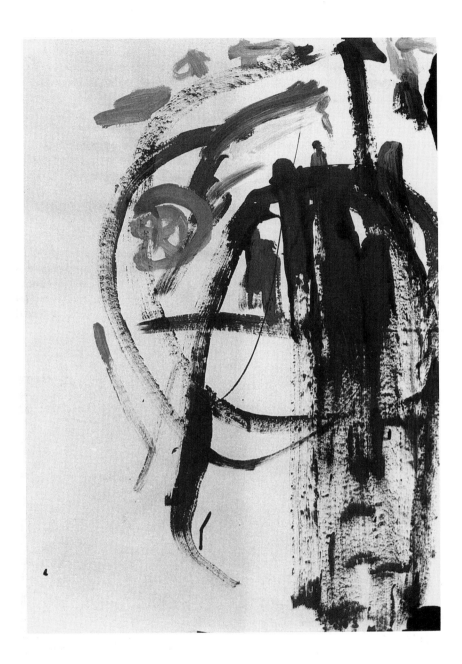

Plate X. A painting by an eight-year-old after a serious road traffic accident. Clinically, he had left-sided neglect, and in a whole series of paintings he never used the left side of the paper

nurses, and others delivering health care. Thompson & Bellenis (1992) have described a joint service with child psychiatrists and health visitors for under-fives which enabled health visitors eventually to manage sleep, habit and behavioural problems themselves, and improve their work in promoting healthy mother–child relationships using, for example, therapeutic groups for depressed mothers.

Another model encourages the exchange of community paediatricians in training and trainee child psychiatrists for attachments to the other service. The community paediatricians can acquire skills in behavioural therapy and family counselling, and the child psychiatrists can increase their knowledge of the mentally well child, educational paediatrics, and social influences on children's behaviour.

Child and adolescent psychiatric consultation should be easily available to community health professionals. Some clinics organise this by using domiciliary visits with a general practitioner, or by having some time available every day for professionals within the community to use for emergency consultation. A good child psychiatric service should be available to the people who need it within their district. In this sense, all child and adolescent psychiatry is liaison work.

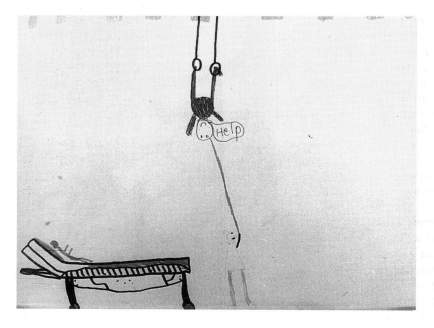

Plate XI. A drawing by a ten-year-old boy who had not been told he had a brain tumour. His picture, with its accurately portrayed hospital bed, shows his feelings of helplessness as he is manipulated by the nurse

The child with a handicap, by David Cottrell

Over the last 20 years major changes have taken place in the services provided for children with a handicap. The decision of the Department of Education and Science in 1970 that children with an intellectual handicap should no longer be regarded as 'ineducable' led to the widespread provision of special day schools for such children. The result has been that today nearly all children with a handicap are cared for in homes by families rather than in institutions. The Sheldon working party (Ministry of Health, 1967) recommended the setting up of a comprehensive diagnostic and therapeutic service for all children with a handicap. Shortly afterwards the Court report (Committee on Child Health Services, 1970) advised that each health district should set up multidisciplinary 'district handicap teams' and stated explicitly that child psychiatric consultation should be available to children and families seen by such services. A review of district handicap teams (Bax & Whitmore, 1991) specifically recommended that each such team should have at least one session per week from a child psychiatrist.

Children with a handicap are at a greater risk of developing psychiatric disorders. In the Isle of Wight study children with mental handicap were between four and seven times more likely to have a psychiatric disorder than the general population, depending upon the severity of the handicap (Rutter *et al*, 1970). Children with a physical handicap, especially where the brain is affected, are also at an increased risk of psychiatric disorder (Seidel *et al*, 1975). The reasons for this involve the complex interaction of individual, family and social factors which are described in greater detail in Chapter 4. The child and adolescent psychiatrist, whose training involves the study of both biological and psychological sciences, is clearly well placed to provide assessment, diagnosis and treatment in such cases. However, there are numerous other professionals (including developmental paediatricians, occupational, speech and physiotherapists, clinical and educational psychologists, teachers, social workers and community nurses) and of course the child's family whose roles are also vital in the care of children with a handicap. When children with a mental handicap were only cared for in institutions, the psychiatrist was often in charge. Now that children are cared for in the community it is important that the psychiatrist recognises that he or she is only one part of a multidisciplinary team of professionals and that the majority of children will not need their services. Nevertheless there is an important role for the psychiatrist and it is the duty of all child mental health services to provide a service for all children, irrespective of whether or not they have a handicap.

The child and adolescent psychiatrist should therefore offer services either as part of, or in close liaison with, the district handicap or child development team. Such liaison includes a combination of assessment, consultation and direct therapeutic work (Evered *et al*, 1989).

Assessment

The increased risk of psychiatric disorder makes the psychiatric viewpoint indispensable in the assessment within the child development team. Children with a handicap have enough difficulties without significant psychiatric disorder going undiagnosed and untreated. As well as conduct and emotional problems throughout childhood and adolescence, of particular importance here is the assessment of possible psychosis in teenagers with mental handicap where lack of communication skills may make diagnosis difficult.

More generally, the psychiatrist acts to remind others of the important psychological consequences for families in coming to terms with the diagnosis of handicap. Most professionals are now aware of the immediate effects of such a diagnosis but it may be necessary, when assessing older children, to remind colleagues that coming to terms with handicap is a process rather than a 'one-off' event. At key points in the family's development further emotional adjustments are necessary and these must be taken into account in assessment. Thus starting a special school, being overtaken in attainments by a younger child, emergent sexuality in adolescence and leaving school are just a few of the events that may reactivate the need for 'coming to terms' with the handicap.

Testament to the difficulties families face is the fact that parents of children with a chronic physical handicap will experience greater marital discord (Sabbeth & Leventhal, 1984). Siblings of some mentally handicapped children are also more likely to have psychiatric disorders (Gath & Gumley, 1987).

More specifically, the child psychiatrist needs to be involved, and indeed may have the major input, in the assessment of those complex conditions where delays or deviance, or both, are evident in attachment behaviour, play, and social and language development. The differential diagnosis in such cases can include generalised learning difficulties either as a result of an inborn deficit or environmental understimulation, specific developmental delays such as receptive language disorder, infantile autism or the effects of severe abuse or neglect. In these cases the key to an accurate diagnosis may be the child psychiatrist's assessment of the child's social and emotional development and functioning in the family and school.

The child psychiatrist may also be asked to participate in the assessment of a child's special educational needs by the local education authority (see below).

Case example

John, aged three, was referred by the clinical medical officer at the local child development team with a request for assessment. The referral described marked delay in language development, severe behaviour problems and a difficulty in getting on with his family and peers. A diagnosis of infantile autism was suggested.

Assessment consisted of a detailed history from John's parents and staff at his day nursery as well as careful observation of his behaviour in the clinic and at the nursery on more than one occasion.

It soon became clear that John came from a warm and caring family, where he received adequate stimulation. Although there was evidence of marked language delay with little use of non-verbal communication such as gesture and no speech at all, a diagnosis of autism was ruled out. John's difficulty in relating to other people seemed to be largely due to frequent temper tantrums which were being managed inconsistently at home and in the nursery and his difficulty in communicating his own needs or understanding those of others. At times he could be a warm and affectionate child who sought cuddles and showed none of the persistent aloofness of the autistic child.

A diagnosis of severe language delay was made and arrangements made for John to attend a local nursery with a specialist language unit. A behaviour modification programme, implemented at home and in the nursery, brought about a rapid diminution in temper tantrums, but progess with his use of language remained slow.

Consultation

Perhaps the most valuable use of psychiatric time is in the provision of consultation to other professionals in the child development team. Creating a climate in which other therapists can go to the psychiatrist to discuss children and their families with an expectation of receiving useful advice and with no fear of being criticised or deskilled is a difficult task and one that has to be worked at. The respect of the rest of the team usually has to be earned. The psychiatrist will have to display a good working knowledge not only of the problems of children with a handicap but of the skills of the different therapists if the consultation relationship is to work. A potential consultant may have to gain credibility by taking on direct work with families before others in the team will go to them for advice about their own work.

Once the consultation relationship is established it has many benefits. Regular meetings allow many cases to be discussed in a relatively short time. Unnecessary referrals can be avoided by enabling other therapists to take fresh directions in their own work, and children who need a psychiatric opinion but who otherwise might have been missed are picked up earlier and referral is facilitated. The psychiatrist's appreciation of psychosocial issues and the need for these to be discussed also plays an important role in staff support within the team.

In addition to consultation within the child development team, the child psychiatrist will find it useful to cultivate links with other professionals who come into contact with children with a handicap. Regular contact with paediatric staff (especially in the local special-care baby unit, where many diagnoses of handicap will be made), with social services and with local schools for children with special needs should all be part of a comprehensive liaison service.

Treatment

The full range of treatments used in child and adolescent psychiatry and described in Chapter 10 are applicable in work with handicapped children and their families. It is important to recognise that the child with a handicap can use individual and group psychotherapeutic methods despite not matching the 'classic' indicators of being articulate and intelligent. Counselling and support groups for parents are helpful and behavioural techniques can be effective in dealing with conduct disorder and self-destructive behaviour in children. Brain injury is not a contra-indication to the use of psychotropic medication.

Case example

Sarah, aged 14, was referred by her general practitioner because of aggressive behaviour at home which had started within the last year and was becoming increasingly difficult for her parents to manage. Sarah was diagnosed as having learning difficulties shortly after birth, although no cause was ever found. She was the youngest of three siblings, her older brother and sister both having left home. On assessment it became clear that most of Sarah's aggressive behaviour appeared in relation to arguments with her parents about going out in the evenings and at weekends to a local youth club and to a school-friend's house. Sarah's parents were reluctant to let her go out without them also being present, fearing that she would not be able to look after herself.

At school, where Sarah was being taught about self-care skills and independent living that year, there were no behaviour problems.

After some initial family meetings, Sarah was offered weekly individual counselling sessions and her parents some meetings together. In these sessions her parents discussed their fears for Sarah's safety and explored with the therapist their feelings about Sarah's disability, something they had not discussed for years. After some months they agreed to allow Sarah out to occasional youth club meetings and when this went well gradually increased her freedom of movement. Her aggressive behaviour gradually decreased.

Through a good liaison relationship, professionals in district handicap teams can make optimum use of the expertise of child and adolescent psychiatrists. Many of the children with a handicap referred to child psychiatrists are not, however, in touch with these handicap teams. Often the difficulties of such children are related to unrealistic parental expectations (in the case of learning difficulties) or lack of appropriate support. The most effective 'treatment' by the psychiatrist is often referral to the appropriate specialists, a referral facilitated by good liaison relationships.

Liaison with education services, by Tony Kaplan

The child and adolescent psychiatrist's relationship with the school is interactive. The school may want help with children they have found difficult to manage or about whose emotional state, behaviour or development they are concerned. The child and adolescent psychiatrist may require the school's help in providing information about a referred child or participation in aspects of treatment agreed with parents. School is the second most important social context for the child after the family, and teachers will often have valuable observations about the child's coping style and strategies, attachments, peer relationships, maturity, educational attainments and special learning difficulties. In the case of teenagers who suffer severe mental disturbance with insidious onset, it is often classmates who notice first.

Working with schools: contexts and maps

The therapeutic system

This system is the network of non-teacher professionals and agencies, working together with or in schools, to enhance the child's emotional well-being in the school in the interests of his or her optimal educational performance and social functioning. The following are included.

(1) The child and adolescent psychiatry department or child and family service (sometimes known as the child guidance service). Members of this team include child and adolescent psychiatrists, clinical (child) psychologists, educational psychologists, child psychotherapists, specialist social workers, and occasionally psychiatric nurses and educational therapists. This is the team that offers most of the direct therapy with children and families but who will also offer consultation to teachers or other professionals.

(2) The school psychological service (sometimes working within the structure of the child guidance service). Educational psychologists (EPs) have a first degree in psychology, a teaching qualification and experience, and have a statutory responsibility to assess children with special educational needs and advise teachers and parents accordingly. In some boroughs they will have an extended direct therapeutic role. Educational psychologists do most of the 'indirect therapeutic work' in schools, consulting to teachers to enhance the therapeutic work teachers do and filtering or facilitating referrals where appropriate. Because they have a foot in the child guidance service and a foot in the school they are invaluable in bridging the world of the child at home and at school, and in ensuring effective communication between the two agencies.

(3) Education welfare service. Education welfare officers (sometimes referred to as educational social workers) have no requirement for formal specialist training, although this is changing. They are predominantly involved with school non-attenders and their families, but may become involved, mainly in a liaison capacity, in cases of child abuse and neglect or other cases of family stress.

(4) The community paediatric service. This is involved in assessing children with special needs, especially physical illness, handicap or developmental delay, and advising parents accordingly. Community paediatricians, community medical officers, school doctors and school nurses fall within this group.

The mainstream school system

In mainstream schools, professionals from the 'therapeutic system' link with or intervene via the conventional hierarchy (directors of education, inspectors/advisers, head teachers, heads of year, class teachers, etc.) or via the professionals who are designated to deal with children with special needs in mainstream schools (including remedial teachers, support teachers, teachers with responsibility for pastoral care, special-needs coordinators and school nurses).

Special-needs school system

This is organised into units, including:

(1) on-site support units, offering more individual attention and small-group work with vulnerable children in mainstream schools
(2) nurture groups, essentially offering the same with or without environmental enrichment for developmentally delayed or emotionally vulnerable young children starting school
(3) off-site units – usually offering brief interventions with children who cannot be managed in mainstream schools, with the intention of returning them to mainstream
(4) tuition units, including the home tuition service, providing education for children excluded from school or not attending for other reasons (illness, pregnancy etc.)
(5) special schools (day or residential/boarding), offering longer-term interventions or in some cases permanent places for children who cannot be managed in mainstream schools, including:
    (a) children with emotional and behavioural disturbances (EBD)
    (b) children with moderate learning difficulties (MLD, previously referred to as educationally subnormal (ESN))
    (c) children with severe learning difficulties (SLD)
    (d) children with highly specific needs including language and communication difficulties, hearing and visual impairments, etc.
    (e) 'delicate' children (including children with chronic physical or mental illness)
(6) hospital schools
(7) schools attached to psychiatric day or in-patient units.

Professionals from this system, and indeed from mainstream schools, will already be doing important therapeutic work with many of the children who are or might be referred to child guidance centres or child psychiatry departments and this must not be undermined. Often liaison or consultation with these professionals will prove to be a valuable adjunct to therapy in the clinic, or may limit the need for involvement of clinic professionals.

Which children do schools want help with?

(1) Children who have emotional and behavioural disturbance sufficient to interfere with their learning, their normal social activity or to disrupt the class.

(2) Children who are difficult to engage in reciprocal communication, with poor social skills or with difficulty in establishing peer relationships: children who are isolated, overly dependent or who show role rigidity, for example with teasing and bullying (as victim or perpetrator), or as clown of the class.

(3) Children with poor school attendance.

The child and adolescent psychiatrist's role with regard to the *school* is to help to maximise the child's potential to learn and to develop socially.

What sort of help?

Assessment ('statementing')

A referral from a teacher or educational welfare officer to a child and adolescent psychiatry service may be for assessment and treatment, and will be dealt with as are other referrals. In addition, following the Warnock report (Department of Education and Science, 1978) there is now an obligation on the education department of the local authority to make a full assessment ('statement') of the educational needs of all children having significant difficulties in school, under section 5 of the Education Act 1981. Warnock systematically reframed 'handicapped' as a mismatch between the child's special needs and the type and setting of the education provided, as an attempt to escape, perhaps too idealistically, the negative effects of labelling. Sociocultural biases remain, although the obligation on education departments to provide resources to maximise the potential of children with special needs has led to some improvements.

The child and adolescent psychiatrist may be asked to contribute towards the full assessment as part of the medical report. The child and adolescent psychiatrist's report will deal with (1) impediments to learning arising out of emotional and behavioural disorder in the child and family, and (2) what special provision may need to be made to ameliorate or overcome this at school. The child and adolescent psychiatrist is not required to advise on placement, which is the responsibility of the special-needs panel, although informal advice may be welcomed. Placement in practice may depend on political biases (e.g. integration versus segregation of children with special needs) and resources.

Consultation

Different models of consultation may coexist.

The expert role (cognition) involves: (1) providing explanation and information, for example regarding the behaviour and predictable thoughts and feelings of children who have been sexually abused or children who are coping with family breakdown or bereavement, (2) giving guidelines on the management in school of children with formal mental illness, or organic states (e.g. following solvent abuse), and (3) prescribing and supervising behaviour modification programmes to be carried out in school.

The facilitative role (process) involves questioning, interpreting or intervening in interactions between the teacher/pupil, teacher/class, teacher/family, teacher/school hierarchy or teacher/school/other agencies (see example below).

The supportive role (affect) is directed towards individual teachers or staff groups, and dealing with those feelings engendered by their work which, if unchecked, will impede performance or interfere with good collaboration (e.g. demoralisation, cynicism, blame, guilt).

The advantage of a child and adolescent psychiatrist as a consultant is that he or she is relatively free of the political or hierarchical constraints of 'in-house' consultants and sufficiently naïve (*vis-à-vis* the educational system) to be allowed to ask impertinent questions, to challenge assumptions, and to provide the voice of authority the teacher may need to risk being creative and decisive.

However, professionals coming into the school will be regarded as outsiders and may generate antagonism and competitiveness unless some simple rules of consultation are followed. Type (see above) and level of consultation (from child-centred to staff-group process) needs to be established and agreed with sensitivity and respect. The active support, if not participation, of the most senior person in the hierarchy is essential (e.g. head teacher). Rules of confidentiality and attendance need to be agreed, as do the time, frequency and place of the meetings. The acceptable level of intervention by the consultant may change over time as trust is established. This will allow the consultant to choose the most appropriate level of intervention (see also Dowling & Osborne, 1985).

Case example 1

A support unit teacher was feeling isolated and overwhelmed by the difficult children sent to her from around the school. She requested consultation from a child and adolescent psychiatrist. At a preliminary meeting the consultant pointed out that class teachers were sending their most *difficult* children to the support unit to have confirmed that it was the child or the family and not the teacher who was to blame for the difficulties. This was apparent in the hostile and rejecting way in which children were sent to the unit. The support unit teacher, in trying to provide an environment and relationship in which these children would succeed in school, did not recognise that her successes meant that her classroom colleagues had failed. Her relationships with her colleagues became competitive. The support unit teacher found herself in sympathy with the feelings of rejection with which the children came, and covertly sided with the pupils against their teachers, not working to help them succeed in *class*, but 'succeeding' with them in the support unit, mirroring for many of the children the rivalry and retaliatory relationships between their parents at home. The more she succeeded, the more difficult they were seen to be in class, and the more rejection they experienced from everyone except her.

The child and adolescent psychiatrist felt that consulting to the support unit teacher alone would enhance negative labelling by the rest of the staff. Both the support teacher and her pupils would be connoted as in need of psychiatric help unless the problem could be owned by the *school* and the contract for consultation came from the school and not the support unit teacher. The child and adolescent psychiatrist requested a meeting with the head teacher, the head of pastoral care and the support unit teacher at which the nature of the split was explored (through questions regarding *procedures* for dealing with difficult pupils); the risks of further enhancing these splits were agreed and new procedures for referral and admission to the support unit in a clearly structured and limited way (not linked to exclusion from class as an ad hoc arrangement) were established. The child and adolescent psychiatrist agreed to consult teachers other than support unit teachers in the school by request. The support unit teacher felt thereafter that her relationships with her colleagues improved and that her work was more manageable and more valued.

Case example 2

In spite of numerous letters home from the teacher about a child's bad behaviour in school, his parents failed to attend meetings with the teacher. The teacher felt hopeless about the child and blamed the parents, citing their non-attendance at meetings as evidence of their parental failure. An alternative hypothesis was proposed by the consultant, that the parents had a poor self-image and were intimidated by the school because of their own educational failure, that they expected to be admonished and blamed by the teachers for their child's school failure and bad behaviour, that they were too afraid to attend meetings, or defended against these feelings by appearing indifferent or arrogant, and that the threatening and unwelcoming tone of the letters by the teacher was adding to this. The teacher was encouraged to acknowledge his feelings of failure in a letter to the parents, to appeal for the parents' help through their expertise with their child and to send reports home of any achievements or progress that the child made. The parents attended the next meeting offered.

Treatment

The school may request specific intervention within the school for a child or a group of children, for example group therapy or behaviour therapy, or they may refer a child for treatment to the child and family service or child psychiatry department when it is felt the child's problems are to do with factors other than the school environment. With regard to the latter it is important to establish that the parents are in agreement with the referral and that the definition of the problem as 'little to do with the school' is accurate. A head teacher blaming the parents for the child not behaving in school and *compelling* the family to see a child and adolescent psychiatrist is bound to lead to failure.

Kolvin *et al* (1981) carried out a comprehensive and controlled study of interventions with children in mainstream schools, which should inform modern practice.

Using the school system as an adjunct to psychiatric treatment

The school may be used as a useful source of information. The Rutter B (Teachers') Questionnaire (Rutter, 1967) is a structured way of doing so.

The school may also be used as an ameliorative influence. Different schools affect different children differently. This has been clearly demonstrated by Rutter *et al* (1979) (see also Chapter 4). Good relationships within the school with both adults and peers may protect children suffering adversity in other domains (Wolkind & Rutter, 1985) and the improvement in peer relationships through group interventions may improve self-esteem and social skills, which would be difficult to achieve by therapy in isolation. Improved educational performance may lead to improved behaviour and mood.

Sometimes it will be necessary, in order to match the child and the school, to suggest a change of school. Sometimes a boarding school placement relieves the child of intolerable stress (e.g. from a mentally ill parent) in an otherwise loving home. Special boarding school placement should not be seen as 'the soft option' alternative to local authority care and placement with foster-parents.

Finally, the teacher may be enlisted as a therapist, counsellor or at least an active supporter of the therapeutic efforts and processes.

Schools and confidentiality

Information about children should be exchanged between the school and the child and adolescent psychiatrist only with the permission of the parent or custodian of the child (and in the case of older children, with their permission too). Parents have the right to refuse this permission or to have control over what information is exchanged without prejudicing the opportunity for therapy. This situation may be circumvented by consulting the family and school representative together. Each party can choose what to say and will know what the other has said. Alternatively the child and adolescent psychiatrist should make it clear to the family that the 'client' is the school or education department, for example with regard to assessments – the family can then choose to withhold information since they have a clear understanding that the interview is not confidential.

It should also be borne in mind when corresponding to schools or the education department that their files are open to parents.

Liaison with social services, by Robert Jezzard

Changes in legislation and clarification of the statutory roles of different agencies, together with more knowledge about factors affecting child development and the escalating demands of work with children who have been sexually abused (Royal College of Psychiatrists, 1988) have all contributed to the increasing liaison between child psychiatric services and social services departments. However, the pace of change has tended to enhance the confusion about the roles and responsibilities of all the contributors to children's services. The knowledge base, the clinical skills and the responsibilities of all professionals working with children overlap. It is therefore incumbent upon child psychiatrists to delineate their role when working in conjunction with social workers and to have a clear understanding of both the extent and the limits of their expertise (Department of Health, 1991b). A child psychiatric opinion, however valid, may be easily discarded by a social services department if it is presented insensitively or if it betrays a lack of awareness of the framework and context in which social workers operate. The interests of a child's future are best served by the child and adolescent psychiatrist who has a full appreciation of all aspects that may influence decision making, including those that relate to the organisation.

Understanding social services

The detailed structure of a social services department will vary from one local authority to another. In all cases the financial resources and broad policies with regard to services provided will be determined by the elected council members of the authority. The service itself will be provided by the employees of that authority and its overall management is in the hands of a director of social services, who is accountable to the chief executive of the council. There are usually several subdivisions of the department, each with specific responsibilities (e.g. child care, residential services, personnel, policy development). Organisation of social work teams with direct contact with the public varies and may be based upon a commitment to a neighbourhood or 'patch' or, as is increasingly also the case, based upon a specialist role (e.g. fostering and adoption, child protection).

Knowledge of the particular structure of a department and the authority, and priorities given to its different employees, increases the effectiveness of another agency in its liaison with it. Hospital social workers are also employees of the local authority social services department and, even if members of a child psychiatric team, are accountable to their employer and not to a Health Service professional. While this may at times produce tension, it is usually the case that mutually acceptable working arrangements can and should be agreed. The roles that such social workers undertake within a child psychiatry service vary considerably and depend upon locally determined expectations.

An understanding of the responsibilities placed upon local authorities and the resources available to them will facilitate liaison with social workers. The Children Act 1989 tries to encompass all the relevant child care legislation in one act but also defines more clearly in section 17 "the general duty of every Local Authority . . ."

"(a) to safeguard and promote the welfare of children within their area who are in need; and
(b) so far as is consistent with that duty, to promote the upbringing of such children by their families".

The act, therefore, encourages work which seeks to prevent or minimise the possibility of a child needing to come into the care of or be accommodated by the local authority. It is clear that child mental health services should be taking steps to liaise closely with social services departments in a preventive capacity. The Children Act goes on to define a "child in need" and this includes those children who may be "significantly impaired" as far as their health (including mental health) and development are concerned. However, this alone will not necessarily be sufficient to guide the child psychiatrist in providing effective advice and recommendations about a child. An appreciation of a social services department's managerial structure, political and financial constraints, available resources, and local policies will help to ensure that the child psychiatric contribution is targeted effectively. Ultimately, therefore, any recommendations will be more valued and will be of greater benefit to the child. This is not to suggest that clinically inappropriate compromises should be made (e.g. if resources are limited) but that a case can be argued more effectively and credibly if the 'system' is fully understood. It is equally in the interests of children that the child psychiatrist should be aware of all issues that are deemed important by a social services department; for example a comment that is perceived to be racist, whether inadvertent or unintentioned, may affect other people's judgements about the opinion being offered.

The law

The Children Act is not the only legal framework that needs to be understood (see Chapter 12). The Mental Health Act 1983, the Education Act 1981 and the White Paper, *Caring for People* (Department of Health, 1989) are all relevant. A working understanding of them is essential for effective liaison work with an agency that has such extensive statutory responsibilities (Black *et al*, 1991). Indeed, such knowledge may at times be essential for sound and ethical practice.

Assessment, planning and treatment

The reasons for referral from social workers vary considerably from case to case and from service to service. For example, an opinion may be sought as to whether a child in the interim care of the local authority following episodes of non-accidental injury should be rehabilitated home to his or her family and whether the family is likely to change sufficiently to prevent recurrence of physical abuse. Another common reason for referral arises from severe and aggressive behavioural disturbance of a young person within residential care. Can this young person be helped by psychiatric intervention? There may be several possible clinical interventions and any single intervention will depend upon many factors.

  In the first example above it may be that a family centre is involved in working with the family, and consultation will clarify the issues. Equally, a full and detailed assessment of the family may be required in order to contribute to the evidence in care proceedings when there is uncertainty as to the best course of action. In the second example, consultation may also play a role, as the young person's disturbance may be as much related to the dynamics of the residential setting as it is to psychopathology. Alternatively, a combination of factors in the young person's life (e.g., specific learning difficulties leading to educational failure, bereavement, sexual abuse) may lead to a recommendation for specific types of child psychiatric treatment.

A preliminary analysis of the referral is the first step. The reason for the referral needs to be clarified, as it may not be immediately evident. This can usefully be done by defining the question(s) being asked (Dare *et al*, 1990). A request for a 'full assessment' that does not define what or who is being assessed, let alone why the assessment is taking place, can lead the clinician into trouble. The response to a referral may vary according to whether the request is from the court for an evaluation of a person's parenting capacity or whether the request is for individual therapy for a 16-year-old in residential care. Time spent on an analysis of the referral followed by careful planning of the intervention will not be wasted. This may involve a preliminary face-to-face consultation with the referrer. At this stage issues such as the legal status of the child, the role of all professionals involved, the requirements for confidentiality, and so on, should be sorted out (Royal College of Psychiatrists, 1988).

Some referrals will ask for assessments of parenting in families with children who are at risk of abuse. Such assessments require meticulous attention to both historical and observational detail (Adcock & White, 1985). There will be requirements to participate at planning meetings, child-protection case conferences and child care reviews, and these contributions need to be anticipated. One skilled intervention at a case conference, if well thought out, may be of great benefit for the child.

The child psychiatrist must consider the long-term needs of a child – in the case of young children particularly, everything should be done to ensure 'permanency'. The concept of permanency has arisen over the last 30 years in recognition of the damaging consequences of leaving children in long-term care without the benefit of a clear plan to achieve stability and consistency of care, preferably within the child's own family or an adoptive family (Shaw, 1988). Familiarity with the advantages and disadvantages of long-term fostering or adoption or residential care is essential (Hersov, 1990). There is a great variation in the usage of all types of child care provision and knowledge based upon local circumstances is insufficient. Applications for secure accommodation orders, in which children can be detained in 'secure' premises for periods defined by a court and for certain legally prescribed reasons, show enormous geographical variation (Millham *et al*, 1978) and factors other than the 'needs' of the young person (Lawson & Lockhart, 1985) play their part in many other child care decisions.

Requests for 'treatment' need to be considered equally carefully. Not infrequently such requests may be inappropriate; for example, the provision of individual therapy when care proceedings have yet to take place may not be desirable if the confidentiality of therapy is compromised by the need to gather evidence. Equally, the uncertainty of the child's future placement and his or her current instability may make the psychotherapeutic task impossible until the child's future is secured. A clear view about the range of treatments available, but also the limits of both the effectiveness and appropriateness of treatment, and its best timing, is helpful information for a social worker.

Consultation

Since Caplan (1964) first described mental health consultation, a wealth of experience has developed about ways in which this can take place. However, there has been little evaluation of its effectiveness for social services. The objectives of consultation may relate to enhancing the general skills, confidence or morale of the consultee, or may be directed at specific child-related issues. Consideration should be given to who is seen (e.g. a field social worker, a group of residential care staff), the setting in which it takes place (e.g. a child psychiatric clinic, a children's home), and whether it is to be a series of contracted sessions or a single consultation. Once again, time will not be wasted if the terms of consultation are negotiated, for example by taking into account the managerial structure of the consultee's organisation and negotiating with an appropriate senior manager; ensure the purposes and aims of the consultation are defined clearly (Steinberg, 1989).

It is essential to understand the different responsibilities of the consultant and the consultee and to differentiate the consultative process from supervision or other types of interprofessional work. There is much to be learned in this regard from the report on 'pindown' in Staffordshire children's homes (Levy & Kahan, 1991). Between 1983 and 1989, a 'system' of control for highly disturbed adolescents resident in four Staffordshire children's homes was in operation. The control mechanisms used were repressive, humiliating and dehumanising and the report described the practice of 'pindown' as falling "decisively outside anything that could be considered as good child care practice. It was in all its manifestations intrinsically unethical, unprofessional and unacceptable." One of the many worrying features of pindown was the fact that it was a structured and institutionalised system of controls which contravened established regulations and yet was allowed to continue in operation. The authors of the report believed that pindown was "likely to have stemmed initially from an ill-digested understanding of behavioural psychology". However, "the regime had no theoretical framework and no safeguards". No advice was sought with regard to the practice of pindown from psychiatric, psychological or educational professionals, but nevertheless a great many professionals working within the child care services of Staffordshire allowed the practice to continue and participated in its operation. There were deficiencies from management down, and despite concerns being voiced within the organisation about pindown, it continued for six years. This collusion with such unethical practice by so many people within an organisation for so long illustrates both the potential hazards for an outside consultant but also the extraordinary responsibility that such a person might have.

While a consultant may not be directly accountable for the work of another agency, the duty to act if unethical or unsatisfactory practice is discovered is clear. Contributions from more than one agency or professional group can help minimise the chances of bad practice becoming institutionalised.

Conclusion

Many of the most troubled children and young people that a child psychiatrist is likely to meet are primarily the responsibility of social services. A good child psychiatric service will play its part, whether by direct work, consultation or training, in helping social services to undertake their task as effectively and benevolently as possible. Mutual understanding of the agencies who are 'working together' is essential.

References

Adcock, M. & White, R. (1985) *Good-Enough Parenting: A Framework for Assessment.* London: British Agencies for Adoption and Fostering.

Bax, M. C. O. & Whitmore, K. (1991) District handicap teams in England: 1983–8. *Archives of Disease in Childhood*, **66**, 656–664.

Bingley, L., Leonard, J., Hensman, S., *et al* (1980) The comprehensive management of children on a paediatric ward – a family approach. *Archives of Disease in Childhood*, **55**, 555–561.

Black, D. (1978) Annotation. The bereaved child. *Journal of Child Psychology and Psychiatry*, **19**, 287–292.

—— (1994) Bereavement. In *Palliative Care for Children* (ed. A. Goldman). London: Oxford University Press (in press).

—— & Urbanowicz, M. A. (1985) Bereaved children – family intervention. In *Recent Research in Developmental Psychopathology* (eds J. Stevenson). Journal of Child Psychology and Psychiatry Book Supplement no. 4. Oxford: Pergamon Press.

——, McFadyen, A. & Broster, G. (1990) Development of a psychiatric liaison service. *Archives of Disease in Childhood*, **65**, 1373–1375.

——, Wolkind, S. & Harris Hendriks, J. (1991) *Child Psychiatry and the Law* (2nd edn). London: Gaskell.

Caplan, G. (1964) *Principles of Preventive Psychiatry.* London: Tavistock.

Committee on Child Health Services (1970) *Fit for the Future* (the Court report), cmnd 6684. London: HMSO.

Dare, J., Goldberg, D. & Walinets, R. (1990) What is the question you need to answer? How consultation can prevent professional systems immobilising families. *Journal of Family Therapy*, **12**, 355–369.

Department of Education and Science (1978) *Report of the Committee of Enquiry into the Education of Handicapped Children and Young People* (the Warnock report). London: HMSO.

Department of Health (1989) *Caring for People: Community Care in the Next Decade and Beyond.* London: HMSO.
—— (1991*a*) *The Welfare of Children and Young People in Hospital.* London: HMSO.
—— (1991*b*) *Working Together under the Children Act 1989. A Guide to Arrangements for Inter-agency Co-operation for the Protection of Children from Abuse.* London: HMSO.
Disasters Working Party (1991) *Disasters: Planning for a Caring Response.* London: HMSO.
Dowling, E. & Osborne, E. (1985) *The Family and the School. A Joint Systems Approach to Problems with Children.* London: Routledge and Kegan Paul.
Eiser, C. (1990) *Chronic Childhood Illness.* Cambridge: Cambridge University Press.
Evered, C. J., Hill, P. D., Hall, D. M., *et al* (1989) Liaison psychiatry in a child development clinic. *Archives of Disease in Childhood,* **64**, 754-758.
Gath, A. & Gumley, D. (1987) Retarded children and their siblings. *Journal of Child Psychology and Psychiatry,* **28**, 715-730.
Hersov, L. (1990) The Seventh Jack Tizard Memorial Lecture. Aspects of adoption. *Journal of Child Psychology and Psychiatry,* **31**, 493-510.
Kolvin, I., Garside, R. F., Nicol, R., *et al* (1981) *Help Starts Here: The Maladjusted Child in the Ordinary School.* London: Tavistock.
Koocher, G. P., O'Malley, J. E., Gogan, J. L., *et al* (1980) Psychological adjustment among pediatric cancer survivors. *Journal of Child Psychology and Psychiatry,* **21**, 163-173.
Lask, B. & Matthew, D. (1979) Childhood asthma, a controlled trial of family psychotherapy. *Archives of Disease in Childhood,* **54**, 116-119.
Lawson, C. W. & Lockhart, D. (1985) The sex distribution of children in care. *Journal of Adolescence,* **8**, 167-181.
Levy, A. & Kahan, B. (1991) *The Pindown Experience and the Protection of Children. The Report of the Staffordshire Child Care Inquiry 1990.* Staffordshire County Council.
Lloyd, G. G. (1980) Liaison psychiatry from a British perspective. *General Hospital Psychiatry,* **2**, 46-51.
Maguire, P., Comaroff, J., Ransell, P. J., *et al* (1979) Psychological and social problems in families of children with leukaemia. In *Topics in Paediatrics, Vol. 1, Haematology and Oncology* (ed. P. H. Morris-Jones). London: Pitman Medical.
Marteau, T., Bloch, S. & Baum, J. (1987) Family life and diabetic control. *Journal of Child Psychology and Psychiatry,* **28**, 823-834.
McFadyen, A., Broster, G. & Black, D. (1991) The impact of a child psychiatry liaison service on patterns of referral. *British Journal of Psychiatry,* **158**, 93-96.
Millham, S., Bullock, R. & Hosie, K. (1978) *Locking Up Children.* Farnborough: Saxon House.
Ministry of Health (1967) *Child Welfare Centres. Report of the Sub-committee* (the Sheldon report). London: HMSO.
Pynoos, R. S. (1986) Witness to violence: the child interview. *Journal of the American Academy of Child Psychiatry,* **25**, 306-319.
Rapoff, M. & Christophersen, E. R. (1982) Compliance of pediatric patients with medical regimes: a review and evaluation. In *Adherence, Compliance and Generalisation in Behavioral Medicine* (ed. R. B. Stuart). New York: Brunner/Mazel.
Royal College of Psychiatrists (1988) Child psychiatric perspectives on the assessment and management of sexually mistreated children. *Bulletin of the Royal College of Psychiatrists,* **12**, 534-540.

Rutter, M. (1967) Children's Behaviour Questionnaire for Completion by Teachers: preliminary findings. *Journal of Child Psychology and Psychiatry*, **8**, 1–11.

——, Tizard, J. & Whitmore, K. (1970) *Education, Health and Behaviour*. London: Longman.

——, Maughan, B., Mortimer, P., *et al* (1979) *15,000 Hours: Secondary Schools and their Effects on Children*. London: Open Books.

Sabbeth, B. & Leventhal, J. (1984) Marital adjustment to chronic childhood illness: a critique of the literature. *Paediatrics*, **73**, 762–767.

Seidel, U. P., Chadwick, O. & Rutter, M. (1975) Psychological disorders in crippled children: a comparative study of children with and without brain damage. *Developmental Medicine and Child Neurology*, **17**, 563–573.

Shaw, M. (1988) *Family Placement for Children in Care: A Guide to the Literature*. London: British Agencies for Adoption and Fostering.

Steinberg, D. (1989) *Inter-professional Consultation*. Oxford: Blackwell Scientific.

Stevenson, J. (1989) The evaluation of collaborative services with health visitors for pre-school children with behaviour problems. In *Health Visitor Based Services for Pre-School Children with Behaviour Problems* (ed. J. Stevenson). Occasional papers no. 2. London: Association for Child Psychology and Psychiatry.

Sumner, M., Dinwiddie, R., Matthew, D. J., *et al* (1991) Loss on a paediatric intensive care unit: parental reactions. *Care of the Critically Ill*, **7**, 64–66.

Thompson, M. J. J. & Bellenis, C. (1992) A joint assesment and treatment service for the under-fives. Work with the health visitors in a child guidance clinic. *ACPP Newsletter*, **14**, 221–227.

Wolkind, S. & Rutter, M. (1985) Socio-cultural factors. In *Child and Adolescent Psychiatry: Modern Approaches* (eds M. Rutter & L. Hersov). London: Blackwell.

Further reading

Hall, D. (1984) *The Child with a Handicap*. Oxford: Blackwell.

K

14 Continuities and discontinuities from childhood to adult life

Ian Goodyer

The influence of the social environment ● *Childhood antecedents of major adult disorder* ● *Outcomes of childhood psychopathology* ● *Conclusion*

There is nothing new or contentious in the proposition that some early childhood experiences influence adult function. Indeed it is apparent that many different life experiences influence the pathways of development from one point in time to another. What is now required, however, is an understanding of the mechanisms and processes by which such experiences operate to influence later behaviour.

This chapter provides an overview of three domains where child–adult links have been sought: firstly, social causation and maintenance of psychopathology; secondly, childhood antecedents of adult-onset disorders; thirdly, continuities and discontinuities between psychiatric disorders in childhood and adulthood.

The influence of the social environment

Adolf Meyer, the eminent adult psychiatrist at Johns Hopkins University, argued for a developmental approach for understanding the ways in which individuals meet key life changes (Meyer, 1951). In the four decades that have passed since then researchers have pursued the task of identifying factors in the environment that increase risk for, or protect individuals from, later disorder (see Rolfe *et al*, 1990). Meyer emphasised the active role of the individual in negotiating and coping with social circumstances.

Concept of risk

What is meant by a risk factor? Put simply, the likelihood of disorder is increased in an individual who is exposed to such a circumstance. This proposes a causal relationship.

A→B

Research has now shown that there are many different types of risk circumstance, both extrinsic and intrinsic to the person. The effects of these are themselves determined by a number of features including the intensity

276

and appraisal of the stimulus, the duration of exposure, the temporal relationship between stimulus and the individual's response, and the condition of the individual at the time.

Quantifying risk

A full discussion of the modern advances in the application of statistical techniques to determine the magnitude of association between a putative causal factor and a subsequent outcome are beyond the scope of this chapter. The reader is strongly advised to follow the principle of consulting a statistician with an interest in psychiatric research when designing a project (for an introduction to this complex but important area see Pickles, 1991). A brief review is provided, however, of the principles that have been used to calculate the magnitude of risk in many published studies to date.

Measuring the association between exposure to a particular factor and the risk of a certain outcome allows researchers to estimate the magnitude of effect of a potentially undesirable environmental circumstance. There have been two commonly employed methods, relative risk and attributable risk.

Relative risk is the ratio of a disease (usually the incidence) among those exposed to the risk compared with those not exposed. Relative risk can be calculated from a fourfold table, as shown in Table 14.1. Relative risk $= ad/bc$.

Using this formula is an appropriate method for calculating the magnitude of association between life events and psychiatric disorder from case-control studies. For example, examination of child and adolescent data shows that one recent undesirable life event increases the risk for psychiatric disorder approximately five times in the 12 months after the event (Goodyer, 1990). When a child is exposed to more than one type of social adversity the magnitude of risk is determined by multiplying together the calculated risks for each circumstance. These tables also show the proportion of individuals who, when exposed to events, do not become ill (i.e. are seen in cell *b*).

Attributable risk per cent is the rate of disease in exposed individuals that can be attributed to the exposure. A relatively precise enumeration of the incidence of the disease in the exposed and non-exposed population is required, making the statistic unsuitable for case-control comparisons but suitable for epidemiological cohort studies. It is derived by subtracting the rate for disease among the non-exposed individuals from those exposed. Attributable risk can be calculated as shown in Table 14.2.

Table 14.1 The calculation of relative risk

Suspected cause	Cases	Controls	Total
Present	*a*	*b*	$a+b$
Absent	*c*	*d*	$c+d$

Relative risk $= ad/bc$.

Table 14.2 The calculation of attributable risk

Suspected cause	Cases	Controls	Total
Present	a	b	$a+b$
Absent	c	d	$c+d$

Attributable risk $\% = \dfrac{ad-bc}{(a+c)\,(c+d)} \times 100$

There are, as yet, no published reports of this estimate for social adversities in young people. In adults, estimates have suggested that perhaps 30–40% of episodes of anxiety and depression could be attributed to recent life events.

Risk factors have been investigated as putative causal factors in the onset of psychiatric disorders, as factors that determine the pathway of individual development, and as precursors to later adult disorder whose effects are latent, that is are not expressed at the time.

Risk: factors, mechanisms

Social adversities such as recent undesirable life events, maternal distress and poor family relationships all carry risk effects for the onset of psychopathology in school-age children (Goodyer *et al*, 1988; Rutter, 1990). Some risk circumstances (e.g. life events) appear to exert relatively short-term effects, over weeks or months. Others (e.g. chronic family difficulties) may exert effects over months or years.

The main discriminating feature between events and difficulties is the degree of exposure. Events are circumscribed, with definable onsets and endings. Difficulties are more ongoing, with poorly defined onsets and end-stages. Different risk circumstances exert psychological effects of different intensities on the individual. In addition, they may exert: (1) *direct effects* on the likelihood of psychopathology occurring, and (2) *cumulative effects* when two or more such risk circumstances occur. In the main, the magnitude of cumulative risk reflects an addition of the known risks carried by each circumstance. In some circumstances, however, there is a synergy which increases the likelihood of disorder, and the magnitude of risk, beyond the known risks for each circumstance (i.e. a multiple risk) (Brown & Harris, 1978; Brown, 1988; Goodyer, 1990).

As well as the magnitude of risk effects, it is equally important to consider their psychological mechanisms, which may vary from one set of risk circumstances to another, even though the risk may be the same or similar for different circumstances. For example, both family and peer group difficulties are pathways for anxiety and depression in school-age children. These two social processes act independently of each other, suggesting different psychological mechanisms accounting for their effects (Goodyer *et al*, 1990).

In other words, a knowledge of one group of circumstances and their mechanisms (i.e. family adversities) does not result in an understanding of the other (difficulties in friendships). Intervention with one process will therefore not alleviate the risk or explain the mechanisms and processes of the other.

Influences of social adversity on child development

Social adversities may adversely influence the normal pathways of child development, increasing the likelihood of psychological difficulties in adult life (Fig. 14.1). Two examples are provided to illustrate that the psychological mechanisms are neither immediately apparent nor the same for different experiences.

Firstly, loss of a parent before 12 (through either death or permanent separation) is associated with later onset of adult depression; the psychological mechanism that accounts for this arises from the subsequent deficiencies in parenting following loss, rather than the loss *per se* (Brown, 1988). This example of a circumscribed event leading to long-term undesirable circumstances indicates how a continuity between adverse events and ongoing difficulties may occur. The risk of such a continuity occurring appears to be increased when a life event is uncontrollable and permanently alters the child's family circumstances. What is not clear, however, is why there appears to be a *latent period*. Of course, 'adult-onset' depression may actually have been experienced

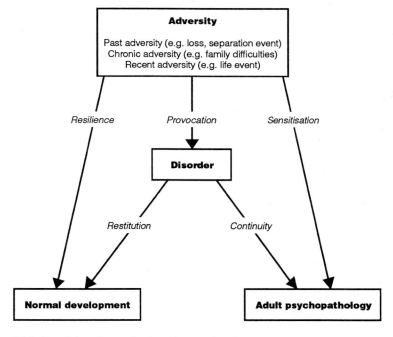

Fig. 14.1 Possible effects of adversity on development.

as recurrent episodes of depression or other psychopathology throughout childhood and adolescence.

Secondly, exposure to chronic aggressive marital disharmony has direct and immediate negative effects on the child's social experiences and '*provokes*' immediate symptoms (Quinton & Rutter, 1988). When adverse life experiences are of sufficient intensity to provoke immediate responses in children, then the disorder itself may exert subsequent effects on the social environment. Behavioural symptoms in the child may then increase the risk of further difficulties between the parents. In these circumstances a continuity of risk circumstances occurs because the parenting difficulties and child's symptoms are interdependent and mutually reinforcing.

The concept of an individual as an active participant in the environment is not new but is often neglected. A clearer understanding of these 'person–environment' interactions would help to predict how and why relationships are influenced by and will influence others (Hinde & Stevenson-Hinde, 1988).

Vulnerability and protection

Vulnerability and protection indicate the presence of modifying effects on risk situations, and may not be apparent until new environmental demands occur which carry a risk to well-being, such as acute undesirable life events. Whether a factor indicates a vulnerability or protective process is not always apparent at first sight.

Firstly, one event or circumstance may be described on a vulnerability/protection continuum: low levels of such a factor render an individual vulnerable and high levels indicate protection. For example, intelligence appears to act as a continuous variable. Lower intelligence is associated with higher rates of psychopathology over a lifetime, while higher intelligence is associated with lower rates. At IQs of less than 50, however, the main effect is *directly* attributed to mechanisms of cerebral dysfunction itself, giving rise to manifold neurodevelopmental and behavioural difficulties. Within the IQ range 70–125, protective effects are not directly related to cerebral mechanisms. In other words, differing levels of the 'factor' intelligence do not explain the underlying mechanisms responsible for vulnerability or protection: the different mechanisms that determine vulnerability or protection at different levels of IQ need to be elucidated as well as determining levels of intelligence *per se*.

Loss and separation constitute a different form of vulnerability and protection from that related to intelligence. It was previously noted that depression is increased in women who lose a parent in childhood, but only in those who subsequently experience poor parenting. It is also clear, however, that loss of parenting is not in itself likely to give rise to later depression – vulnerabilities of this kind have no or only modest effects on their own. It is likely only when a further adverse life event or difficulty arises (Brown & Harris, 1978; Brown, 1988). Some women, however, after parental loss retain adequate parenting through another source. Under these conditions, they appear *protected* from depression. Vulnerability is conferred in the *absence* of parenting. Here then there is a continuity of vulnerability and protection depending not explicitly on the loss event, but on its consequences.

Restitution and enhancement

Loss of a parent results in an undesirable and permanent alteration in a child's life and introduces a new, adverse developmental pathway. Later psychopathology is not, however, an inescapable fate for all individuals who experience such early loss or even later separations (Quinton *et al*, 1984). Positive social processes may arise which vulnerable individuals may make use of to renegotiate current circumstances and experiences. Planning ahead, avoiding social circumstances which would increase risk, choosing or finding adequate relations in adulthood are all examples of how a negative developmental pathway can be ameliorated.

These restorative processes are a consequence of desirable environmental conditions. The implications are that such new and desirable social experiences can in vulnerable persons influence thoughts, feelings and behaviour.

Perhaps psychological treatments themselves can be considered as restorative. A long-term psychotherapeutic relationship may restore self-esteem and self-efficacy; a brief conversational model (cognitive–behavioural or brief psychodynamic psychotherapy) may promote the better use of the environment in a person's life, for example improving personal relations or social or work achievements.

On the other hand, processes may occur which maintain the undesirable trajectory, although they are not able to worsen it. In school-age children and adolescents, for example, the absence of good friendships provokes anxiety and depressive disorder. By contrast, an absence of social achievement (defined as success in school, sports, creative or community activities) has no such direct effect. A substantial interactive effect for anxious and depressive disorder was noted, however, in those children who report an absence of good friendships and subsequently experience no social achievements (Goodyer *et al*, 1990). This *adverse social enhancing mechanism* was also specific for peer-group social processes, as no such interaction for the absence of social achievements was found with family adversities. The findings suggest that family and social adversities exert substantial independent effects on developmental trajectory and subsequent risk for adult disorder.

In summary, some risk circumstances exert direct effects on disorder at all ages and can be termed 'provoking agents'. Vulnerability and protective mechanisms and processes exert indirect effects by amplifying or ameliorating the effects of provoking agents. Later restorative processes may reduce or remove adverse effects and return a person to an adaptive developmental trajectory. Later enhancing factors may consolidate or maintain adverse developmental trajectories.

Psychopathology and social relationships

The provoking causal effects of adverse life experiences for psychopathology also have implications for subsequent social development. While much remains to be discovered, there is some preliminary evidence that major depression has a greater adverse effect on subsequent peer relations than anxiety disorders, even if the two disorders arise in individuals exposed to the same type of potentially causal life events and difficulties (Puig-Antich *et al*, 1985; Goodyer *et al*, 1991). This effect of depression may occur even if family adversities improve. In other words, depressive symptoms increase the likelihood of further adverse experiences in the social domain *but not* in the family domain.

This is because there is a *chaining of effects*, whereby the symptoms of depression increase the risk of subsequent friendship difficulties which in turn lead either to further episodes or increased duration of depressive disorder.

Relapsing psychopathological conditions during the school-age years may occur: (1) because of persisting undesirable interactions between environment and child behaviour, as in coercive parent–child relationships and conduct disorder (Patterson & Dishion, 1988), or (2) because the trajectory of social development has been altered adversely by an episode of psychiatric disorder such as described above for major depression and subsequent friendships (Goodyer *et al*, 1991).

Resilience

Resilience can simply be defined as individual differences in response to social difficulties. In almost every investigation of 'children at risk', findings indicate that there are individuals exposed to the putative risk factor who remain well. Even in the presence of multiple family or social adversities, some children appear resilient (Garmezy, 1985; Goodyer *et al*, 1988, 1990; Rutter, 1989, 1990).

Studies of stress-resistant children have indicated that three broad sets of variables operate to promote resilience:

(1) self-esteem, sociability and autonomy
(2) family cohesion, warmth and an absence of parental discord
(3) social support systems that encourage personal effort and coping.

Clearly, these broad domains must be dissected to find the mechanisms and processes that determine resilience in some individuals faced with social adversities. Why is it that some individuals remain well while others give up hope in the face of the same or similar adversities? This is a fundamental question facing current and future research.

Childhood antecedents of major adult disorder

Schizophrenia

Schizophrenia has a prevalence of 1% in adults between 18 and 65 years of age. The search for genetic factors using twin-adoption and family studies has gained momentum in recent years. The relatively infrequent onset of the condition under 14 years of age has led researchers to consider three developmentally related questions. (1) Are there behavioural precursors to schizophrenia that are detectable in at-risk populations such as the offspring of schizophrenics? (2) What factors in young people govern the later onset of schizophrenic symptoms? (3) Are there discernible factors in the early environment that deter or decrease the risk of adult-onset disorder?

The 'at-risk research strategy' of the last two decades has used a number of methods to determine the premorbid childhood status of schizophrenics. Follow-up and catch-up studies (the latter using retrospective collection of information from proven cases) can be summarised as follows.

(1) A significant proportion of adult-onset schizophrenics are atypical in behaviour during childhood, but there is no specific pattern of behaviour that predicts later onset of schizophrenia – the full range of emotional and behavioural symptoms have been described as occurring in the childhood of schizophrenics.

(2) In particular, simple shyness has no relation to symptom onset, schizoid-type personality traits are found frequently in non-schizophrenic adults, and only a minority of schizophrenics were schizoid as children.

(3) There are no other significant personality or temperamental characteristics that predict later-onset schizophrenia.

(4) The childhood IQs of schizophrenics are sometimes (but not always) lower than those of their siblings. These findings may be related to neurophysiological vulnerabilities such as abnormalities of eye tracking, and neuropsychological deficiencies such as inattention and abnormalities of information processing on experimental performance tasks.

(5) Earlier onset and premorbid difficulties are more common in males than in females, suggesting there is something potentially protective about female sex. Males are more likely than females to suffer from all forms of pervasive developmental difficulties. The male vulnerability may be expressed through increased 'neurological organicity'.

(6) Many schizophrenics grow up with impoverished family relations, but these environmental effects are clearly non-specific. High expressed emotion (Leff, 1989) may precipitate episodes of disorder. High expressed emotion is not however confined to families of schizophrenics and may not result in episodes of disorder in all circumstances.

In summary, there are no specific developmental factors or processes which predict the later onset of schizophrenia. It is encouraging to note that children with one or two parents with schizophrenia, reared apart from their biological parents, may escape their adverse developmental trajectory.

It is likely that further research will determine developmental continuities for particular subgroups of schizophrenics. Males with neurophysiological and neurocognitive deficits in childhood may be one such group. Developmental dysplasia of the temporal areas of the cortex may underlie such deficits and merits further study. Advances in brain imaging and molecular genetics make elucidation significantly more likely.

It is equally apparent, however, that there are discontinuities between the early environment and later schizophrenia, and all types of schizophrenia will not be explained by intrinsic neurocognitive deficits, adverse social development or chronic adversities within family life.

Major depression

As noted above, parental loss in early childhood increases the risk in some individuals for major depressive disorder in adult life (Brown & Harris, 1978; Bowlby, 1980; Brown, 1988); while the precise mechanisms of this effect are yet to be confirmed, for some individuals it is the lack of adequate parental care following loss that is important. This lack of care appears more important for the onset of unipolar rather than bipolar disorders, and there may be mediating cognitive processes between parental loss/lack of care and depression. It has been postulated, for example, that individuals who experience early parental loss have lower self-esteem as adults than those who do not. The prediction from this postulate is that when such individuals are exposed to stressful conditions as adults they are more likely to blame themselves and perceive any consequent difficulties as their fault, thus increasing the risk of depression. Not all adults with low self-esteem experienced parental loss in childhood and low self-esteem has yet to be shown as a specific prerequisite for all forms of unipolar depression.

Clearly there is a continuity between some childhood adversities and some forms of unipolar adult depression. There are however many other aetiological models. It seems increasingly likely that depressive subtypes will emerge, some with a developmental aetiology (of which parental loss/lack of care may be one) and many without.

Adult deviant behaviour

The classic longitudinal study of Robins (1966) charts the continuities between antisocial behaviour in childhood and later deviant behaviour in adults. The links and chains in this process appear to be in the continuous exposure of children to deviant behaviour in their families. Thus divorce, criminality, alcoholism and psychopathy are all significantly more likely in children from deprived and disadvantaged homes. The term 'cycle of disadvantage' captured the repeated intergenerational patterns of maladjustment that have been documented in numerous studies of deviant behaviour in family life (e.g. Kolvin *et al*, 1983).

Studies are required to discriminate high-risk and low-risk groups of children since mechanisms and processes predicting adjustment may be different both within and between these populations. So far, protection appears to involve reducing the effect of risk circumstances and providing social opportunities for improved self-esteem. The evidence also indicates that personal qualities in the child substantially influence his or her ability to make best use of such opportunities.

The evolution of psychopathological conditions from childhood to adulthood emphasises individual differences in outcome. The second section of this chapter notes that not all forms of the same disorder arise from developmental processes. For some children early onset heralds a chronic relapsing course but others recover, with no apparent sequelae. We lack the necessary information to determine which cases are most likely to show a continuity of disorder into adult life. Intrinsic factors may be important mediators in risk circumstances and contribute to the observed individual differences in the nature and outcome of psychiatric conditions. The contribution of neurodevelopmental, temperamental and cognitive factors to the nature of psychopathology remains poorly understood. Research must consider the physiological aspects of development concurrently with social adversities in relation to the onset nature and outcome of psychiatric disorder.

Finally, mechanisms resulting in an adverse developmental trajectory must be delineated, as must those that redirect children to a more adaptive path.

References

Bowlby, J. (1980) *Attachment and Loss, Vol. 3, Sadness and Depression*. London: Hogarth Press.

Brown, G. W. (1988) Early loss of parent and depression in adult life. In *Handbook of Life Stress, Cognition and Health* (eds S. Fisher & J. Reason). Chichester: Wiley.

—— & Harris, T. (1978) *The Social Origins of Depression*. London: Tavistock.

Christie, K. A., Burke, J. D., Regier, D. A., *et al* (1988) Epidemiologic evidence for early onset of mental disorders and higher risk of drug abuse in young adults. *American Journal of Psychiatry*, **145**, 971–975.

Garmezy, N. (1985) Stress-resistant children – the search for protective factors. In *Recent Advances in Developmental Psychopathology* (ed J. Stevenson). Oxford: Pergamon.

Goodyer, I. M. (1990) *Life Experiences, Development and Childhood Psychopathology*. Chichester: Wiley.

——, Wright, C. & Altham, P. M. E. (1988) Maternal adversity and recent stressful life events in childhood and adolescence. *Journal of Child Psychology and Psychiatry*, **29**, 651–657.

——, —— & —— (1990) Recent adversities and achievements in anxious and depressed school-age children. *Journal of Child Psychology and Psychiatry*, **31**, 1063–1077.

——, —— & —— (1991) Social influences on the course of anxious and depressive disorders in school-age children. *British Journal of Psychiatry*, **158**, 676–684.

Harrington, R. C., Fudge, H., Rutter, M., *et al* (1990) Adult outcome of childhood and adolescent depression. 1. Psychiatric status. *Archives of General Psychiatry*, **47**, 465–473.

Hinde, R. A. & Stevenson-Hinde, J. (eds) (1988) *Relationships Within Families*. Oxford: Clarendon Press.

Kolvin, I., Miller, F. W., Garside, R. F., *et al* (1983) A longitudinal study of deprivation: life cycle changes in one generation – implications for the next generation. In *Epidemiological Approaches to Child Psychiatry, Vol. 2* (eds M. H. Schmidt & H. Remschmidt). Stuttgart: George Thieme.

Leff, J. P. (1989) Controversial issues and growing points in research on relatives' expressed emotion. *International Journal of Social Psychiatry*, **35**, 133–145.

Meyer, A. (1951) The life chart and obligation of specifying positive data in psychopathological diagnosis. In *The Collected Papers of Adolf Meyer, Vol. III* (ed. E. E. Winters). Baltimore: Johns Hopkins University Press.

Patterson, G. R. & Dishion, T. J. (1988) Multilevel family process models: traits, interactions and relationships. In *Relationships Within Families* (eds R. A. Hinde & J. Stevenson-Hinde). Oxford: Clarendon Press.

Pickles, A. (1991) The analysis of change in longitudinal studies of development. *Journal of Child Psychology and Psychiatry*, **32**, 571–580.

Puig-Antich, J., Lukens, E. & Davies, M. (1985) Psychosocial functioning in prepubertal major depressive disorders. 1. Interpersonal relationships during the depressive episode. *Archives of General Psychiatry*, **42**, 500–507.

Quinton, D., Rutter, M. & Liddle, C. (1984) Institutional rearing, parenting difficulties and marital support. *Psychological Medicine*, **14**, 107–124.

—— & —— (1988) *Parental Breakdown: The Making and Breaking of Intergenerational Links*. Aldershot, Gower.

Richman, N., Stevenson, J. & Graham, P. (1982) *Pre-school to School: A Behavioural Study*. London: Academic Press.

Robins, L. N. (1966) *Deviant Children Grown Up: A Sociological and Psychiatric Study of Sociopathic Personality*. Baltimore: Williams and Wilkins.

—— (1991) Conduct disorder. *Journal of Child Psychology and Psychiatry*, **32**, 193–212.

——, Helyer, J. E., Weissman, M. M., *et al* (1984) Lifetime prevalence of specific psychiatric disorders in three sites. *Archives of General Psychiatry*, **41**, 959–958.

Rolfe, J., Masten, A. S., Cicchetti, D., *et al* (eds) (1990) *Risk and Protective Factors in the Development of Psychopathology*. Cambridge: Cambridge University Press.

Rutter, M. (ed.) (1989) *Studies of Psychosocial Risk: the Power of Longitudinal Data*. Cambridge: Cambridge University Press.

—— (1990) Psychosocial resilience and protective mechanisms. In *Risk and Protective Factors in the Development of Psychopathology* (eds J. Rolfe, A. S. Masten, D. Cicchetti, *et al*), pp. 181–214. Cambridge: Cambridge University Press.

Weissman, M. M., Warner, V., Wickramaratne, P., *et al* (1988) Early onset major depression in parents and their children. *Journal of Affective Disorders*, **15**, 269–277.

Zeitlin, H. (1987) *The Natural History of Psychiatric Disorder in Childhood*. Institute of Psychiatry Monograph no. 29. Oxford: Oxford University Press.

Index

Compiled by Linda English